Nephrology: Case Studies

Nephrology: Case Studies

Edited by **Barbara Mayer**

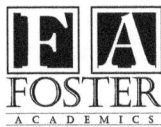

FA

FOSTER
ACADEMICS

New Jersey

Published by Foster Academics,
61 Van Reypen Street,
Jersey City, NJ 07306, USA
www.fosteracademics.com

Nephrology: Case Studies
Edited by Barbara Mayer

International Standard Book Number: 978-1-63242-436-5 (Hardback)

Printed in the United States of America.

Contents

Preface

This book has been an outcome of determined endeavour from a group of educationists in the field. The primary objective was to involve a broad spectrum of professionals from diverse cultural background involved in the field for developing new researches. The book not only targets students but also scholars pursuing higher research for further enhancement of the theoretical and practical applications of the subject.

Optimal functioning of kidneys is essential for leading a healthy life. These maintain and regulate the fluid, electrolyte and acid-base concentration in the body. Nephrology is concerned with diagnosing and finding cure for diseases of the kidneys. This book is a collective contribution of a renowned group of international experts. It aims to equip students and experts with the advanced topics and upcoming concepts in this area. Case studies from multiple countries have been discussed in this book, in order to provide it a global perspective. Nephrologists, researchers and students associated with this field will find this book extremely beneficial.

It was an honour to edit such a profound book and also a challenging task to compile and examine all the relevant data for accuracy and originality. I wish to acknowledge the efforts of the contributors for submitting such brilliant and diverse chapters in the field and for endlessly working for the completion of the book. Last, but not the least; I thank my family for being a constant source of support in all my research endeavours.

Editor

Ceftriaxone-Induced Acute Encephalopathy in a Peritoneal Dialysis Patient

Sami Safadi, Michael Mao, and John J. Dillon

Division of Nephrology and Hypertension, Mayo Clinic, 200 1st Street SW, Rochester, MN 55905, USA

Correspondence should be addressed to Sami Safadi; safadi.sami@mayo.edu

Academic Editor: Bernard Jaar

Encephalopathy is a rare side effect of third and fourth generation cephalosporins. Renal failure and preexisting neurological disease are notable risk factors. Recognition is important as discontinuing the offending agent usually resolves symptoms. We present a case of acute encephalopathy in a patient with end stage renal disease (ESRD) treated with peritoneal dialysis (PD) who received intravenous ceftriaxone for peritonitis. This case illustrates the potential severe neurologic effects of cephalosporins, which are recommended by international guidelines as first-line antimicrobial therapy for spontaneous bacterial peritonitis.

1. Introduction

Encephalopathy is a rare side effect of cephalosporins. It is more common in fourth generation cephalosporins [1, 2]. However, it has been reported in third generation cephalosporins as well [3]. Predisposing risk factors include kidney impairment and preexisting neurological disease. We show here a case of acute reversible encephalopathy in a patient with end stage renal disease who received intravenous ceftriaxone for peritonitis. The case highlights key issues with diagnosing and managing this side effect of cephalosporins.

2. Case Presentation

A 37-year-old female, receiving PD for ESRD due to lupus nephritis, presented with *Yersinia enterocolitica* peritonitis. She has been on PD for 4 years. She performed continuous cycling peritoneal dialysis nightly. Her PD prescription included 6 exchanges, 1700 mL each, over 9 hours, and a one-day dwell of 500 mL. She used 1.5% dextrose for all exchanges. Her dry weight was 45 kg. Her medication regimen consisted of a metoprolol, sevelamer carbonate, darbepoetin, mycophenolate mofetil, and a low dose prednisone. On exam, her abdomen was soft and nontender. PD exit site was clean with no discharge or erythema.

She was initially treated with intraperitoneal ceftazidime (125 mL/L). Two days later, she was hospitalized for possible sepsis as her PD cultures grew *Yersinia enterocolitica*. She was switched to intravenous ceftriaxone (2 grams daily). PD was continued. She defervesced quickly and remained hemodynamically stable and her blood cultures were negative. After 3 days of intravenous ceftriaxone, the patient developed agitation, paranoia, and visual hallucinations. The neurological examination was nonfocal. An EEG (Figure 1) showed background moderate diffuse nonspecific slowing without epileptogenic activity. An MRI showed cerebral and cerebellar volume loss but no focal findings to account for the patient's symptoms. She was not receiving any pain medications or centrally acting agents at the time. Furthermore, hallucinations occurred a few hours after ceftriaxone infusions, so ceftriaxone was suspected. The symptoms resolved completely, within 36 hours, after ceftriaxone was switched to ciprofloxacin.

3. Discussion

Adverse drug reactions (ADRs) are a serious problem in modern health care. A meta-analysis of prospective studies from US hospitals revealed an overall incidence of 6.7% for serious ADRs (requiring hospitalization or resulting in permanent disability or death), 0.32% for fatal ADRs, and

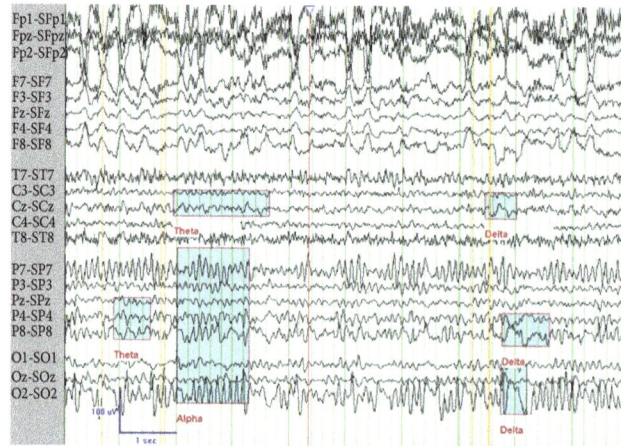

FIGURE 1: Awake EEG using transverse Laplacian montage, showing normal 9 Hz alpha rhythm in the posterior head regions, as well as abnormal 5-6 Hz theta and 2–4 Hz delta slowing seen diffusely but most prominent in the right posterior temporal (P8), parietal (P4), and occipital (O2) head regions.

15.1% for all-severity ADRs [4]. This study further illustrated the clinical impact by showing that, in 1994, 106,000 deaths were estimated to be caused by ADRs in the United States, placing fatal ADRs as the fifth leading cause of death. The majority of ADRs (76.2%) were dose-dependent reactions [4].

Among the many potential reactions to drugs, delirium is a well-known side effect that can lead to increased hospital duration and patient morbidity and mortality. Elderly hospitalized patients, who often may already have multiple risk factors for delirium, such as fluid, electrolyte, metabolic, and sensory/environmental disturbances, are at particularly increased risk when drug toxicity is added to the mix [5]. Chronic kidney disease (CKD) patients share many of the same identified risks for delirium and encephalopathy as elderly hospitalized patients. In addition, they are at a higher risk for fluid, electrolyte, and metabolic abnormalities. Furthermore, the pharmacokinetic and pharmacodynamic parameters of many drugs are altered in CKD [6, 7]. Unfortunately, drug dosing in CKD is often not performed correctly, with inadequate adjustments for renal impairment in 19–67% of hospitalized patients and 42% of long-term care residents [8, 9]. In the ambulatory setting, among nondialysis CKD patients receiving antibiotics, 66% of medications were dosed erroneously [10]. A retrospective observational study showed that necessary renal dose adjustments were not performed for 81% of medications [6]. Among patients with baseline risk factors for delirium and drug toxicity, multiple acute concomitant contributing insults, and inadequate renal drug adjustments, it is no surprise that delirium is a prevalent complication with medications such as narcotics, benzodiazepines, anticholinergic drugs, methyldopa, and nonsteroidal anti-inflammatory agents [5].

This case report however highlights an unusual etiology of delirium and encephalopathy from a common third generation cephalosporin that is currently recommended in the International Society for Peritoneal Dialysis (ISPD)

guidelines as a first-line empiric antibiotic for peritonitis, with treatment duration potentially lasting for 14–21 days [11]. It is further worth noting that antimicrobials constituted the majority of the 81% of medications that were not adequately adjusted for CKD in the retrospective, observational study above [6]. Hence, it is worthwhile to raise awareness of the potential for cephalosporin neurotoxicity, especially in this vulnerable population, as it is a dose-dependent effect and rapid recognition of the offending agent would allow rapid recovery [12]. CNS side effects of cephalosporins have also been described in prior case reports that identified renal failure and prior central nervous disease as important risk factors for cephalosporin encephalopathy, often occurring with generalized triphasic waves on EEG [1, 3, 13].

There have been five peritoneal dialysis patients reported in the literature with cefepime-associated encephalopathy [2]. Ceftriaxone-associated encephalopathy has been previously described with CKD [3]; however, to our knowledge, ceftriaxone-associated encephalopathy in peritoneal dialysis has not been described.

Ceftriaxone has a long elimination half-life ranging between 5.8 and 8.7 hours. Between 33 and 67 percent of a dose is excreted in the urine as unchanged drug, and the remainder is secreted in the bile and ultimately is found in the feces as microbiologically inactive compounds [14]. Minimal alterations in the pharmacokinetics of ceftriaxone were, however, observed in patients with renal impairment compared with healthy adult subjects. The average elimination half-life of ceftriaxone is 14.7 hours in patients on hemodialysis and 15.7 hours in patients with severe renal impairment (creatinine clearance 5 to 15 mL/min) [15]. Thus, according to the manufacturer, no adjustment in ceftriaxone dose is needed in renal impairment. They recommend, however, not to exceed 2 grams per day with combined renal and hepatic impairment.

There is a paucity of data regarding the pharmacokinetics of ceftriaxone in PD. However, ceftriaxone seems to exhibit similar pharmacokinetics in hemodialysis and PD patients [16]. Overall, the drug is removed poorly by both modalities. In PD patients with peritonitis, intraperitoneal ceftriaxone administration is preferred as it provides higher concentrations in the peritoneal space. Systemic absorption through the peritoneal membrane is estimated at 40% in patients without peritonitis [17]. The absorption may be higher in peritonitis as ongoing inflammation increases the permeability of the peritoneal membrane. One study looked at the pharmacokinetics of ceftriaxone in CAPD in 8 patients without peritonitis. A single 1.0 g IP dose during a 4-hour dwell time led to serum and dialysate concentrations of ceftriaxone above the minimum inhibitory concentration for susceptible pathogens for 24 hours. The ISPD guidelines recommend a once daily intraperitoneal dose of 1 to 1.5 grams for most cephalosporins in intermittent PD [11]. For continuous PD, half of the dose is given as a loading dose, and the rest is divided over the other exchanges. They, however, do not refer to ceftriaxone specifically.

Our patient had small body size which poses the question whether the drug dose was relatively overestimated for her. However, according to the manufacturer, no weight adjustments are required for ceftriaxone. We also performed a drug interaction analysis using the Micromedex 2.0 drug interaction tool, and this did not reveal any significant interaction with the other medications that our patient was receiving that would alter the pharmacokinetics of ceftriaxone. It is also worth noting that she was not taking any pain medications or centrally acting drugs that can potentially contribute to her altered mental status.

The proposed pathophysiologic mechanisms for cephalosporin CNS effects include inhibition of γ-aminobutyric acid (GABA) release from nerve terminals, competitive inhibition of GABA binding to receptor sites, and increased excitatory amino acids [18]. The resulting clinical effects include confusion, hallucinations, cognitive disturbances, delirium, agitation, myoclonus, tremors, convulsions, nonconvulsive status epilepticus, and coma [1, 19]. The temporal pattern of cephalosporin neurotoxicity is an average latency of 1–10 days after drug initiation with regression of all neurological symptoms within 2–7 days after drug cessation [12, 19].

Aside from appropriate renal dosage adjustments and optimization of other mitigating etiologies, there are limited options for reducing the risk for cephalosporin-induced encephalopathy. Genetic studies still have limited applicability in daily clinical practice due to cost and feasibility. Prior studies have identified age, gender, number of medications, alcohol intake, comorbidities, and factors that alter drug distribution or metabolism (heart failure, renal insufficiency, and hepatic insufficiency) as predictors for ADR [20]. More CKD-specific clinical prediction tools for ADR have been attempted using logistic regression formulated risk scores that include age 65 or greater, female sex, conservatively managed ESRD, vascular disease, CRP levels, albumin levels, and eight or greater medications during hospitalization [20]. In daily clinical practice, a high index of suspicion for cephalosporin-induced encephalopathy among vulnerable populations, with immediate cessation of therapy, may still be the most practical approach to limiting this severe ADR.

Conflict of Interests

The authors declare that there is no conflict of interests regarding the publication of this paper.

References

[1] A. McNally, A. Pithie, and D. Jardine, "Cefepime: a rare cause of encephalopathy," Internal Medicine Journal, vol. 42, no. 6, pp. 732–733, 2012.

[2] C.-J. Lin, S.-P. Chen, S.-J. Wang, and J.-L. Fuh, "Cefepime-related encephalopathy in peritoneal dialysis patients," Journal of the Chinese Medical Association, vol. 74, no. 2, pp. 87–90, 2011.

[3] R. Roncon-Albuquerque Jr., I. Pires, R. Martins, R. Real, G. Sousa, and P. von Hafe, "Ceftriaxone-induced acute reversible encephalopathy in a patient treated for a urinary tract infection," Netherlands Journal of Medicine, vol. 67, no. 2, pp. 72–75, 2009.

[4] J. Lazarou, B. H. Pomeranz, and P. N. Corey, "Incidence of adverse drug reactions in hospitalized patients: a meta- analysis of prospective studies," The Journal of the American Medical Association, vol. 279, no. 15, pp. 1200–1205, 1998.

[5] J. Francis, D. Martin, and W. N. Kapoor, "A prospective study of delirium in hospitalized elderly," Journal of the American Medical Association, vol. 263, no. 8, pp. 1097–1101, 1990.

[6] A. Prajapati and B. Ganguly, "Appropriateness of drug dose and frequency in patients with renal dysfunction in a tertiary care hospital: a cross-sectional study," Journal of Pharmacy and Bioallied Sciences, vol. 5, no. 2, pp. 136–140, 2013.

[7] R. K. Verbeeck and F. T. Musuamba, "Pharmacokinetics and dosage adjustment in patients with renal dysfunction," European Journal of Clinical Pharmacology, vol. 65, no. 8, pp. 757–773, 2009.

[8] A. Papaioannou, J.-A. Clarke, G. Campbell, and M. Bedard, "Assessment of adherence to renal dosing guidelines in long-term care facilities," Journal of the American Geriatrics Society, vol. 48, no. 11, pp. 1470–1473, 2000.

[9] C. L. Long, M. A. Raebel, D. W. Price, and D. J. Magid, "Compliance with dosing guidelines in patients with chronic kidney disease," Annals of Pharmacotherapy, vol. 38, no. 5, pp. 853–858, 2004.

[10] A. Farag, A. X. Garg, L. Li, and A. K. Jain, "Dosing errors in prescribed antibiotics for older persons with CKD: a retrospective time series analysis," American Journal of Kidney Diseases, vol. 63, no. 3, pp. 422–428, 2014.

[11] P. K.-T. Li, C. C. Szeto, B. Piraino et al., "Peritoneal dialysis-related infections recommendations: 2010 update," Peritoneal Dialysis International, vol. 30, no. 4, pp. 393–423, 2010.

[12] G. Calandra, E. Lydick, J. Carrigan, L. Weiss, and H. Guess, "Factors predisposing to seizures in seriously Ill infected patients receiving antibiotics: experience with imipenem/cilastatin," American Journal of Medicine, vol. 84, no. 5, pp. 911–918, 1988.

[13] J. R. Koup, E. Keller, H. Neumann, and K. Stoeckel, "Ceftriaxone pharmacokinetics during peritoneal dialysis," European Journal of Clinical Pharmacology, vol. 30, no. 3, pp. 303–307, 1986.

[14] I. H. Patel and S. A. Kaplan, "Pharmacokinetic profile of ceftriaxone in man," The American Journal of Medicine, vol. 77, no. 4C, pp. 17–25, 1984.

[15] R. Pharmaceuticals, Ceftriaxone Sodium Powder for Injection, vol. 4, Product Information, 2013.

[16] T. Y. Ti, L. Fortin, J. H. Kreeft, D. S. East, R. I. Ogilvie, and P. J. Somerville, "Kinetic disposition of intravenous ceftriaxone in normal subjects and patients with renal failure on hemodialysis or peritoneal dialysis," *Antimicrobial Agents and Chemotherapy*, vol. 25, no. 1, pp. 83–87, 1984.

[17] H. Albin, J. M. Ragnaud, F. Demotes-Mainard, G. Vinçon, M. Couzineau, and C. Wone, "Pharmacokinetics of intravenous and intraperitoneal ceftriaxone in chronic ambulatory peritoneal dialysis," *European Journal of Clinical Pharmacology*, vol. 31, no. 4, pp. 479–483, 1986.

[18] A. de Sarro, D. Ammendola, M. Zappala, S. Grasso, and G. B. de Sarro, "Relationship between structure and convulsant properties of some β-lactam antibiotics following intracerebroventricular microinjection in rats," *Antimicrobial Agents and Chemotherapy*, vol. 39, no. 1, pp. 232–237, 1995.

[19] G. K. Dakdouki and G. N. Al-War, "Cefepime-induced encephalopathy," *International Journal of Infectious Diseases*, vol. 8, no. 1, pp. 59–61, 2004.

[20] F. S. Sharif-Askari, S. A. S. Sulaiman, N. S. Sharif-Askari, and A. A. S. Hussain, "Development of an adverse drug reaction risk assessment score among hospitalized patients with chronic kidney disease," *PLoS ONE*, vol. 9, no. 4, Article ID e95991, 2014.

Levamisole/Cocaine Induced Systemic Vasculitis and Immune Complex Glomerulonephritis

Lohit Garg,[1] Sagar Gupta,[2] Abhishek Swami,[3] and Ping Zhang[4]

[1]Department of Internal Medicine, Oakland University William Beaumont School of Medicine, Royal Oak, MI 48073, USA
[2]Department of Nephrology, Washington University in St. Louis, St. Louis, MO 63130, USA
[3]Department of Nephrology, Oakland University William Beaumont School of Medicine, Royal Oak, MI 48073, USA
[4]Department of Pathology, William Beaumont Hospital, Royal Oak, MI 48073, USA

Correspondence should be addressed to Lohit Garg; lohit.garg@beaumont.edu

Academic Editor: Ze'ev Korzets

Levamisole is an antihelminthic and immunomodulator medication that was banned by the USFDA in 1998. It has been increasingly used to adulterate cocaine due to its psychotropic effects and morphological properties. Adverse reactions including cutaneous vasculitis, thrombocytopenia, and agranulocytosis have been well described. Despite systemic vasculitis in this setting, renal involvement is uncommon. We report here a case of ANCA positive systemic vasculitis with biopsy proven immune complex mediated glomerulonephritis likely secondary to levamisole/cocaine. A 40-year-old Caucasian male with no past medical history presented with 3-week history of fatigue, skin rash, joint pains, painful oral lesions, oliguria, hematuria, worsening dyspnea on exertion, and progressive lower extremity edema. He had a history of regular tobacco and cocaine use. Lab testing revealed severe anemia, marked azotemia, deranged electrolytes, and 4.7 gm proteinuria. Rheumatologic testing revealed hypocomplementemia, borderline ANA, myeloperoxidase antibody, and positive atypical p-ANCA. Infectious and other autoimmune workup was negative. Kidney biopsy was consistent with immune mediated glomerulonephritis and showed mesangial proliferation and immune complex deposition consisting of IgG, IgM, and complement. High dose corticosteroids and discontinuing cocaine use resulted in marked improvement in rash, mucocutaneous lesions, and arthritis. There was no renal recovery and he remained hemodialysis dependent.

1. Introduction

Levamisole is an antihelminthic and immunomodulator medication previously used to treat steroid resistant nephrotic syndrome in pediatric population and also as adjuvant chemotherapy for colorectal and breast cancer [1, 2]. It was banned by USFDA in 1998 due to serious side effects including nonspecific rash, thrombocytopenia, and agranulocytosis. It was associated with reversible cutaneous vasculitis with earliest cases reported in 1970s [3, 4]. Particularly striking feature in these cases was purpura involving the ear. More recently, it has increasingly been used as a cutting agent in cocaine especially in the United States. Nearly 69% of cocaine samples seized by the Drug Enforcement Administration (DEA) in 2008-2009 tested positive for adulteration [5]. Renal involvement in the form of glomerulonephritis is relatively uncommon. We describe here a case of ANCA positive systemic vasculitis with biopsy proven immune complex mediated glomerulonephritis secondary to levamisole/cocaine, a rare entity.

2. Case Presentation

A 40-year-old Caucasian male with no past medical history presented to the emergency room with one-week history of progressive shortness of breath on exertion. He also complained of palpitations, fatigue, and orthopnea. In addition, he complained of progressive lower extremity swelling for the last 3 weeks and multiple painful ulcerations on his tongue and in his mouth for 2 weeks. History was also notable for multiple joint pains for 6 months. He was diagnosed with Lyme's disease and was treated with high dose doxycycline for

TABLE 1: Lab results.

Variable	Result on admission (reference range)	Result at discharge (reference range)
White cell count	12.7 (3.5–10.1)	5.7 (3.5–10.1)
Neutrophils %	10.8 (1.6–7.2)	4.6 (1.6–7.2)
Lymphocytes %	1.4 (1.1–4.0)	0.8 (1.1–4.0)
Eosinophils %	0.1 (0.0–0.4)	0.0 (0.0–0.4)
Basophils %	0.1 (0.0–0.1)	0.0 (0.0–0.1)
Monocytes %	0.3 (0.0–0.9)	0.3 (0.0–0.9)
Hemoglobin, g/dL	6.1 (13.5–17.0)	9.4 (13.5–17.0)
Platelet count	334 (150–400)	267 (150–400)
Sodium mmol/L	120 (135–145)	138 (135–145)
Potassium mmol/L	6.9 (3.5–5.2)	4.6 (3.5–5.2)
Chloride mmol/L	87 (95–107)	100 (95–107)
Carbon dioxide mmol/L	10 (21–31)	24 (21–31)
Blood urea nitrogen mg/dL	195 (8–22)	67 (8–22)
Creatinine mg/dL	20.83 (0.60–1.40)*	6.77 (0.60–1.40)
Calcium mg/dL	5.6 (8.5–10.5)	8.6 (8.5–10.5)
Phosphorus mg/dL	20.2 (2.3–4.3)	5.8 (2.3–4.3)
Aspartate aminotransferase, U/L	721 (10–37)	39 (10–37)
Alanine aminotransferase, U/L	252 (9–47)	62 (9–47)
Alkaline phosphatase, U/L	146 (30–110)	113 (30–110)
Total bilirubin, mg/dL	0.8 (0.3–1.2)	0.3 (0.3–1.2)
Albumin, g/dL	2.9 (3.5–5.1)	3.4 (3.5–5.1)
Protein, g/dL	5.3 (6.4–8.6)	5.3 (6.4–8.6)
International normalized ratio	1.7	1.1
Partial thromboplastin time, sec	44.1 (25.0–32.0)	28.8 (25.0–32.0)
Urine protein/creatinine ratio	4.7 (0.0–0.2)	
Urinalysis	3+ protein, 2+ blood, 10–20 RBC, and Hyaline and RBC cast	
ESR, mm/hr	61 (0–20)	
CRP mg/dL	7.4 (0.0–1.0)	
Complement C3, mg/dL	42 (70–176)	
Complement C4, mg/dL	7.7 (12.1–42.9)	
Anti-nuclear antibodies, IU/mL	<1 : 160 (<1 : 160)	Negative (<1 : 160)
Anti-double-stranded DNA, IU/mL	6.6 (0.0–29.9)	
Anti-neutrophil cytoplasmic antibody	1 : 640 p-ANCA (<1 : 20)	
Anti-SSA, U	0.9 (<20)	
Myeloperoxidase antibody, U	2.8 (<0.4)	
Proteinase-3 auto antibody, U	0.4 (<0.4)	
Cryoglobulin screen	Negative	

TABLE 1: Continued.

Variable	Result on admission (reference range)	Result at discharge (reference range)
Lupus anticoagulant	Negative	
Serum and protein electrophoresis	Negative for monoclonal antibodies	
Tuberculin skin test	Negative	
HIV-1 and HIV-2 antibodies	Negative	
Acute hepatitis panel	Negative for hepatitis B and hepatitis C	
Rapid plasma reagin	Negative	
Histoplasma urine antigen	Negative	
Blood and urine cultures	Negative	

*No serum creatinine values were available prior to admission.

2 months. Two months prior to admission, he noticed diffuse nonitchy rash on his chest, back, abdomen, arms, and legs that subsequently resolved. One month prior to admission, he noticed decreased urine output and dark colored urine. There was no history of fever, chills, weight loss, night sweats, cough, chest pain, or hemoptysis. He denied having any dry eyes, oral ulcers, photosensitivity, abdominal pain, hematuria, dysuria, or neurologic symptoms.

Medications included doxycycline and ibuprofen. He had history of long standing tobacco abuse, alcohol use, and regular cocaine use. He denied having any tattoos, sick contacts, recent travel, or environmental or occupational exposure.

On examination, he was afebrile, tachycardic, tachypneic, and hypoxic on room air. The tongue had hyperkeratotic, hyperpigmented papules. There were scattered erythematous maculopapular lesions on the chest. He had bilateral lower extremity edema with skin changes suggestive of chronic venous stasis and prominent symmetric synovitis of metacarpophalangeal and wrist joints. Chest auscultation revealed diffuse rales bilaterally. Cardiovascular, abdominal, and neurologic examinations were unremarkable.

Lab results are shown in Table 1. Notable lab abnormalities included anemia and severe azotemia with multiple electrolyte abnormalities (no records of prior serum creatinine values). Urinalysis showed significant hematuria and proteinuria. Urine protein/creatinine ratio was 4.7. Acute phase reactants ESR and CRP were elevated. BNP and PTH were also elevated. Rheumatologic testing revealed borderline ANA, positive atypical p-ANCA (1 : 640), and positive anti-myeloperoxidase antibodies. Complement levels (C3 and C4) were low. Remainder of the rheumatologic workup was negative. Chest X-ray showed pulmonary edema. Urine screen for drugs returned positive for cocaine and levamisole. Unfortunately quantification of levamisole could not be performed on time and resulted negative.

Kidney biopsy showed diffuse tubulointerstitial fibrosis with the majority of glomeruli globally sclerosed. Few intact

(a)

(b)

(c)

(d)

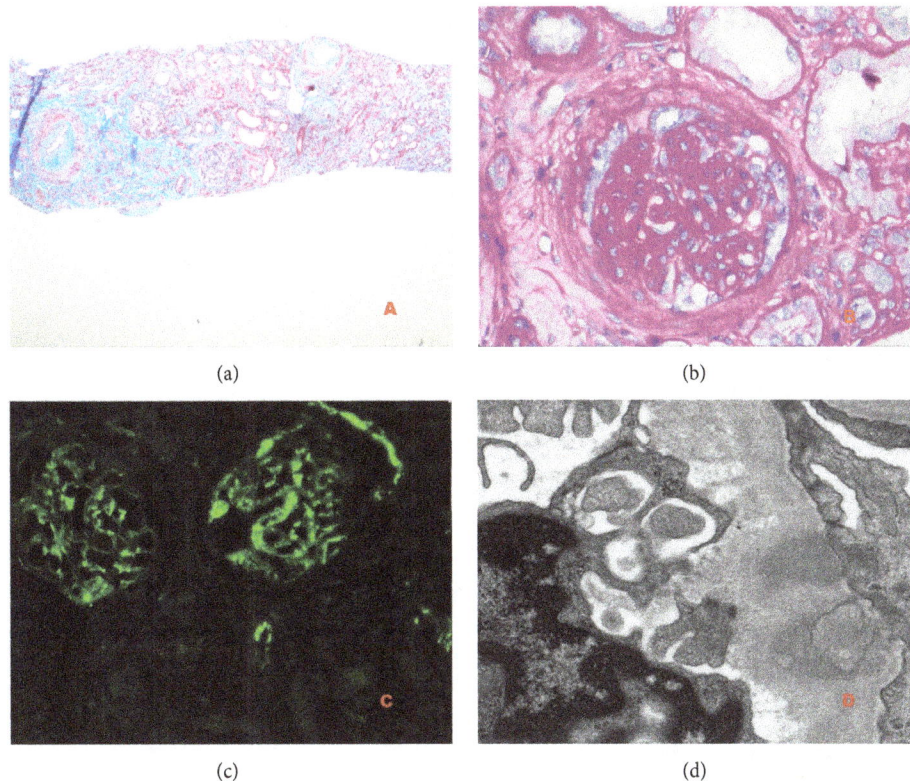

FIGURE 1: (a) Masson trichrome stain (100x) revealed severe interstitial fibrosis, thickened arterioles, and mild proliferation of glomeruli. (b) PAS stain (600x) showed mild mesangial proliferation and segmental sclerosis. No extra capillary crescent or necrosis was identified. Six of 10 glomeruli were globally sclerosed. (c) IF showed 2-3+ IgG and C3 deposit mainly in mesangium and also along the capillary loops. (d) Electron microscopy showed intramembranous and subepithelial electron dense deposits with occasional subendothelial and mesangial deposits. There were segmental foot process effacement and focal mesangial interposition.

glomeruli showed mesangial proliferation and immune complex deposition consisting of IgG, IgM, and complement in mesangial and endocapillary distribution. It was consistent with immune mediated glomerulonephritis (Figure 1). Skin biopsy of the rash was consistent with leukocytoclastic vasculitis.

Given the clinical, laboratory, and pathologic findings, we concluded that the ANCA associated systemic vasculitis and immune complex mediated glomerulonephritis were secondary to levamisole/cocaine use.

3. Clinical Course

He required mechanical ventilation for acute hypoxic and hypercarbic respiratory failure. He was placed on continuous renal replacement therapy for severe azotemia with multiple electrolyte abnormalities including hyperkalemia. He was started on high dose steroids with marked improvement in his rash, mucocutaneous lesions, and arthritis. There was no renal recovery and he remained hemodialysis dependent. He was discharged on prednisone 40 mg daily, slowly tapered, and stopped after 3 months with resolution of arthritis and skin rash. Repeat rheumatologic workup was negative for ANCA after 3 months of steroid therapy and cocaine abstinence. He is currently undergoing intermittent hemodialysis and is awaiting renal transplant.

4. Discussion

Levamisole contamination of cocaine has become a widespread health problem. In 2009, nearly two-thirds of cocaine samples seized by the DEA in the US [5] were found to be contaminated with levamisole. It is thought to potentiate the psychotropic effect of the illicit drug by increasing dopamine in the brain, acts as a bulking agent, and is morphologically difficult to recognize as an adulterant. It continues to gain medical attention as more and more cases of adverse effects of levamisole are being reported.

Earliest cases of levamisole induced necrotizing cutaneous vasculitis were reported in 1970s by Scheinberg et al. and Macfarlane and Bacon [3, 4]. Segal et al. reported levamisole induced arthritis in patients treated with levamisole as immunomodulator for Crohn's disease [6]. Strazzula et al. reported multiple cases of purpuric skin lesions in levamisole exposed patients that required less aggressive strategies than what is used for primary ANCA associated vasculitis [7]. Most of these patients tested positive for anticardiolipin antibodies, ANA, p-ANCA, or c-ANCA, all of which resolved after drug withdrawal.

Cocaine itself has been associated with ANCA positive cutaneous vasculitis but systemic organs are rarely affected [8, 9]. The contamination with levamisole adds an additional compounding factor and toxicity can occur with snorting, smoking, or intravenous use. Most of the affected individuals are chronic, habitual users suggesting large cumulative, dose dependent response [10–14].

First description of levamisole induced nephropathy was as early as in 1978 when Hansen et al. described a case of rheumatoid arthritis treated with levamisole developing a pruritic rash, leukopenia, thrombocytopenia, and proteinuria [15]. Kidney biopsy revealed granular mesangial deposits of IgA, IgG, IgM, and C3. Zwang et al. described a similar presentation with arthritis, neutropenia, purpuric rash, and acute kidney injury that had also urinalysis consistent with proteinuria but no red blood cells or cast [16]. Díaz et al. also reported cutaneous vasculitis, leukopenia, renal failure, and nephrotic proteinuria in their patient abusing intravenous cocaine [17]. Unfortunately no renal biopsies were performed in these patients. McGrath et al. in their case series of 30 patients with ANCA positivity associated with levamisole-contaminated cocaine use found 8 patients to have abnormal urinalysis with dipstick proteinuria, hematuria, or the presence of cellular casts on microscopy [18]. Two of these developed severe acute kidney injury and one underwent renal biopsy; however, that revealed pauci-immune focal necrotizing and crescentic glomerulonephritis. The mechanism in the pathogenesis of levamisole/cocaine induced ANCA positive systemic vasculitis and immune complex glomerulonephritis is unclear.

Renal involvement is relatively uncommon with ANCA positive vasculitis caused by levamisole/cocaine. To the best of our knowledge, this may be the second reported case with biopsy proven immune complex mediated glomerulonephritis. Rheumatologic workup in our patient was positive for atypical p-ANCA, myeloperoxidase antibody, and hypocomplementemia. In the presence of adequate exposure, these abnormalities are now increasingly recognized as very specific for levamisole-adulterated cocaine exposure [18–20].

5. Conclusion

This case illustrates the growing issue of cocaine abuse and levamisole contamination. Levamisole induced vasculitis is a diagnosis of exclusion but should be considered in cocaine users presenting with vasculitis, arthralgia, leukopenia, and positive ANCA titers after excluding infections and other idiopathic vasculitides. Timely recognition of this clinical entity is important to avoid misdiagnosis and unnecessary prolonged treatment with harmful cytotoxic agents as discontinuation of cocaine use could result in resolution of symptoms.

Abbreviations

ANA: Antinuclear antibody
p-ANCA: Perinuclear anti-neutrophilic
          cytoplasmic antibody
USFDA: US Food and Drug Administration
ESR: Erythrocyte sedimentation rate
C-RP: C-reactive protein
BNP: B-natriuretic peptide

PTH: Parathyroid hormone
Anti-MPO: Anti-myeloperoxidase antibody.

Conflict of Interests

All the authors have no conflict of interests and nothing to disclose.

Authors' Contribution

All authors have contributed to this paper and reviewed, and approved the current form of the paper to be submitted.

References

[1] A. A. Eddy and J. M. Symons, "Nephrotic syndrome in childhood," *The Lancet*, vol. 362, no. 9384, pp. 629–639, 2003.

[2] T. J. Hobday and C. Erlichman, "Adjuvant therapy of colon cancer: a review," *Clinical Colorectal Cancer*, vol. 1, no. 4, pp. 230–236, 2002.

[3] M. A. Scheinberg, J. B. Gomes Bezerra, F. A. Almeida, and L. A. Silveira, "Cutaneous necrotising vasculitis induced by levamisole," *British Medical Journal*, vol. 1, article 408, 1978.

[4] D. G. Macfarlane and P. A. Bacon, "Levamisole-induced vasculitis due to circulating immune complexes," *British Medical Journal*, vol. 1, no. 6110, pp. 407–408, 1978.

[5] J. A. Buchanan, K. Heard, C. Burbach, M. L. Wilson, and R. Dart, "Prevalence of levamisole in urine toxicology screens positive for cocaine in an inner-city hospital," *The Journal of the American Medical Association*, vol. 305, no. 16, pp. 1657–1658, 2011.

[6] A. W. Segal, S. F. Pugh, A. J. Levi, and G. Loewi, "Levamisole-induced arthritis in Crohn's disease," *The British Medical Journal*, vol. 2, no. 6086, article 555, 1977.

[7] L. Strazzula, K. K. Brown, J. C. Brieva et al., "Levamisole toxicity mimicking autoimmune disease," *Journal of the American Academy of Dermatology*, vol. 69, no. 6, pp. 954–959, 2013.

[8] D. R. Friedman and S. D. Wolfsthal, "Cocaine-induced pseudovasculitis," *Mayo Clinic Proceedings*, vol. 80, no. 5, pp. 671–673, 2005.

[9] G. F. L. Hofbauer, J. Hafner, and R. M. Trueb, "Urticarial vasculitis following cocaine use," *British Journal of Dermatology*, vol. 141, no. 3, pp. 600–601, 1999.

[10] N. M. G. Walsh, P. J. Green, R. W. Burlingame, S. Pasternak, and J. G. Hanly, "Cocaine-related retiform purpura: evidence to incriminate the adulterant, levamisole," *Journal of Cutaneous Pathology*, vol. 37, no. 12, pp. 1212–1219, 2010.

[11] J. M. Waller, J. D. Feramisco, L. Alberta-Wszolek, T. H. McCalmont, and L. P. Fox, "Cocaine-associated retiform purpura and neutropenia: is levamisole the culprit?" *Journal of the American Academy of Dermatology*, vol. 63, no. 3, pp. 530–535, 2010.

[12] M. Bradford, B. Rosenberg, J. Moreno, and G. Dumyati, "Bilateral necrosis of earlobes and cheeks: another complication of cocaine contaminated with levamisole," *Annals of Internal Medicine*, vol. 152, no. 11, pp. 758–759, 2010.

[13] J. A. Buchanan, J. A. Vogel, and A. M. Eberhardt, "Levamisole-induced occlusive necrotizing vasculitis of the ears after use of cocaine contaminated with levamisole," *Journal of Medical Toxicology*, vol. 7, no. 1, pp. 83–84, 2011.

[14] E. K. Farhat, T. T. Muirhead, M. L. Chaffins, and M. C. Douglass, "Levamisole-induced cutaneous necrosis mimicking coagulopathy," *Archives of Dermatology*, vol. 146, no. 11, pp. 1320–1321, 2010.

[15] T. M. Hansen, J. Petersen, P. Halberg et al., "Levamisole-induced nephropathy," *The Lancet*, vol. 2, no. 8092, p. 737, 1978.

[16] N. A. Zwang, L. B. Van Wagner, and S. Rose, "A case of Levamisole-induced systemic vasculitis and cocaine-induced midline destructive lesion: a case report," *Journal of Clinical Rheumatology*, vol. 17, no. 4, pp. 197–200, 2011.

[17] H. Á. Díaz, A. I. M. Callejo, J. F. G. Rodríguez, L. R. Pazos, I. G. Buela, and A. M. B. Barrera, "ANCA-positive vasculitis induced by levamisole-adulterated cocaine and nephrotic syndrome: the kidney as an unusual target," *American Journal of Case Reports*, vol. 14, pp. 557–561, 2013.

[18] M. M. McGrath, T. Isakova, H. G. Rennke, A. M. Mottola, K. A. Laliberte, and J. L. Niles, "Contaminated cocaine and antineutrophil cytoplasmic antibody-associated disease," *Clinical Journal of the American Society of Nephrology*, vol. 6, no. 12, pp. 2799–2805, 2011.

[19] J. Graf, K. Lynch, C.-L. Yeh et al., "Purpura, cutaneous necrosis, and antineutrophil cytoplasmic antibodies associated with levamisole-adulterated cocaine," *Arthritis and Rheumatism*, vol. 63, no. 12, pp. 3998–4001, 2011.

[20] W. F. Pendergraft and J. L. Niles, "Trojan horses: drug culprits associated with antineutrophil cytoplasmic autoantibody (ANCA) vasculitis," *Current Opinion in Rheumatology*, vol. 26, no. 1, pp. 42–49, 2014.

An Unusual Initial Presentation of Lupus Nephritis as a Renal Mass

Remi Goupil,[1] Annie-Claire Nadeau-Fredette,[1] Virginie Royal,[2] Alexandre Dugas,[3] and Jean-Philippe Lafrance[1,4,5]

[1]Nephrology Division, Hôpital Maisonneuve-Rosemont, Montreal, QC, Canada H1T 2M4
[2]Pathology Department, Hôpital Maisonneuve-Rosemont, Montreal, QC, Canada H1T 2M4
[3]Radiology Division, Hôpital Maisonneuve-Rosemont, Montreal, QC, Canada H1T 2M4
[4]Medicine Department, Universite de Montreal, Montreal, QC, Canada H3T 1J4
[5]Centre de Recherche Hôpital Maisonneuve-Rosemont, Montreal, QC, Canada H1T 2M4

Correspondence should be addressed to Jean-Philippe Lafrance; jean-philippe.lafrance@umontreal.ca

Academic Editor: Kouichi Hirayama

Lupus nephritis is a frequent manifestation of systemic lupus erythematous. Lupus nephritis usually presents with abnormal urinalysis, proteinuria, and/or renal insufficiency. We report a case of a 48-year-old woman who underwent partial nephrectomy for a fortuitously discovered solid enhancing left kidney mass. No neoplastic cells were found in the biopsy specimen; however, the pathology findings were compatible with immune complex glomerulonephritis with a predominantly membranous distribution, a pattern suggestive of lupus nephritis. The mass effect was apparently due to a dense interstitial lymphocytic infiltrate resulting in a pseudotumor. Further investigation revealed microscopic hematuria with a normal kidney function and no significant proteinuria. Antinuclear antibodies were negative, although anti-DNA and anti-SSA/Rho antibodies were positive. A diagnosis of probable silent lupus nephritis was made and the patient was followed up without immunosuppressive treatment. After two years of follow-up, she did not progress to overt disease. To our knowledge, this represents the first case of lupus nephritis with an initial presentation as a renal mass.

1. Introduction

Lupus nephritis (LN) carries one of the highest morbidity and mortality risks of systemic lupus erythematous (SLE). Usually, LN will be suspected in the presence of active urine sediment, proteinuria, and/or renal insufficiency and confirmed by kidney biopsy. This report describes an unusual case of LN diagnosed fortuitously after a partial nephrectomy for a solid renal lesion.

2. Case Presentation

A 48-year-old woman with abdominal pain was diagnosed with acute cholecystitis based on findings on a computed tomography (CT) scan and ultrasound. The CT scan also showed a 15 × 17 mm homogeneous, enhancing left renal lesion without fat or calcium contents (Figure 1(a)). Magnetic resonance imaging (MRI) revealed a focal left renal iso/mildly hypointense T1 and T2 lesion, with diffusion restriction, and a mild to moderate homogeneous enhancement, without fat content (Figures 1(b) and 1(c)). The differential diagnosis included papillary neoplasm of the kidney, focal lymphomatous infiltration, focal pyelonephritis, and pseudotumoral sarcoidosis. The patient underwent a partial left nephrectomy for a neoplasm suspicion. Pathology evaluation did not show any neoplastic cells but rather a focal and dense lymphocytic infiltrate resulting in a pseudotumor (Figure 1(d)). This interstitial infiltrate was predominantly composed of mature T lymphocyte, with fewer B lymphocytes, and rare plasmocytes, without IgG4 overexpression. Light microscopic evaluation of the glomeruli showed features of membranous glomerulonephritis with diffusely thickened glomerular basal membranes (GBM). Jones' silver stain revealed vacuolisation and spike appearance of the GBM. Few glomeruli showed

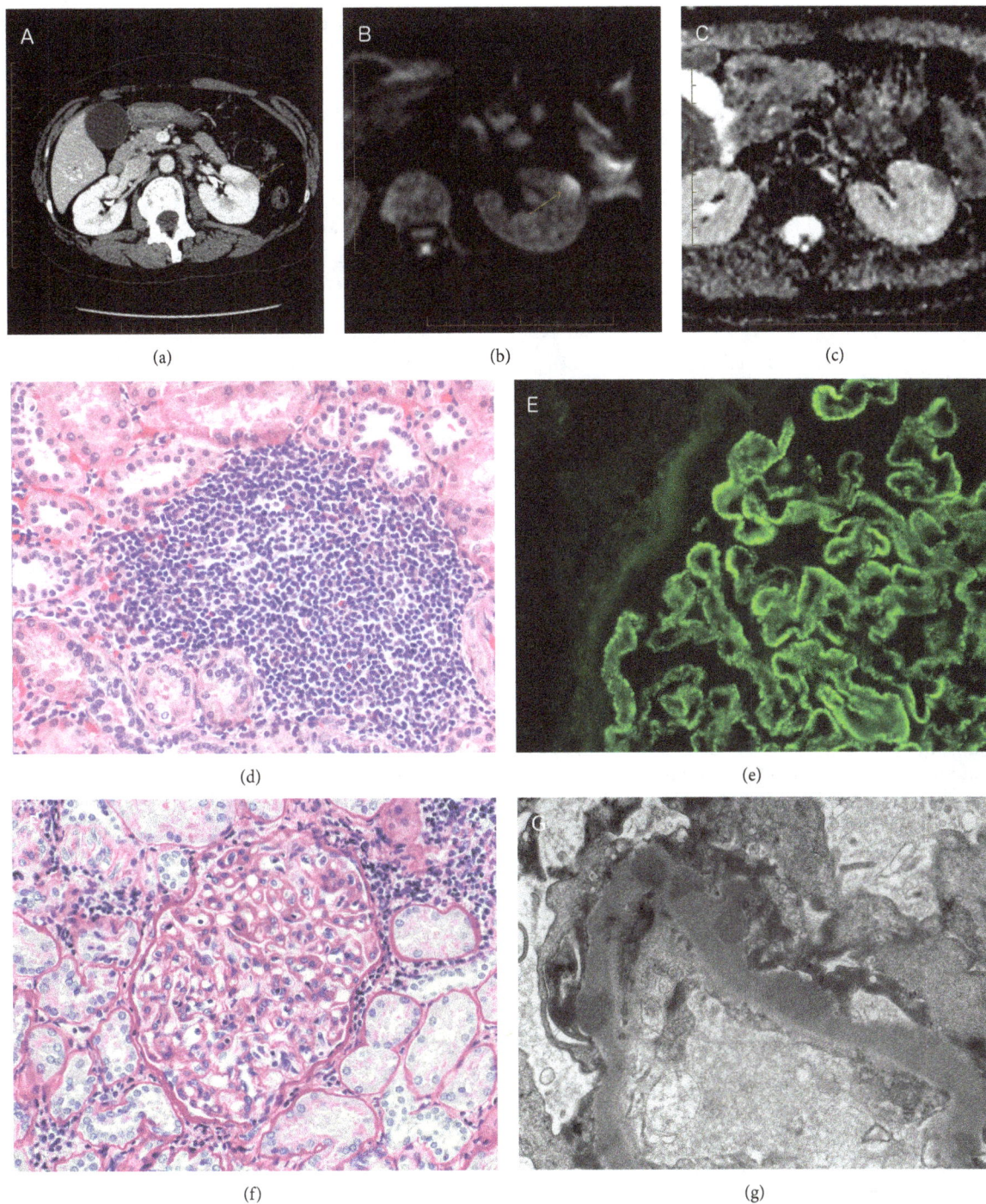

FIGURE 1: Radiologic and pathologic presentation of the renal lesion. (a) CT scan image showing a homogeneous, enhancing left renal lesion. (b) Diffusion renal magnetic resonance imaging (MRI) image of the same left renal lesion. (c) Apparent diffusion coefficient (ADC) MRI image. (d) Light microscopy with periodic acid-Schiff staining showing a lymphocytic infiltration. (e) Granular positivity of C1q on the glomerular basement membrane by immunofluorescence. (f) Higher magnification of endocapillary hypercellularity. (g) Electronic microscopy showing subepithelial deposits on the glomerular basal membrane.

a focal endocapillary hypercellularity and two presented fibrocellular crescents. Necrosis was not seen. Immunofluorescence microscopy showed granular positivity along the GBM and mesangium for IgG (3+, on 0–3 scale), IgA (3+), IgM (1+), C3 (3+), C1q (2+), Kappa (3+), and Lambda (3+) (Figure 1(e)). Testing for IgG subclasses was uninterpretable, and testing for anti-PLA2R was not performed. Electron microscopy showed numerous subepithelial and mesangial deposits and rare small subendothelial deposits (Figure 1(g)). There were no extraglomerular deposits, and tubuloreticular

TABLE 1: Investigation results at time of partial nephrectomy specimen and subsequent kidney biopsy after 12 months of clinical follow-up.

Investigation	Results	
	Partial nephrectomy	Biopsy
Serum creatinine	60 μmol/L	61 μmol/L
Microscopic hematuria	3–5 red blood cells per field	3–5 red blood cells per field
Urinary albumin/creatinine ratio	7.6 mg/mmol	10 mg/mmol
ANA titer	<1 : 80	<1 : 80
Anti-DNA	424×10^3 IU/L	$<55 \times 10^3$ IU/L
Anti-SSA/Rho	10.4 IU/L	—
Anti-SSB/La	15.9 IU/L	—
C3 complement	1.22 g/L	1.08 g/L
C4 complement	0.15 g/L	0.19 g/L
Serum IgG	28.7 g/L	—
IgG4 subclass	0.6 g/L	—

inclusions were not seen. Thus, a diagnosis of immune complex glomerulonephritis with a predominant membranous distribution was made, a pattern suggestive of lupus nephritis [1].

On further evaluation, the patient denied any symptoms which could have been related to SLE and physical examination was noncontributory. Past personal and familial medical history were noncontributory, without known autoimmune or renal conditions. Laboratory tests were as follows (Table 1): creatinine 60 μmol/L, microscopic hematuria (3–5 red blood cells (RBC) per field on multiple occasions and 6–10 RBC per field once), absence of urinary casts, urine albumin-to-creatinine ratio 7.6 mg/mmol (normal < 3.4), negative antinuclear antibodies (ANA), anti-DNA 424×10^3 IU/L (normal < 55×10^3), anti-SSA/Rho and anti-SSB/La 10.4 and 15.9 IU/L, respectively (normal < 8.0), normal C3, lower limit of normal C4, serum IgG 28.7 g/L (normal 5.5–16.3), IgG4 subclass 0.6 g/L (normal 0.07–0.88), and negative HIV, hepatitis B and C viruses testing.

Considering the absence of major signs of disease activity, the patient was first observed without treatment. During the subsequent 12 months, the patient remained asymptomatic with persistent microscopic hematuria and microalbuminuria (Table 1). In order to clarify prognostic and to determine treatment indication, a right kidney biopsy was performed (11 glomeruli were obtained). The pathology confirmed an immune complex glomerulonephritis with a predominantly membranous distribution, with immunofixation showing deposition of IgG, IgA, IgM, C3, and C1q, but without any signs of focal proliferation. The patient was further observed without immunosuppressive therapy. Eighteen months after initial diagnosis, she reported arthralgia in both hands and was referred to a rheumatologist. She had no physical signs of lupus-related arthritis and, as hematuria and albuminuria had disappeared and both ANA and anti-DNA levels were

negative, it was decided to continue observation without treatment.

3. Discussion

To our knowledge, this is the first description of a lupus nephritis diagnosed in the context of a renal lesion suggestive of malignancy. In the partial nephrectomy specimen, no tumorous or neoplastic cells were found but only features compatible with LN. IgG4 renal disease was considered as it may also present as inflammatory mass and membranous nephropathy, but IgG4 serum levels and immunostaining on the biopsy were not in favour of this diagnosis [2]. Renal disease in SLE is usually not associated with renal masses but, in this case, it appears it was the result of a dense lymphocytic infiltrate.

According to the Systemic Lupus International Collaborating Clinics (SLICC) group, biopsy-proven LN in presence of ANA or anti-DNA antibodies is now sufficient to make a diagnosis of SLE [3]. Renal involvement is frequent among SLE patients and presentation is highly variable [4]. True prevalence of renal-limited SLE is not well described, as this disease is usually accompanied by systemic manifestations on diagnosis or can herald the arrival of clinical SLE. However, cases of LN with negative serologies and without subsequent development of systemic involvement have been described [5].

Silent LN is usually defined as biopsy-proven LN without any renal clinical evidence of disease activity [6]. In silent LN, renal pathology usually shows isolated mesangial disease, although it can also demonstrate focal of diffuse proliferative disease. In a series of 86 SLE patients without clinical signs of renal involvement, 15 percent had class III or IV nephritis and 10 percent had class V membranous nephritis [7]. Prognosis of silent LN ranges from benign renal evolution to progression into a clinically active disease [7, 8].

This case of lupus nephritis is unusual because of its initial manifestation as a malignancy-suspected renal mass. The evolution suggests a case of early silent LN. Prevalence, prognosis, and usefulness of immunosuppressive treatment in similar cases remain unclear as this condition would usually not warrant a kidney biopsy. Further studies are needed to better characterize silent LN.

Key Message

Lupus nephritis can present itself as a solid mass suggestive of neoplasm.

Ethical Approval

Publication of this case report was approved by the Director of the professional services at Maisonneuve-Rosemont Hospital.

Consent

The patient described in the case report had given informed consent for the case report to be published.

Conflict of Interests

The authors have nothing to declare.

References

[1] J. J. Weening, V. D. D'Agati, M. M. Schwartz et al., "The classification of glomerulonephritis in systemic lupus erythematosus revisited," *Kidney International*, vol. 65, pp. 521–530, 2004.

[2] L. D. Cornell, " IgG4-related kidney disease," *Current Opinion in Nephrology and Hypertension*, vol. 21, pp. 279–288, 2012.

[3] M. Petri, A. M. Orbai, G. S. Alarcón et al., "Derivation and validation of the Systemic Lupus International Collaborating Clinics classification criteria for systemic lupus erythematosus," *Arthritis & Rheumatology*, vol. 64, no. 8, pp. 2677–2686, 2012.

[4] N. Kasitanon, L. S. Magder, and M. Petri, "Predictors of survival in systemic lupus erythematosus," *Medicine*, vol. 85, no. 3, pp. 147–156, 2006.

[5] A. Huerta, A. S. Bomback, V. Liakopoulos et al., "Renal-limited 'lupus-like' nephritis," *Nephrology Dialysis Transplantation*, vol. 27, no. 6, pp. 2337–2342, 2012.

[6] M. E. Zabaleta-Lanz, L. E. Muñoz, F. J. Tapanes et al., "Further description of early clinically silent lupus nephritis," *Lupus*, vol. 15, no. 12, pp. 845–851, 2006.

[7] D. Wakasugi, T. Gono, Y. Kawaguchi et al., "Frequency of class III and IV nephritis in systemic lupus erythematosus without clinical renal involvement: an analysis of predictive measures," *The Journal of Rheumatology*, vol. 39, no. 1, pp. 79–85, 2012.

[8] M. R. Gonzalez-Crespo, J. I. Lopez-Fernandez, G. Usera, M. J. Poveda, and J. J. Gomez- Reino, "Outcome of silent lupus nephritis," *Seminars in Arthritis and Rheumatism*, vol. 26, no. 1, pp. 468–476, 1996.

4

Common Iliac Artery Thrombosis following Pelvic Surgery Resulting in Kidney Allograft Failure Successfully Treated by Percutaneous Transluminal Angioplasty with Balloon-Expandable Covered Stent

Maheswara S. Golla, Subasit Acharjee, Bertrand L. Jaber, and Lawrence A. Garcia

Department of Medicine, St. Elizabeth's Medical Center, Department of Medicine, Tufts University School of Medicine, Boston, MA 02135, USA

Correspondence should be addressed to Lawrence A. Garcia; lawrence.garcia@steward.org

Academic Editor: Helmut H. Schiffl

We report the case of a 66-year-old woman who developed acute kidney allograft failure due to thrombotic occlusion of the common iliac artery after hysterectomy requiring emergent allograft rescue. She underwent percutaneous transluminal angioplasty with endovascular balloon expandable covered stent graft placement in the right common iliac artery. Although there are a handful of case reports of acute limb ischemia secondary to acute common iliac artery thrombosis, this is the first case reported in the literature resulting in successful kidney allograft rescue following pelvic surgery.

1. Background

Arterial thrombosis causing late acute kidney allograft failure is extremely rare. Pelvic or abdominal surgeries may place kidney allografts implanted in the pelvis at risk for injury [1]. In the literature of pelvic surgery complications, injury to the common iliac artery or external iliac artery has been reported, and required either surgical or endovascular repair [2–4]. We report a case that may represent the first in the literature of a kidney allograft rescue following pelvic surgery.

2. Case Presentation

A 66-year-old woman with end-stage renal disease in the setting of type-2 diabetes mellitus, hypertension, kidney stones, and renal artery stenosis had received an unrelated living-donor kidney transplant 7 years earlier. She also had a history of chronic obstructive pulmonary disease, coronary artery disease, heart failure with preserved left ventricular ejection fraction, and atrial fibrillation (on rivaroxaban, an orally active direct factor Xa inhibitor) for which she had undergone atrioventricular nodal ablation and insertion of a permanent pacemaker. She presented with excessive uterine bleeding. The workup demonstrated a pelvic mass and fluid-filled uterus. She underwent an elective hysteroscopy with dilation and curettage, which revealed pyometra. The intraoperative course was complicated by bleeding and uterine perforation requiring total abdominal hysterectomy and bilateral salpingooophorectomy. She lost 300 mL of blood and received intraoperatively 3.2 liters of crystalloids. There was no documented intraoperative hypotension. Pulses were equally palpable in both lower extremities before and after surgery. The patient developed anuria in the immediate postoperative period, and furosemide (40 mg) was administered intravenously with no response. The patient was reintubated for acute respiratory failure, and her anuria persisted.

3. Investigations

The urology service was initially consulted, and the patient underwent a cystoscopy with retrograde ureterogram, which revealed normal iodinated contrast filling and caliber of

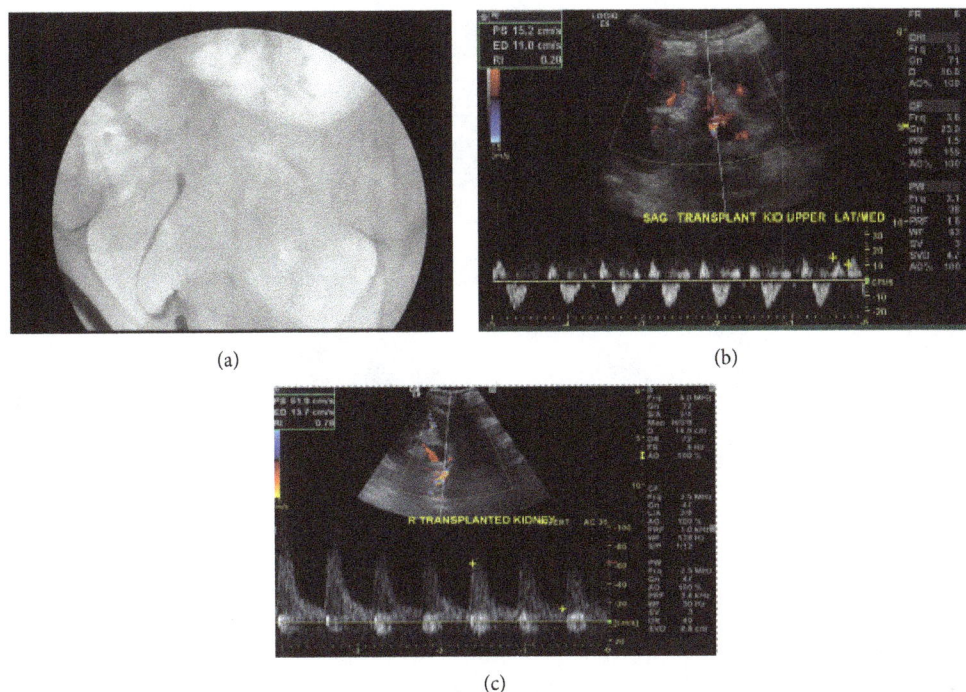

(a)

(b)

(c)

FIGURE 1: Retrograde pyelography of the kidney allograft showing patency of the ureter, pelvis, and calyces (a). Preprocedural color Doppler of kidney allograft showing renal arterial flow reversal during diastolic phase (b), with normalization of arterial flow pattern on day 1 after the intervention (c).

the ureter and intrarenal collective system of the kidney allograft (Figure 1(a)). The nephrology service was consulted approximately 4 hours from the onset of anuria and recommended a Duplex ultrasound of the kidney allograft to assess the renal vasculature. The study demonstrated reversal of flow within multiple renal arterial branches during diastole (Figure 1(b)), which was suspicious for either arterial or venous occlusive disease. Of note, the patient was receiving tacrolimus and vancomycin, and both serum trough levels were therapeutic. The patient was initiated on systemic anticoagulation.

The vascular medicine service was consulted immediately, and emergent iliac and renal angiography was performed within 6 hours from the onset of anuria. Iliac angiography revealed a thrombus obstructing 99% of the proximal right common iliac artery (Figure 2(a)). The length of the arterial segment involved was 50 mm. The anastomosis of the kidney allograft to the right common iliac artery was patent and free of disease. There was no evidence of iliac vein trauma or disruption to account for the anuria.

4. Treatment

We performed the intervention through retrograde right common femoral artery in an intraluminal position. The culprit lesion was located at the origin of the right common iliac artery, which was 50 mm in length. The lesion was crossed intraluminally by a 0.035″ Terumo guide wire. A 5 × 40 mm Admiral Xtreme (Medtronic, Inc.) balloon was advanced over the guide wire on to the lesion

and predilated by two inflations with a maximum pressure of 14 atmospheres (Figures 2(c) and 2(d)). A 7 × 59 mm iCast covered stent (Atrium Medical Corporation, Hudson, NH), a balloon-expandable stainless steel encapsulated stent, was then deployed in the right common iliac artery. To control sandwiched thrombi (thrombi in between the vessel wall and covered stent) prolapse from the edge of the stent to the intraluminal area and to cover the edge of the culprit lesion completely, we deployed a second 7 × 22 mm iCast stent more distally (Figure 2(e)). Both stents were postdilated with a 8 × 40 mm Dorado PTA balloon (Bard Peripheral Vascular, Inc., Tempe, AZ) (Figure 2(e)) to minimize in-stent restenosis and stent thrombosis. There was no residual stenosis and the pressure gradient dropped to zero with normal flow noted through the iliac artery and the kidney allograft artery (Figure 2(f)). We used a total of 80 mL of Iohexol (Omnipaque, GE Healthcare) due to the unavailability of carbon dioxide for the angiogram during the intervention.

5. Outcome and Follow-Up

Following the procedure, the anuria began to resolve within hours and corrected overnight. The serum creatinine level, which had peaked at 3.3 mg/dL, declined and returned to the baseline value of 0.9 mg/dL over two weeks (Figure 3).

One week after the intervention, a repeat Duplex ultrasound of the right common iliac artery revealed normal flow and patent stents (Figure 1(c)). There was normal Doppler flow to the kidney allograft. The patient remained

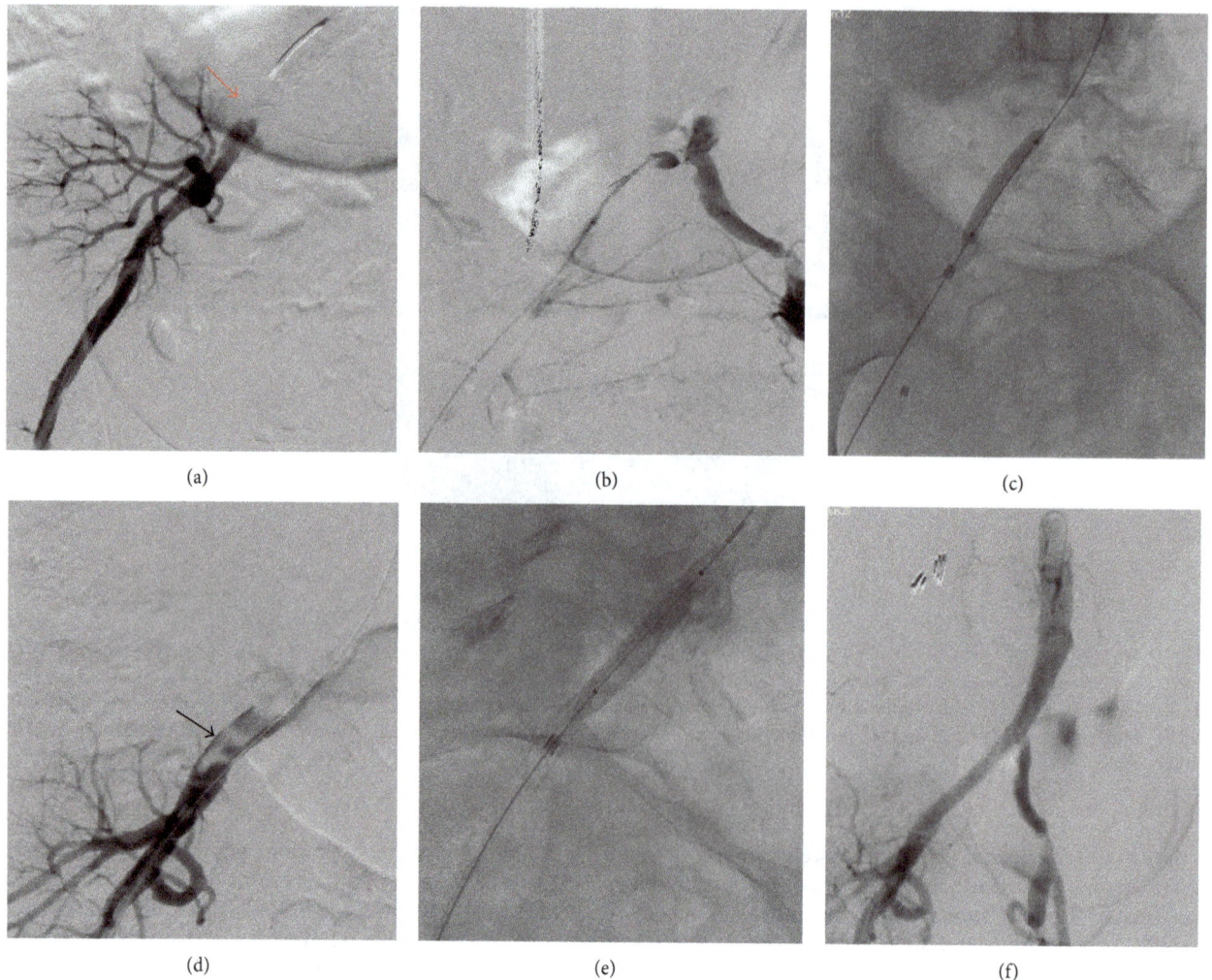

FIGURE 2: Aortoiliac and femoral angiogram showing complete occlusion (red arrow) of the right common iliac artery proximal to the kidney allograft anastomosis (a). Collaterals from the left iliac and femoral arteries feeding right-sided vessels below the occlusion (b). Balloon angioplasty of the right common iliac artery (c). Partial recanalization and visible floating thrombus (black arrow) of the right common iliac artery after balloon angioplasty (d). Balloon assisted covered stent (iCast) deployment and postdilation of the stent (e). Postintervention angiogram shows normal flow to the kidney allograft (f).

asymptomatic and her serum creatinine obtained at 8 months of follow-up was 1.0 mg/dL.

6. Discussion

Late kidney allograft failure after pelvic surgery is extremely rare. To our knowledge, this is the first case to report the successful rescue of a kidney allograft after pelvic surgery by endovascular intervention. One similar case was reported in 1990, although the kidney allograft was completely thrombosed and infarcted [1]. A handful of iliac artery injury cases have been reported following pelvic surgeries [2–4]. The etiology of vascular complications can be classified as thrombotic and embolic and from other causes (external or internal compression or injury). Thrombosis may arise as a complication of intraoperative manipulation of vital structures [1–4]. In our case, Doppler arterial scan of the allograft renal artery showed "flow reversal in diastole,"

which may be a consequence of either arterial obstruction or venous obstruction/occlusion similar to a phlegmatic limb (Figure 1(a)). The angiogram revealed right common iliac artery subtotal occlusion with evident thrombus (Figure 2(a)) but a patent renal allograft anastomosis. Hence, this late acute allograft failure was attributed to decreased perfusion pressure to the kidney allograft secondary to acute arterial inflow obstruction. Prompt intervention within the 6 hours after initial anuria successfully rescued the renal allograft.

The Covered versus Balloon-Expandable Stent Trial (COBEST), a multicenter, randomized, controlled trial involving iliac arteries in patients with severe aortoiliac occlusive disease, showed that covered stents had a significantly better primary patency for Trans-Atlantic Inter-Society Consensus (TASC) C and D lesions compared with the noncovered stents [5]. Among the balloon-expandable covered stents, iCast stents are approved in the US for aortoiliac occlusions or stenotic disease. In our case, the patient

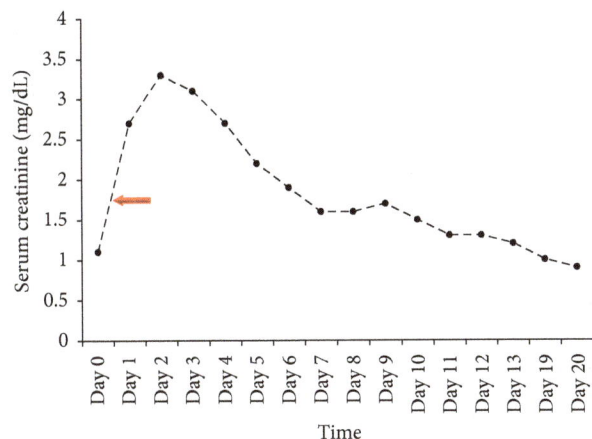

FIGURE 3: Time course of the serum creatinine in relation to the pelvic surgery (day 0) and the endovascular intervention (red arrow: time of intervention).

underwent balloon angioplasty with iCast stenting to the right common iliac artery. The patient remains symptom-free 8 months after the intervention, with an excellent kidney allograft function.

Conflict of Interests

The authors declare that they have no conflict of interests regarding the publication of this paper.

References

[1] J. M. McCarthy, C. K. Yeung, and P. A. Keown, "Late renal-artery thrombosis after transplantation associated with intraoperative abdominopelvic compression," *The New England Journal of Medicine*, vol. 323, no. 26, article 1845, 1990.

[2] J. A. Akoh, "Transplant nephrectomy," *World Journal of Transplantation*, vol. 1, no. 1, pp. 4–12, 2011.

[3] J.-C. Shih, K.-L. Liu, and M.-K. Shyu, "Temporary balloon occlusion of the common iliac artery: new approach to bleeding control during cesarean hysterectomy for placenta percreta," *American Journal of Obstetrics and Gynecology*, vol. 193, no. 5, pp. 1756–1758, 2005.

[4] L. Canaud, K. Hireche, F. Joyeux et al., "Endovascular repair of aorto-iliac artery injuries after lumbar-spine surgery," *European Journal of Vascular and Endovascular Surgery*, vol. 42, no. 2, pp. 167–171, 2011.

[5] B. P. Mwipatayi, S. Thomas, J. Wong et al., "A comparison of covered vs bare expandable stents for the treatment of aortoiliac occlusive disease," *Journal of Vascular Surgery*, vol. 54, no. 6, pp. 1561–1570, 2011.

5

Successful Antiviral Triple Therapy in a Longstanding Refractory Hepatitis C Virus Infection with an Acute Kidney Injury

David Callau Monje,[1] Niko Braun,[1] Joerg Latus,[1] Kerstin Amann,[2] Mark Dominik Alscher,[1] and Martin Kimmel[1]

[1] *Department of Internal Medicine, Division of Nephrology, Robert-Bosch-Hospital, Auerbach Street 110, 70179 Stuttgart, Germany*
[2] *Department of Pathology, Erlangen University Hospital, Krankenhaus Street 8-10, 91054 Erlangen, Germany*

Correspondence should be addressed to David Callau Monje; david.callaumonje@rbk.de

Academic Editor: Ichiei Narita

Introduction. The HCV infection is a common disease with many chronically infected patients worldwide. So far, the standard therapy of a chronic HCV infection consisted of interferon as single therapy or in combination with ribavirin. After approval of the two protease inhibitors, boceprevir and telaprevir, the standard therapy for patients with genotype 1 changed. In patients with acute kidney injury (AKI) these therapies are not approved and have so far not been evaluated in studies. *Case Report.* In April 2012, a 58-year-old female was admitted due to a cryoglobulin-positive chronic HCV infection which had been treated with interferon and ribavirin. Currently, the patient was admitted because of severe complications with an acute kidney injury. We treated our patient successfully with a boceprevir based triple therapy. *Conclusion.* Limited data suggests that a therapy with ribavirin in patients with AKI seems to be safe under close monitoring. Our patient was treated successfully with a protease inhibitor based triple therapy. Nevertheless, it is necessary to plan an interventional study to evaluate the exact risk-benefit profile of triple therapy regimens in patients with AKI and hepatitis C.

1. Introduction

HCV infection is a very common disease with about 170 million chronically infected patients worldwide. Once a chronic infection develops, it is associated with high morbidity and mortality due to hepatic and extrahepatic involvement. Extrahepatic manifestations are a common phenomenon and are present in approximately 40% of all patients with chronic HCV infection [1]. These extrahepatic symptoms often manifest in a dermatologic, autoimmune, renal, or hematologic manner. Proofs of cryoglobulins are one of the most common findings in chronic HCV infection. Approximately 50% of all patients with chronic HCV infection are positive for cryoglobulins and, in case of an essential cryoglobulinemia in more than 90% of all cases, a chronic HCV infection is detectable [2].

So far the standard therapy of a chronic HCV infection consisted of pegylated or regular interferon alfa as a single therapy or in combination with ribavirin. After approval of the two protease inhibitors, boceprevir and telaprevir, in 2011, the standard therapy for patients with a genotype 1 changed. Triple therapy protocols were developed by maintaining the standard therapy containing of interferon alfa and ribavirin, by adding one of the new protease inhibitors. With these triple therapies, a relevant increase in sustained virologic response (SVR) rates was observed; SVR is defined as a negative HCV-RNA 24 weeks after cessation of antiviral therapy. The SVR rates in therapy naive patients increased from 40% to 67-68% [3] and, in formerly treated patients, from 21% to 59–66% [4].

In patients with chronic kidney disease (CKD) and a glomerular filtration rate (GFR) of less than 50 mL/min, these therapies are not approved due to a contraindication of ribavirin and have so far not been evaluated in studies. KDIGO (Kidney Disease: Improving Global Outcomes) recommends, in case of an HCV-associated glomerulopathy with a decreased GFR, a monotherapy with pegylated interferon alfa [5]. In the most recent German guidelines for chronic HCV infection there is a grade B recommendation for a therapy with standard or pegylated interferon alfa as a monotherapy or in combination with low-dose ribavirin with controls of the blood count in close intervals [6]. This recommendation concurs to the results of a multicenter study, where pegylated interferon was used successfully in combination with low-dose ribavirin in patients with Hepatitis C infection receiving hemodialysis [7]. In one single-center study, the triple therapies were safely used in patients with CKD [8]. So far, no data exists about the use of a triple therapy in patients with acute kidney injury and cryoglobulinemic vasculitis.

2. Case Report

In April 2012, a 58-year-old female was admitted to our hospital due to a cryoglobulin-positive chronic HCV infection. The chronic HCV infection (genotype 1b) was first diagnosed in July 2007 and was treated according to guidelines from September 2007 over 24 weeks with pegylated interferon alfa and ribavirin. In the course of the therapy, a considerable drop of HCV-RNA in the blood occurred, but the HCV-RNA never dropped below the detection threshold (partial nonresponse). The antiviral therapy was, therefore, stopped according to the guidelines after 24 weeks.

Currently, the patient was admitted because of a dramatic decline in the general state of health. She complained about shortness of breath, peripheral edema, and an increase in body weight.

The examination revealed edema at the lower and upper limbs as well as anasarca. Furthermore, vasculitic skin efflorescences were found at the lower legs.

Laboratory tests showed an increased erythrocyte sedimentation rate (65 mm/h, norm 1–30 mm/h) and the serum creatinine was increased to 1,8 mg/dL (norm 0,5–1,2 mg/dL) according to an estimated GFR (MDRD equation) of 30 mL/min. A nephrotic syndrome with a proteinuria of 6,9 g/24 h, a serum albumin of 2,2 g/dL (norm 3,5–5,0 g/dL), and elevated lipids (LDL 272 mg/dL, norm 100–150 mg/dL) was diagnosed. Liver function tests were within normal range, but HCV-RNA was positive with 5 million copies/mL. Complement factors C3 (75 mg/dL, norm 90–180 mg/dL) and C4 (2,7 mg/dL, norm 10,0–40,0 mg/dL) were decreased and cryoglobulins (type IgM) were positive. A liver ultrasound showed sonographic signs of a beginning liver cirrhosis.

After recompensation with loop diuretics with a decrease in body weight of 9 kg, we performed a kidney biopsy. Histological workup showed a severe diffuse membranoproliferative glomerulonephritis (MPGN) type 1 with a discrete extracapillary proliferative component and a diffuse tubulointerstitial damage (Figure 1). The immunofluorescence study revealed granular deposits of IgG, IgM, and C3c alongside the glomerular basement membrane while IgA was negative.

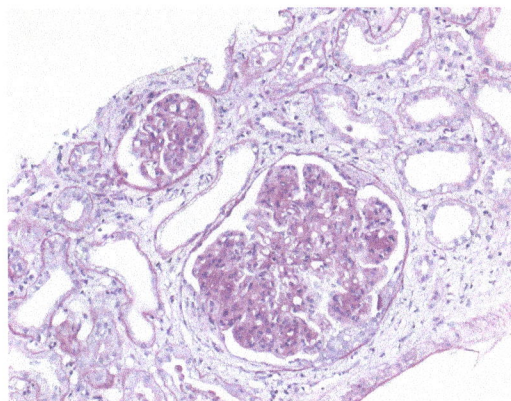

FIGURE 1: PAS stained renal biopsy of our patient showing the characteristic histologic features of a MPGN type 1 (thickening of the basement membrane, diffuse mesangial expansion, and proliferation). Furthermore, a discrete extracapillary proliferative component and a diffuse tubulointerstitial damage were present.

The final electron microscopy confirmed the diagnosis and showed a partially doubled glomerular basement membrane with interposition of mesangial cells, fusion of the podocyte foot processes, and intracapillary proliferation.

Because of a severe chronic HCV infection with hepatic and extrahepatic manifestations, we decided to treat our patient with a boceprevir based triple therapy. We initiated the therapy with a 4-week lead-in phase with pegylated interferon alfa 2a and ribavirin. Due to renal impairment, we decreased the interferon dose to 135 μg weekly and the ribavirin dose to 200 mg daily. After control of the virologic response and decrease of the HCV-RNA to 6.000 IU/mL, we added boceprevir 800 mg 3 times daily. Due to the beginning liver cirrhosis, the triple therapy was continued for a total of 48 weeks.

During the antiviral therapy, the administration of erythropoetin was necessary due to anemia. After 10 weeks of therapy duration, the viral load and the cryoglobulins were negative for the first time. The creatinine level dropped within the normal range and the proteinuria declined from initially 12.5 g protein/g creatinine to 0.4 g protein/g creatinine (Figure 2).

The triple therapy was discontinued after a total therapy duration of 48 weeks. HCV-RNA remained negative during the whole surveillance and a SVR was declared 24 weeks after cessation of therapy.

3. Discussion

Our patient received an appropriate antiviral therapy with a partial nonresponse in the past. Currently, we diagnosed a chronic HCV infection with severe hepatic and extrahepatic manifestations with acute kidney injury. In general, KDIGO suggested that all patients with renal impairment and HCV infection should be evaluated for antiviral therapy [9]. The decision whether to treat or not should be based on the potential benefits and risks of therapy. Because of the severity of the hepatic and extrahepatic manifestations in our patient

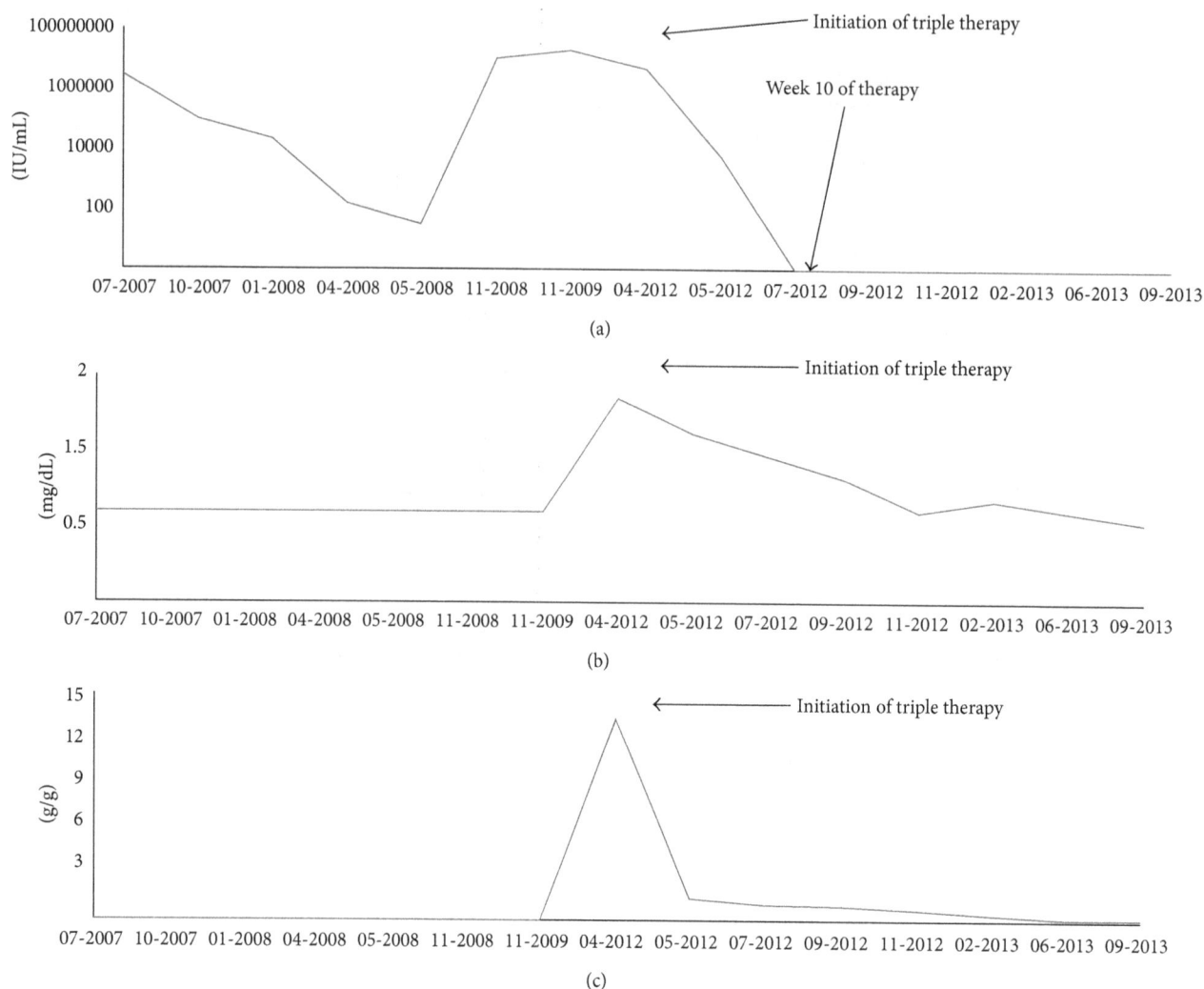

FIGURE 2: Trend of crucial laboratory parameters. (a) HCV-RNA blood levels in IU/mL. After initiation of triple therapy, the levels fell continuously and were negative for the first time after 10 weeks of therapy. (b) Serum creatinine blood levels in mg/dL. At admission, the creatinine was considerably elevated and fell constantly after start of therapy. (c) Proteinuria in g protein/g creatinine. Quickly after initiation of antiviral therapy, proteinuria decreased dramatically and remained low over the whole time of surveillance.

and a partial nonresponse to interferon alfa and ribavirin, we chose a new triple therapy regimen adding boceprevir to pegylated interferon alfa and ribavirin. With this decision, we followed an expert recommendation about retherapy in patients with partial virologic response in patients without renal impairment [10].

Concerning the weekly doses of pegylated interferon alfa, we followed the German HCV guidelines which recommend 90–135 μg weekly [6] which is in line with a recommendation in a recently published review about Hepatitis C therapy in patients with renal impairment [11]. Most of the studies which investigated the use of pegylated interferon alfa in patients with impaired kidney function used 135 μg weekly [12]. However, there was only one randomized study with 85 patients which compared 90 μg to 135 μg weekly and detected so far no differences in SVR [13]. Given that most studies investigated 135 μg weekly, we chose 135 μg pegylated interferon alfa as weekly dose.

In terms of ribavirin, the guidelines recommend an initial dose of 200 mg every other day with increase of doses to a maximum of 200–400 mg daily in patients with renal impairment [6]. We chose 200 mg as starting dose with respect to studies in dialysis patients [14].

Our patient developed anemia without a hemolytic component; therefore, an erythropoetin therapy was initiated.

4. Conclusion

In summary, growing data suggests that a therapy with ribavirin in patients with renal impairment seems to be safe under close monitoring. Our patient with severe renal and extrarenal manifestations was treated successfully (normalization of kidney function, dropped proteinuria, and restitution of vasculitic skin findings) with a protease inhibitor based triple therapy and still has an SVR 30 weeks after cessation of antiviral therapy.

Nevertheless, it is necessary to plan an interventional study to evaluate the exact risk-benefit profile of a triple therapy regimen in patients with acute kidney injury and hepatitis C. Till then the triple therapies could be administered to such patients only on an individual case decision.

Disclosure

The case report was presented on the ASN 2013 (Atlanta, USA, poster presentation).

Conflict of Interests

D. Callau Monje, N. Braun, J. Latus, K. Amann, M. D. Alscher, and M. Kimmel hereby declare that no conflicts of interests exist and that there was no funding/support.

References

[1] P. Cacoub, C. Renou, E. Rosenthal et al., "Extrahepatic manifestations associated with hepatitis C virus infection. A prospective multicenter study of 321 patients. The GERMIVIC. Groupe d'Etude et de Recherche en Medecine Interne et Maladies Infectieuses sur le Virus de l'Hepatite C," *Medicine*, vol. 79, no. 1, pp. 47–56, 2000.

[2] F. Lunel, L. Musset, P. Cacoub et al., "Cryoglobulinemia in chronic liver diseases: role of hepatitis C virus and liver damage," *Gastroenterology*, vol. 106, no. 5, pp. 1291–1300, 1994.

[3] F. Poordad, J. McCone Jr., B. R. Bacon et al., "Boceprevir for untreated chronic HCV genotype 1 infection," *The New England Journal of Medicine*, vol. 364, no. 13, pp. 1195–1206, 2011.

[4] B. R. Bacon, S. C. Gordon, E. Lawitz et al., "Boceprevir for previously treated chronic HCV genotype 1 infection," *The New England Journal of Medicine*, vol. 364, no. 13, pp. 1207–1217, 2011.

[5] A. Covic, D. Abramowicz, A. Bruchfeld et al., "Endorsement of the Kidney Disease Improving Global Outcomes (KDIGO) hepatitis C guidelines: a European Renal Best Practice (ERBP) position statement," *Nephrology Dialysis Transplantation*, vol. 24, no. 3, pp. 719–727, 2009.

[6] C. Sarrazin, T. Berg, R. S. Ross et al., "Prophylaxis, diagnosis and therapy of Hepatitis C Virus (HCV) infection: the German guidelines on the management of HCV infection," *Zeitschrift fur Gastroenterologie*, vol. 48, no. 2, pp. 289–351, 2010.

[7] C. H. Liu, C. F. Huang, C. J. Liu et al., "Pegylated interferon-α2a with or without low-dose ribavirin for treatment-naive patients with hepatitis C virus genotype 1 receiving hemodialysis: a randomized trial," *Annals of Internal Medicine*, vol. 159, no. 11, pp. 729–738, 2013.

[8] D. Saadoun, M. Resche Rigon, V. Thibault et al., "Peg-IFNα/ribavirin/protease inhibitor combination in hepatitis C virus associated mixed cryoglobulinemia vasculitis: results at week 24," *Annals of the Rheumatic Diseases*, vol. 73, no. 5, pp. 831–837, 2014.

[9] L. Alric, E. Plaisier, S. Thébault et al., "Influence of antiviral therapy in hepatitis C virus-associated cryoglobulinemic MPGN," *American Journal of Kidney Diseases*, vol. 43, no. 4, pp. 617–623, 2004.

[10] C. Sarrazin, T. Berg, M. Cornberg et al., "Expert opinion on Boceprevir- and Telaprevir-based triple therapies of chronic hepatitis C," *Zeitschrift fur Gastroenterologie*, vol. 50, no. 1, pp. 57–72, 2012.

[11] F. Fabrizi, A. Aghemo, and P. Messa, "Hepatitis C treatment in patients with kidney disease," *Kidney International*, vol. 84, pp. 874–879, 2013.

[12] T. Casanovas-Taltavull, C. Baliellas, M. Llobet et al., "Preliminary results of treatment with pegylated interferon alpha 2A for chronic hepatitis C virus in kidney transplant candidates on hemodialysis," *Transplantation Proceedings*, vol. 39, no. 7, pp. 2125–2127, 2007.

[13] M. W. Russo, R. Ghalib, S. Sigal, and V. Joshi, "Randomized trial of pegylated interferon α-2b monotherapy in haemodialysis patients with chronic hepatitis C," *Nephrology Dialysis Transplantation*, vol. 21, no. 2, pp. 437–443, 2006.

[14] A. Bruchfeld, K. Lindahl, O. Reichard, T. Carlsson, and R. Schvarcz, "Pegylated interferon and ribavirin treatment for hepatitis C in haemodialysis patients," *Journal of Viral Hepatitis*, vol. 13, no. 5, pp. 316–321, 2006.

A Case of Chronic Ethylene Glycol Intoxication Presenting without Classic Metabolic Derangements

Stephanie M. Toth-Manikowski,[1] **Hanni Menn-Josephy,**[2] **and Jasvinder Bhatia**[2]

[1] *Department of Medicine, Boston Medical Center, 72 East Concord Street, Evans 124, Boston, MA 02118, USA*
[2] *Renal Section, Boston University School of Medicine, 650 Albany Street, Rm 504, Boston, MA 02118, USA*

Correspondence should be addressed to Stephanie M. Toth-Manikowski; stephaniemtoth@gmail.com

Academic Editor: Yen-Ling Chiu

Acute ethylene glycol ingestion classically presents with high anion gap acidosis, elevated osmolar gap, altered mental status, and acute renal failure. However, chronic ingestion of ethylene glycol is a challenging diagnosis that can present as acute kidney injury with subtle physical findings and without the classic metabolic derangements. We present a case of chronic ethylene glycol ingestion in a patient who presented with acute kidney injury and repeated denials of an exposure history. Kidney biopsy was critical to the elucidation of the cause of his worsening renal function.

1. Introduction

Ethylene glycol is a colorless, odorless, sweet-tasting chemical found in products such as automotive antifreeze, windshield wiper fluid, solvents, cleaners, and other industrial products. Ingestion can lead to central nervous system depression, organ dysfunction, and ultimately death if left untreated [1].

In the acute setting of ethylene glycol ingestion, diagnosis in an intoxicated individual is confirmed by profound anion gap metabolic acidosis, elevated osmolar gap, and elevated ethylene glycol level. However, chronic ingestion of small amounts of ethylene glycol presents a diagnostic conundrum because laboratory derangements are often absent and physical symptoms can be mild. To date, very few case reports describe chronic ethylene glycol ingestion.

A review of the literature demonstrates common themes in chronic ethylene glycol ingestion. Patients present with acute kidney injury and a mildly elevated anion gap that resolve with minimal intervention [2, 3]. They describe abdominal discomfort that ranges from nausea, vomiting, and diarrhea to abdominal cramping [1, 3–5]. Cases are also notable for a prior history of substance abuse or a history of depression [1–3, 6].

We present a case of chronic ethylene glycol ingestion in a patient who presented with unexplained acute kidney injury, abdominal complaints, and anion gap acidosis which resolved quickly with supportive therapy. Ultimately, kidney biopsy was essential in revealing the etiology of his worsening renal function. This case illustrates the need for a high index of suspicion of intoxication despite the lack of history, minimal symptoms, and lack of classic lab abnormalities.

2. Case Presentation

A 41-year-old man with a history of hypertension, migraines, stroke, and depression presented to the emergency department complaining of five days of abdominal pain, nausea, and vomiting. Initial workup in the emergency room revealed a creatinine elevation of $696\,\mu$mol/L (7.9 mg/dL) from a baseline of $80\,\mu$mol/L (0.9 mg/dL) six weeks before. His anion gap was elevated to 19, but otherwise there were no electrolyte abnormalities. His ABG were indicative of combined metabolic acidosis and mild respiratory acidosis. The pH was 7.28, with HCO^3 of 14.7 mmol/L (mEq/L) and PCO^2 of 32 mmHg. The patient was not hypoxic at that time. The Ca level of the patient on the day of his admission was 9.2 mg/dL, with ionized calcium of 4.6 mg/dL. During his hospital stay, his calcium level was checked on a daily basis and was always at the normal range. His physical exam was unremarkable and his vital signs were stable. He reported

(a)

(b)

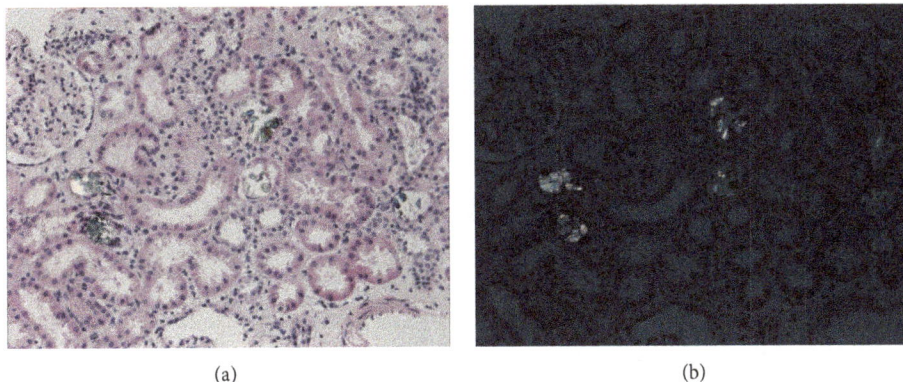

FIGURE 1: (a) Tubules packed with oxalate crystals. H&E staining, 20x magnification. (b) Birefringent oxalate crystals. H&E staining, 20x magnification, using polarized light.

taking atenolol for hypertension, topiramate for migraines, and clopidogrel and simvastatin for his history of stroke. He denied any tobacco, alcohol, or illicit drug use and he denied a family history of renal disease.

On admission, the patient was oliguric and was given normal saline at 200 mL/hour. Within 24 hours, his urine output had increased to >100 cc/hour and anion gap had normalized. Despite these improvements, his creatinine continued to rise, peaking at 1,370.2 μmol/L (15.5 mg/dL). Urine sediment showed nonpigmented granular casts without cellular casts or crystals. A renal ultrasound revealed normal sized kidneys without hydronephrosis or nephrolithiasis. A renal magnetic resonance angiogram was notable for loss of renal corticomedullary differentiation but was otherwise unremarkable. Complement levels were normal, and serologies for ANA, anti-GBM, ANCA, HIV, and hepatitis A, B, and C were negative. Serum and urine immunofixation were also unremarkable.

During his hospitalization, the patient continued to complain of abdominal pain. A computed tomography scan of his abdomen was performed but did not demonstrate an intra-abdominal process to explain his persistent pain. In an effort to further work up his acute kidney injury, the patient underwent kidney biopsy.

A core sample submitted for microscopy revealed multiple tubules packed with birefringent oxalate crystals (Figures 1(a) and 1(b)). The tubules revealed degenerative changes of the epithelium, characterized by distention of the lumen, a low cuboidal epithelial lining, and vacuolization of the cytoplasm. The interstitium showed mild focal inflammation, with infiltrates composed primarily of mononuclear elements. There were no signs of active glomerulitis and the basement membranes appeared normal in thickness. On immunofluorescence, there was no glomerular or tubulointerstitial staining for immunoglobulins A (IgA), G (IgG), and M (IgM), C1q, C3, albumin, fibrin-related antigens, or κ and λ light chains. On electron microscopy, rare irregular electron densities are observed in the subendothelium in isolated capillaries, thought to represent entrapment of macromolecules rather than immune complexes.

A diagnosis of extensive oxalate crystal deposition in the tubules was made with associated signs of acute tubular

injury and mild focal interstitial inflammation indicative of a hyperoxaluric state.

The patient was confronted about ingestion of ethylene glycol but he adamantly denied any intentional ingestions. With supportive care, the patient's kidney function gradually improved and the metabolic acidosis resolved. Upon discharge, the patient was no longer oliguric and had a creatinine of 380 μmol/L (4.3 mg/dL).

He was seen one week later in renal clinic and reported persistent abdominal discomfort and nausea since discharge. The issue of ethylene glycol was once again raised, but the patient again denied any intentional toxic ingestions. A renal follow-up appointment, one month after his hospital admission, revealed a normalized creatinine of 106 μmol/L (1.2 mg/dL) and normal anion and osmolar gaps. An outpatient esophagogastroduodenoscopy for the persistent abdominal pain did not reveal a source for his continued discomfort.

Seven months after his initial admission to the hospital, the patient was brought to the emergency room after being found unresponsive in a hotel room. He had recently ingested ethylene glycol and various pills in an attempt to end his life. His mental status was altered. Laboratory values revealed HCO^3 of 5 mmol/L (mEq/L) and creatinine of 159 μmol/L (1.8 mg/dL). He had an anion gap of 25 and an osmolar gap of 45. Urine sediment revealed calcium oxalate crystals, and his ethylene glycol level was 94 mg/dL (15.2 mmol/L). The patient was intubated. Emergent hemodialysis and fomepizole were started for ethylene glycol toxicity. His creatinine peaked at 689.5 μmol/L (7.8 mg/dL). Upon extubation, he reported chronic ingestion of small amounts of ethylene glycol over the past several months, including the time period prior to his initial hospital admission. His creatinine on hospital discharge was 353.6 μmol/L (4 mg/dL). He was discharged to a psychiatric facility and, unfortunately, was lost to outpatient followup.

3. Discussion

In the United States, 5,400 ethylene glycol exposures were reported to poison control centers in 2005; 700 of them were intentional ingestions [7]. Like other alcohols, ethylene glycol is rapidly and completely absorbed after oral ingestion and reaches peak serum concentrations within one to two hours [8]. Within 12–24 hours, it is metabolized to its toxic metabolites, glycolic acid, glyoxylic acid, and oxalate. At this point, an anion gap remains because of the presence of the metabolites, but the osmolar gap has resolved [9, 10].

Therefore, a delay in presentation may lead to the absence of an osmolar gap. Similarly, ingestion of small amounts of ethylene glycol may present with only a mild anion gap. Together, these observations can lead a clinician away from suspecting ethylene glycol ingestion.

Whereas ethylene glycol poisoning is a well-known clinical entity characterized by neurologic, pulmonary, and cardiovascular symptoms, chronic ethylene glycol ingestion is less common and does not have classic clinical findings [10]. In hindsight, our patient's admitting symptoms were related to chronic ethylene glycol ingestion, a diagnosis that became evident only after the kidney biopsy was performed and his subsequent suicide attempt. In reviewing the literature, we have noted a few common presenting themes that may aid the clinician in making a presumptive diagnosis of chronic ethylene glycol ingestion when laboratory findings are inconclusive and biopsy is not immediately indicated.

Patients generally describe abdominal discomfort that ranges from nausea, vomiting, and diarrhea to abdominal cramping [1, 3–6, 11]. In addition, medical history may be notable for substance abuse or mood disorders [1–3, 6]. Initial laboratory results may be notable for acute kidney injury and anion gap metabolic acidosis that resolves with minimal medical intervention [1–3]. An osmolar gap may not always be present especially if ethylene glycol ingestion is minimal and presentation to a healthcare setting is delayed [1, 11, 12]. Urine analysis may also be unremarkable [1–3].

In summary, diagnosing chronic ethylene glycol ingestion is not straightforward. Our patient presented with vague abdominal complaints, acute kidney injury, and anion gap metabolic acidosis which improved quickly and were attributed to volume depletion and acute kidney injury. Ultimately, a renal biopsy revealing oxalate crystal deposition was critical to making the diagnosis. Despite the biopsy results, our patient continued to deny intentional ingestion of ethylene glycol and only after his suicide attempt did he admit repeatedly ingesting small amounts. This case underscores the importance of keeping a high level of clinical suspicion for chronic ethylene glycol ingestion despite a lack of exposure history and significant laboratory gaps, particularly in high risk patients with a history of depression, abdominal pain, and unexplained acute kidney injury.

Conflict of Interests

The authors declare that there is no conflict of interests regarding the publication of this paper.

References

[1] S. Moossavi, N. K. Wadhwa, and E. P. Nord, "Recurrent severe anion gap metabolic acidosis secondary to episodic ethylene glycol intoxication," *Clinical Nephrology*, vol. 60, no. 3, pp. 205–210, 2003.

[2] M. B. DeSilva and P. S. Mueller, "Renal consequences of long-term, low-dose intentional ingestion of ethylene glycol," *Renal Failure*, vol. 31, no. 7, pp. 586–588, 2009.

[3] C. Bigaillon, H. Thefenne, S. Samy et al., "Intoxication par l'éthylène glycol: réflexion à propos d'un cas," *Annales de Biologie Clinique*, vol. 65, no. 4, pp. 437–442, 2007.

[4] W. Kaiser, H.-G. Steinmauer, G. Biesenbach, O. Janko, and J. Zazgornik, "Chronic ethylene glycol intoxication," *Deutsche Medizinische Wochenschrift*, vol. 118, no. 17, pp. 622–626, 1993.

[5] T. Liberek, J. Sliwarska, K. Czurak, A. Perkowska-Ptasinska, E. Weber, and B. Rutkowski, "Prolonged renal failure in the course of atypical ethylene glycol intoxication," *Acta Biochimica Polonica*, vol. 60, no. 4, pp. 661–663, 2013.

[6] A. F. Eder, C. M. Mcgrath, Y. G. Dowdy et al., "Ethylene glycol poisoning: toxicokinetic and analytical factors affecting laboratory diagnosis," *Clinical Chemistry*, vol. 44, no. 1, pp. 168–177, 1998.

[7] M. W. Lai, W. Klein-Schwartz, G. C. Rodgers et al., "2005 Annual report of the American association of poison control centers' national poisoning and exposure database," *Clinical Toxicology*, vol. 44, no. 6-7, pp. 803–932, 2006.

[8] M. L. A. Sivilotti and J. F. Winchester, "Methanol and ethylene glycol poisoning," in *UpToDate*, S. J. Traub and M. B. Ewald, Eds., Waltham, Mass, USA, 2012.

[9] R. Hess, M. J. Bartels, and L. H. Pottenger, "Ethylene glycol: an estimate of tolerable levels of exposure based on a review of animal and human data," *Archives of Toxicology*, vol. 78, no. 12, pp. 671–680, 2004.

[10] J. A. Kraut and I. Kurtz, "Toxic alcohol ingestions: clinical features, diagnosis, and management," *Clinical Journal of the American Society of Nephrology*, vol. 3, no. 1, pp. 208–225, 2008.

[11] B. Darchy, L. Abruzzese, O. Pitiot, B. Figuoredo, and Y. Domart, "Delayed admission for ethylene glycol poisoning: lack of elevated serum osmol gap," *Intensive Care Medicine*, vol. 25, no. 8, pp. 859–861, 1999.

[12] T. Alhamad, J. Blandon, A. T. Meza, J. E. Bilbao, and G. T. Hernandez, "Acute kidney injury with oxalate deposition in a patient with a high anion gap metabolic acidosis and a normal osmolal gap," *Journal of Nephropathology*, vol. 2, no. 2, pp. 139–143, 2013.

Pulmonary Limited MPO-ANCA Microscopic Polyangiitis and Idiopathic Lung Fibrosis in a Patient with a Diagnosis of IgA Nephropathy

Alwin Tilanus,[1] Patricia Van der Niepen,[2] Caroline Geers,[3] and Karl Martin Wissing[2]

[1]Departamento de Medicina Interna/Infectologia, Hospital General de Medellin Luz Castro de Gutiérrez,
 Carrera 48 # 32- 102, Medellin, Colombia
[2]Departement Interne Geneeskunde/Nefrologie, Universitair Ziekenhuis Brussel, Laarbeeklaan 101, 1090 Brussels, Belgium
[3]Departement Anatomo-Pathologie, Universitair Ziekenhuis Brussel, Laarbeeklaan 101, 1090 Brussels, Belgium

Correspondence should be addressed to Alwin Tilanus; alwintilanus@hotmail.com

Academic Editor: Mahzuz Karim

We present a case of a male patient with chronic renal insufficiency, due to crescentic glomerulonephritis with IgA deposits, who successively developed (idiopathic) thrombocytopenic purpura (ITP) and MPO-ANCA microscopic polyangiitis (MPA) with pulmonary fibrosis. The patient presented with cough, weight loss, and dyspnea on exertion. CT imaging and pulmonary function tests were compatible with interstitial pneumonitis with pulmonary fibrosis. Laboratory results showed high MPO-ANCA titers; the urinary sediment was bland. The patient was treated successfully with cyclophosphamide and methyl-prednisolone. This unique case illustrates the diagnostic and therapeutic challenges of an unusual presentation of microscopic polyangiitis presenting first as isolated kidney disease with recurrence in the form of pneumonitis without renal involvement, in association with renal IgA deposits and ITP as coexisting autoimmune conditions.

1. Introduction

The association between pulmonary fibrosis (PF) and Myeloperoxidase Anti-Neutrophil Cytoplasmic Antibodies (MPO-ANCAs) positivity has been reported in several small retrospective case-series, but the pathologic mechanism remains unclear [1]. In published case series [2–8] most patients were men with an average age of about 70 years, presenting typically with dry cough and dyspnea.

In a large proportion of cases, the diagnosis of MPO-ANCA vasculitis was preceded months to years by the diagnosis of PF or signs of interstitial pneumonia. During follow-up prognosis is unfavorable due to respiratory failure [2–8].

MPO-ANCAs have been reported in 7% to 33% of patients with interstitial pneumonia and idiopathic pulmonary fibrosis. Along the same line pulmonary fibrosis has been detected in one-third of a cohort of patients with p-ANCA-MPO [5, 7, 9].

Studies of patients with ANCA-positive and ANCA-negative PF demonstrated no significant differences between these clinical entities regarding symptoms, pulmonary function tests, and CT scanning [1, 5]. In most patients, more than one organ is affected, most frequently the kidney.

Here we report a unique case of MPO-ANCA microscopic polyangiitis affecting primarily the lung in a patient with a history of MPO-ANCA microscopic polyangiitis with renal-limited vasculitis and coexisting IgA deposits as well as idiopathic thrombocytopenic purpura (ITP).

2. Case Report

A 71-year-old man was admitted in June 2012 because of progressive dyspnea on exertion, dry cough, progressive weight loss of approximately 20 kg in 3 months, and edema of the lower extremities.

He had a complex medical history of autoimmune diseases including chronic kidney disease from a biopsy-proven

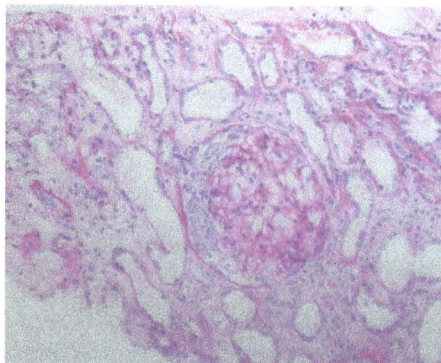

FIGURE 1: Periodic acid-Schiff stained histologic preparation with an overview of the renal parenchyma. The glomerulus shows a cellular crescent. The glomerular tuft shows mesangial hypercellularity. Tubular cells are damaged with regenerative features (PAS, ×200).

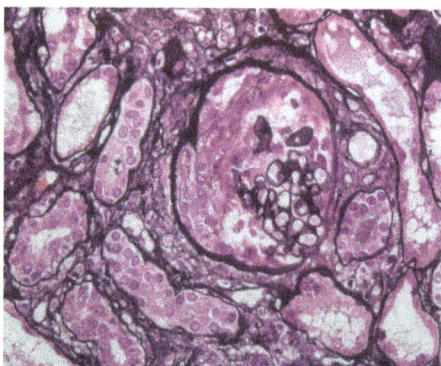

FIGURE 2: The methenamine silver stain shows fibrinoid necrosis with early crescent formation in the urinary space (Jones methenamine silver, ×400).

crescentic glomerulonephritis with MPO-ANCA and coexistent glomerular IgA deposits in 2007 and idiopathic thrombocytopenic purpura (ITP) in 2011. The patient had never smoked.

In December 2007 he was hospitalized because of acute renal failure with serum creatinine >1060 μmol/liter, oliguria, microscopic hematuria (250 RBC/μL), and proteinuria (1.3 g/day). Furthermore, he had an inflammatory syndrome (CRP 194 mg/liter) and very high ANCA (>1/5120) and anti-MPO (2337 IU/mL) titers.

Renal biopsy (2007) showed necrotizing crescentic glomerulonephritis (Figures 1 and 2) with significant IgA deposits (not shown in figure).

The patient received a diagnosis of severe IgA nephropathy with crescentic glomerulonephritis and was initially treated with high dose corticosteroids and hemodialysis. His kidney function progressively recovered and he was able to stop dialysis therapy after 3 months. Between June 2008 and 2011 serum creatinine values stabilized at values between 206 and 252 μmol/liter with maintenance methyl-prednisolone of approximately 8 mg every other day. Microscopic hematuria and proteinuria resolved and anti-MPO antibodies decreased from 2337 IU/mL to 208 IU/mL by April 2009.

In October 2011 the patient was hospitalized for epistaxis and severe thrombocytopenia $7 * 10^3/mm^3$ in the absence of anemia or leucopenia. The patient had no clinical signs of recurring renal disease or vasculitis and anti-MPO ANCA had further decreased to 45 IU/mL. Bone marrow examination was performed with diagnosis of idiopathic thrombocytopenia. Platelets rapidly normalized after short course of intravenous methyl-prednisolone followed by increased doses of maintenance steroids.

Interstitial pneumonia with beginning pulmonary fibrosis was diagnosed in November 2011 during evaluation for progressive dyspnea. A Broncho Alveolar Lavage (BAL) (performed under corticoid treatment) showed no abnormalities.

During the following six months his clinical condition progressively worsened in spite of treatment with high dose steroids and the patient was hospitalized several times for corticosteroid-induced diabetes, herpes zoster infection, and cellulitis of the right leg.

When admitted in June 2012 he appeared severely ill, wheelchair bound, with symmetric muscle wasting and loss of strength and resting dyspnea. He was profoundly anorectic with a loss of 27 kg since October 2011 and of 16 kg during the two month before admission. The examination of the chest revealed normal heart tones and bibasal fine lung crackles with oxygen saturation at 93%. Examination of the abdomen was unremarkable. Venous insufficiency and slight pitting edema were present at both lower limbs.

Laboratory examination showed a normocytic anemia Hb 7.0 g/dL, normal leukocyte count, an elevated C-reactive protein (CRP 246 mg/liter), and erythrocyte sedimentation rate (ESR 99 mm/h). Serum creatinine was stable at 203 μmol/liter; the urinary sediment showed no red or white blood cells and no casts; no proteinuria was detected. The patient had normal levels of eosinophils.

As compared to December 2011 and in spite of high dose steroids, p-ANCA titers had increased from 1/80 to 1/640 U/mL and MPO antibodies were above the upper limit of the titration curve of the test.

During the same period, spirometry showed a remarkable worsening of the restrictive pattern with forced expiratory volume in 1 second (FEV1) decreasing from 1.99 L to 0.71 L and diminishing carbon monoxide (CO) diffusion capacity of the lung.

CT scan of the thorax was classified as usual interstitial pneumonia (UIP) with reticular infiltrates and honeycombing predominantly in the subpleural areas of the lower lobes, without possibility to differentiate between idiopathic pulmonary fibrosis and fibrosis secondary to vasculitis on radiological grounds (Figure 3). Giant vessel vasculitis was excluded by PET-CT scan (though performed under corticosteroid treatment). A biopsy of the nasal mucosa showed nonspecific inflammation without signs of vasculitis or granulomatous lesions. There were no signs of active renal disease with a bland urinary sediment and absence of proteinuria as well as a stable but decreased renal function (CKD stage 3B).

Because of inflammation in the blood and a sputum culture positive for Moraxella/Proteus, the patient was treated with amoxicillin/clavulanic acid. This treatment was complicated by the development of an extensive erythematous

TABLE 1: Change of p-ANCA, MPO, spirometry, and CT scanning characteristics in the period from December 2011 to October 2012.

	Period		
	December 2011	June 2012	October 2012 (after 5 cycles of cyclophosphamide)
p-ANCA	1/180	1/640	1/320
MPO (IU/L)	45	>134[1]	44
Spirometry			
FVC (forced vital capacity) (liters)	2.51 (58% of PV[2])	0.84 (20% of PV)	2.23 (52% of PV)
Forced expiratory volume 1 second (FEV1) (liters)	1.99 (61% of PV)	0.71 (22% of PV)	1.63 (50% of PV)
FEC/FVC %	79 (74% of PV)	84% (74% of PV)	73% (74% of PV)
VC (vital capacity) (liters)	2.51 (56% of PV)	0.98 (22% of PV)	2.23 (50% of PV)
TLC (total lung capacity) (liters)	3.84 (51% of PV)	Not measured	3.96 (53% of PV)
RV (residual volume) (liters)	1.33 (49% of PV)	Not measured	1.73 (63% of PV)
DLCO (diffusing capacity of the lung for carbon monoxide) (mL/mmHg/min)	9.2 (32% of PV)	Not measured	7.6 (27% of PV)
CT scanning	Interstitial pneumonia/idiopathic lung fibrosis	Interstitial pneumonia/idiopathic lung fibrosis	Unchanged (permanent damage)

[1] Protocolled as >134 IU (above upper limit of test range).
[2] PV: Predicted Value.

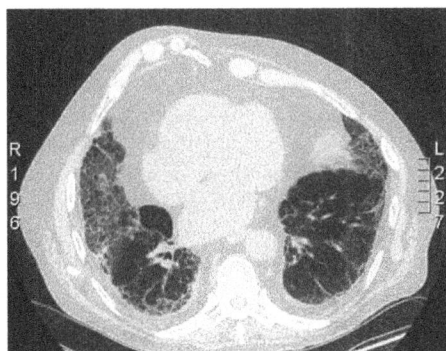

FIGURE 3: CT scan (prior to treatment) showing diffuse pulmonary fibrosis (honeycombing) and bilateral pleural fluid collection.

skin rash spreading over the entire body. Skin biopsies showed diffuse infiltrates with eosinophils and neutrophils and were protocoled as drug-induced rash. Antibiotic treatment was changed to moxifloxacine and 32 mg/day methylprednisolone with improvement of the rash. At that time the patient was considered too ill to undergo open lung biopsy for a formal histological diagnosis of fibrosis and/or vasculitis. In the context of increasing ANCA, an inflammatory syndrome as well as anorexia and severe weight loss microscopic polyangiitis with rapidly progressive pulmonary fibrosis was considered as sufficiently likely to justify the initiation of combination therapy with intravenous cyclophosphamide and high dose oral corticosteroids according to the CYCLOPS protocol [10].

Within days after the first cycle of cyclophosphamide we observed remarkable clinical improvement with decrease in dyspnea, increased appetite, and improved gait.

After 5 cycles of IV cyclophosphamide, pANCA/MPO titers decreased from 1/640 to 1/320 and 134 to 44 U/mL,

respectively, and inflammatory parameters normalized. Furthermore, FEV1 significantly improved from 0.71 to 1.63 L, Table 1. The CT scan showed no changes. The patient was last seen at the outpatient clinic in December 2012 with a serum creatinine of 190 μmol/L, hemoglobin levels of 11.4 g/dL, and a CRP of 8.6 mg/L. Weight increased from 81 to 91 kg during the 6 months after starting cyclophosphamide and the patient was again able to walk without assistance. He received a maintenance immunosuppression with azathioprine and Medrol 4 mg/day and no longer returned for follow-up at our unit.

3. Discussion

The present case is characterized by both the unusual association of several autoimmune conditions and a sequential and atypical presentation of microscopic polyangiitis, with selective damage of first the kidneys and subsequently the lungs without recurring of kidney disease. The initial presentation of our patient with rapidly progressive renal failure, high titers of MPO-ANCA, and crescentic glomerulonephritis with fibrinoid necrosis was clearly suggestive of renal-limited microscopic polyangiitis. The patient received a diagnosis of aggressive IgA nephropathy at this moment because of the presence of mesangial IgA deposits. Similar to our patient, several reports have described patients with (crescentic) IgA nephropathy in the presence of positive ANCAs [11–14]. It is unclear whether IgA nephropathy precedes ANCA positivity or if mesangial inflammation due to IgA deposits creates an inflammatory microenvironment that triggers vasculitis. Similar to our patient the clinical presentation is in general characterized by rapid loss of renal function and requires aggressive immunosuppressive therapy combining cyclophosphamide and steroids. Although our patient ultimately entered remission and was able to stop dialysis therapy, in retrospect we have to conclude that he should have been treated for MPA at the first presentation of his disease.

Thrombotic and thrombocytopenic purpura (TTP) has been described in rare patients with ANCA-associated vasculitis [15–17]; there has been, to the best of our knowledge, no previous report on the association between idiopathic thrombocytopenic purpura and ANCA-associated vasculitis. The relation of ITP with vasculitis in our patient is not clear because it occurred at a moment when MPO-ANCA titers were low but ITP was also rapidly followed by recurrence of vasculitis in the form of pulmonary fibrosis. Severe thrombocytopenia rapidly responded to high dose steroids and did not recur during the rest of follow-up.

Our patient developed progressive interstitial pneumonitis and pulmonary fibrosis that was first diagnosed approximately one month after the development of ITP and occurred in spite of the administration of high dose steroids for ITP and initially without increase in MPO-ANCA and other signs of MPA. The link with ANCA vasculitis was made only 6 months later when the patient had developed severe systemic disease in the form of anorexia, wasting, anemia, and an inflammatory syndrome in the context of high MPO-ANCA titers. Surprisingly, although MPA had initially presented as renal limited disease, the recurrence occurred without any signs of renal involvement. The presentation of our patient is compatible with the largest series published up to now which reported a predominance of older male patients with MPO-ANCA among those developing PF and a majority presenting with a typical UIP pattern on CT scans [8]. Homma et al. examined 31 patients diagnosed as having PF with positive MPO-ANCA. In 11 autopsied patients the histopathological features of the diseased lung tissues were compatible with the usual interstitial pneumonia pattern. Vasculitis in bronchial arteries and/or pulmonary arterioles was confirmed in only five patients [6]. Hervier et al. reported low diagnostic yield of 3 transbronchial biopsies which showed only fibrosis and no vasculitis [4]. On the contrary a large series of patients with open lung biopsy (25) or autopsy (2) provided a correct diagnosis of vasculitis in 21 of 27 ANCA positive patients (78%), capillaritis being the most common lesion [18]. In the present patient we decided against transbronchial biopsy because of the low diagnostic yield and against open lung biopsy because the patient was considered too ill to undergo surgery. The treating physicians had also decided that systemic inflammation with anorexia and wasting in the context of high titers of MPO-ANCA were a justification of standard treatment of MPA irrespective of the results of an eventual open lung biopsy.

The pathologic mechanism of pulmonary fibrosis and positive MPO-ANCA remains unclear [1]. There is evidence that infection and certain drugs can stimulate ANCA-MPO/PR3 antibody production [19]. Infection can prime and activate neutrophils by circulating inflammatory cytokines. Subsequent translocation of ANCA antigens (e.g., MPO/PR3) to the cell surface of neutrophils and expression of adhesion molecules by endothelial cells result in cell adhesion, release of reactive oxygen species, vasculitis, and endothelial apoptosis [20]. Chan et al. described a case of MPO-ANCA microscopic vasculitis following a suppurative wound infection in a cancer patient [21]. Infectious events in our patient

(cellulitis right leg, pneumonia) might have triggered MPO-ANCA titers increase. Takato et al. described a case of an MPO-ANCA positive PF patient in which a Mycoplasma infection triggered the elevation of MPO-ANCA titers and the development of a crescentic glomerulonephritis [22].

When examining the published case series [2–8], prognosis was typically worse when PF was associated with MPO-ANCA positivity especially when eosinophilia was present [4]. The MPO-ANCA antibodies could lead to pulmonary capillaritis which might result in (subclinical) alveolar hemorrhage and finally fibrosis [23–26]. Nozu et al. suggested that there is some evidence that corticosteroid therapy is more effective in ANCA positive patients and that survival tends to be better when the MPO titers were low (<50 IU/L) [5]. Nevertheless, and similar to the initial clinical presentation of our patient who developed fibrosis before increasing MPO titers, the development of PF has been reported to precede increase in MPO-ANCA positivity. In about half of the patients the diagnosis of PF precedes the diagnosis of vasculitis [8]. Therefore the opposite theory that PF could result in MPO-ANCA production and be a trigger for the development or recurrence of MPA cannot be discarded [4, 7]. The reported lack of clear correlation between MPO-ANCA titers and severity of PF also question the unique role of ANCA in the disease process [6].

Although in our case the lungs were the only vital organ affected, other organs might have been subsequently damaged during disease progression as previously reported by Hiromura et al. In this report, four patients with MPO-ANCA positive idiopathic pulmonary fibrosis subsequently developed rapidly progressive glomerulonephritis [27].

Our patient was treated according to the vasculitis guidelines (CYCLOPS protocol [10]) with rapid clinical improvement. Renal function improved and MPO-ANCA titers decreased significantly. A control spirometry after 5 cycles of cyclophosphamide showed a remarkable improvement in total lung volume and FEV1. However, a control pulmonary CT scan was unchanged, indicating that most lung tissue damage was irreversible.

Since high (e.g., >50 IU/mL) MPO-ANCA titers in a patient with PF carry a worse prognosis and risk of evolution to MPA, every patient with (idiopathic) PF should be screened for MPO-ANCA positivity. When positive, we propose to look for underlying infections, treat them as necessary, and start treatment with cyclophosphamide/corticosteroids, even without prior lung biopsy.

Conflict of Interests

The authors declare that they have no conflict of interests.

References

[1] H. Yamada, "ANCA: associated lung fibrosis," *Seminars in Respiratory and Critical Care Medicine*, vol. 32, no. 3, pp. 322–327, 2011.

[2] G. M. Eschun, S. N. Mink, and S. Sharma, "Pulmonary interstitial fibrosis as a presenting manifestation in perinuclear

antineutrophilic cytoplasmic antibody microscopic polyangiitis," *Chest*, vol. 123, no. 1, pp. 297–301, 2003.

[3] G. Foulon, P. Delaval, D. Valeyre et al., "ANCA-associated lung fibrosis: analysis of 17 patients," *Respiratory Medicine*, vol. 102, no. 10, pp. 1392–1398, 2008.

[4] B. Hervier, C. Pagnoux, C. Agard et al., "Pulmonary fibrosis associated with ANCA-positive vasculitides. Retrospective study of 12 cases and review of the literature," *Annals of the Rheumatic Diseases*, vol. 68, no. 3, pp. 404–407, 2009.

[5] T. Nozu, M. Kondo, K. Suzuki, J. Tamaoki, and A. Nagai, "A comparison of the clinical features of ANCA-positive and ANCA-negative idiopathic pulmonary fibrosis patients," *Respiration*, vol. 77, no. 4, pp. 407–415, 2009.

[6] S. Homma, H. Matsushita, and K. Nakata, "Pulmonary fibrosis in myeloperoxidase antineutrophil cytoplasmic antibody-associated vasculitides," *Respirology*, vol. 9, no. 2, pp. 190–196, 2004.

[7] G. E. Tzelepis, M. Kokosi, A. Tzioufas et al., "Prevalence and outcome of pulmonary fibrosis in microscopic polyangiitis," *European Respiratory Journal*, vol. 36, no. 1, pp. 116–121, 2010.

[8] C. Comarmond, B. Crestani, A. Tazi et al., "Pulmonary fibrosis in antineutrophil cytoplasmic antibodies (ANCA)-associated vasculitis: a series of 49 patients and review of the literature," *Medicine*, vol. 93, no. 24, pp. 340–349, 2014.

[9] A. Shiraki, M. Ando, J. Shindoh et al., "Prevalence of myeloperoxidase-anti-neutrophil cytoplasmic antibody (MPO-ANCA) in patients with interstitial pneumonia," *Nihon Kokyuki Gakkai Zasshi*, vol. 45, no. 12, pp. 921–926, 2007.

[10] K. De Groot, L. Harper, D. R. W. Jayne et al., "Pulse versus daily oral cyclophosphamide for induction of remission in antineutrophil cytoplasmic antibody-associated vasculitis: a randomized trial," *Annals of Internal Medicine*, vol. 150, no. 10, pp. 670–680, 2009.

[11] M. Haas, J. Jafri, S. M. Bartosh, S. L. Karp, S. G. Adler, and S. M. Meehan, "ANCA-associated crescentic glomerulonephritis with mesangial IgA deposits," *The American Journal of Kidney Diseases*, vol. 36, no. 4, pp. 709–718, 2000.

[12] S. L. Lui, K. W. Chan, P. S. Yip, T. M. Chan, K. N. Lai, and W. K. Lo, "Simultaneous occurrence of diabetic glomerulosclerosis, IgA nephropathy, crescentic glomerulonephritis, and myeloperoxidase-antineutrophil cytoplasmic antibody seropositivity in a Chinese patient," *American Journal of Kidney Diseases*, vol. 40, no. 4, pp. e14.1–e14.4, 2002.

[13] J. Ara, J. Bonet, R. Rodríguez, E. Mirapeix, I. Agraz, and R. Romero, "IgA nephropathy with crescentic glomerulonephritis and ANCA positive," *Nefrologia*, vol. 25, no. 6, pp. 712–717, 2005.

[14] C. Bantis, M. Stangou, C. Schlaugat et al., "Is presence of ANCA in crescentic IgA nephropathy a coincidence or novel clinical entity? A case series," *The American Journal of Kidney Diseases*, vol. 55, no. 2, pp. 259–268, 2010.

[15] V. Agrawal, C. K. Vaidya, J. Ye et al., "Concomitant thrombotic thrombocytopenic purpura and ANCA-associated vasculitis in an adolescent," *Pediatric Nephrology*, vol. 26, no. 8, pp. 1317–1320, 2011.

[16] H. Watanabe, W. Kitagawa, K. Suzuki et al., "Thrombotic thrombocytopenic purpura in a patient with rapidly progressive glomerulonephritis with both anti-glomerular basement membrane antibodies and myeloperoxidase anti-neutrophil cytoplasmic antibodies," *Clinical and Experimental Nephrology*, vol. 14, no. 6, pp. 598–601, 2010.

[17] K. Nagai, T. Kotani, T. Takeuchi et al., "Successful treatment of thrombotic thrombocytopenic purpura with repeated plasma exchange in a patient with microscopic polyangitis," *Modern Rheumatology*, vol. 18, no. 6, pp. 643–646, 2008.

[18] P. B. Gaudin, F. B. Askin, R. J. Falk, and J. C. Jennette, "The pathologic spectrum of pulmonary lesions in patients with antineutrophil cytoplasmic autoantibodies specific for anti-proteinase 3 and anti-myeloperoxidase," *American Journal of Clinical Pathology*, vol. 104, no. 1, pp. 7–16, 1995.

[19] E. Csernok, P. Lamprecht, and W. L. Gross, "Clinical and immunological features of drug-induced and infection-induced proteinase 3-antineutrophil cytoplasmic antibodies and myeloperoxidase-antineutrophil cytoplasmic antibodies and vasculitis," *Current Opinion in Rheumatology*, vol. 22, no. 1, pp. 43–48, 2010.

[20] C. G. M. Kallenberg, "Pathogenesis of ANCA-associated vasculitides," *Annals of the Rheumatic Diseases*, vol. 70, supplement 1, pp. i59–i63, 2011.

[21] B. Chan, V. d'Intini, and J. Savige, "Anti-neutrophil cytoplasmic antibody (ANCA)-associated microscopic polyangiitis following a suppurative wound infection," *Nephrology Dialysis Transplantation*, vol. 21, no. 10, pp. 2993–2994, 2006.

[22] H. Takato, M. Yasui, Y. Waseda, N. Sakai, T. Wada, and M. Fujimura, "A case of microscopic polyangiitis following mycoplasma infection in a patient with MPO-ANCA positive pulmonary fibrosis," *Allergology International*, vol. 60, no. 1, pp. 93–96, 2011.

[23] A. Schnabel, M. Reuter, E. Csernok, C. Richter, and W. L. Gross, "Subclinical alveolar bleeding in pulmonary vasculitides: correlation with indices of disease activity," *European Respiratory Journal*, vol. 14, no. 1, pp. 118–124, 1999.

[24] J.-F. Cordier and V. Cottin, "Alveolar hemorrhage in vasculitis: primary and secondary," *Seminars in Respiratory and Critical Care Medicine*, vol. 32, no. 3, pp. 310–321, 2011.

[25] P. Manganelli, P. Fietta, M. Carotti, A. Pesci, and F. Salaffi, "Respiratory system involvement in systemic vasculitides," *Clinical and Experimental Rheumatology*, vol. 24, no. 2, pp. S48–S59, 2006.

[26] J. Birnbaum, S. Danoff, F. B. Askin, and J. H. Stone, "Microscopic polyangiitis presenting as a 'pulmonary-muscle' syndrome: is subclinical alveolar hemorrhage the mechanism of pulmonary fibrosis?" *Arthritis and Rheumatism*, vol. 56, no. 6, pp. 2065–2071, 2007.

[27] K. Hiromura, Y. Nojima, T. Kitahara et al., "Four cases of anti-myeloperoxidase antibody-related rapidly progressive glomerulonephritis during the course of idiopathic pulmonary fibrosis," *Clinical Nephrology*, vol. 53, no. 5, pp. 384–389, 2000.

Dabigatran-Related Nephropathy in a Patient with Undiagnosed IgA Nephropathy

Rachele Escoli,[1] **Paulo Santos,**[1] **Sequeira Andrade,**[1] **and Fernanda Carvalho**[2]

[1]*Department of Nephrology, Centro Hospitalar do Médio Tejo, 2350-754 Torres Novas, Portugal*
[2]*Department of Nephrology, Centro Hospitalar de Lisboa Central, Hospital Curry Cabral, 1069-166 Lisbon, Portugal*

Correspondence should be addressed to Rachele Escoli; rachele_escoli@hotmail.com

Academic Editor: Yoshihide Fujigaki

Dabigatran is a direct thrombin inhibitor used as an alternative to warfarin for long term anticoagulation. Warfarin-related nephropathy is an increasingly recognized entity, but recent evidence suggests that dabigatran can cause a WRN-like syndrome. We describe a case of a biopsy-proven anticoagulant nephropathy related to dabigatran in a patient with IgA nephropathy and propose that, despite the base glomerular disease, acute kidney injury was due to tubular obstruction by red blood cells and heme-associated tubular injury, and through a mechanism involving inhibition of anticoagulation cascade and barrier abnormalities caused by molecular mechanisms.

1. Introduction

Anticoagulant therapy plays a central role in the prevention and treatment of venous and arterial thromboembolic diseases. Recently, several oral anticoagulants were approved, including the direct thrombin inhibitors such as dabigatran. It has a quick onset of action, results in a predictable anticoagulation response, and does not require routine laboratory monitoring. However, concerns have been raised since there is no antidote for treatment of secondary hemorrhages. We report a case of a 69-year-old woman with a biopsy-proven anticoagulant nephropathy related to dabigatran and discuss the diagnostic and management approach.

2. Case Presentation

A 69-year-old white female with a past history of hypertension presented with nausea, vomiting, and oliguria. The patient had been in her usual state of health until 2 weeks earlier, when she developed palpitations that prompted her to seek medical care. New-onset atrial fibrillation was diagnosed. After reversing into sinus rhythm with amiodarone, she was discharged with a prescription of dabigatran 110 mg twice daily (Pradaxa Boehringer). At this time serum

creatinine was 1,5 mg/dL (corresponding to an estimated glomerular filtration rate [eGFR] of 35,2 mL/min/1,73 m^2 as calculated by the CKD-EPI [Chronic Kidney Disease Epidemiology Collaboration] equation). Two weeks later she started vomiting and having oliguria and was sent to our medical facilities. She denied additional complaints and was on dabigatran 100 mg twice a day during the previous two weeks.

The patient's medical history included arterial hypertension medicated with ramipril. On admission blood pressure was 212/98 mmHg, pulse rate was 98 heart beats per minute, and she was oliguric. The physical examination revealed hydrated mucosa with no respiratory distress, crackles in bilateral lung fields, and mild lower-extremity edema. Laboratory results showed the following: serum urea was 230 mg/dL, serum creatinine was 8 mg/dL, hemoglobin was 9.1 g/dL, white blood cell count was $14.7 \times 10^3/\mu L$ with 86% of PMN and 0.2% of eosinophils, platelet count was $369 \times 10^3/\mu L$, prothrombin time (PT) was 25.3 seconds with international normalized ratio (INR) of 2.3, activated partial thromboplastin time (aPTT) was 68 seconds, LDH was 531 IU/L, and C-reactive protein was 7.1 mg/dL. A random urine specimen revealed that leukocytes were 500/μL, proteins were 100 mg/dL, and hemoglobin was 1 mg/dL. Urine

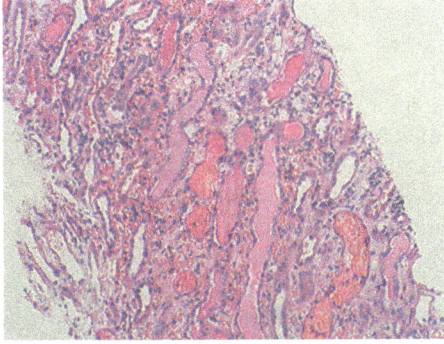

FIGURE 1: Prominent interstitial hemorrhage and intratubular casts (haematoxylin/eosin staining, magnification 100x).

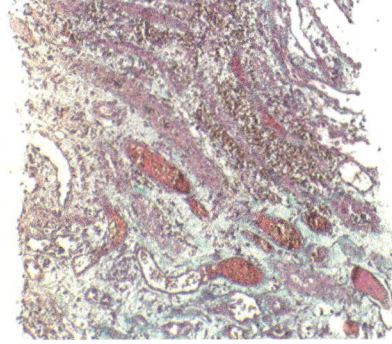

FIGURE 2: Interstitial hemorrhage (Masson's trichrome, magnification 100x).

sediment had hematuria (>100 red blood cells (RBC)/high-power field) and leukocyturia (6 leukocytes/high-power field) without dysmorphic red blood cells or red blood casts. Renal ultrasound suggested globular kidneys with regular shape but hyperechogenic cortical parenchyma without hydronephrosis. The patient was then transferred to the Nephrology Department. Due to oliguric acute renal failure she started hemodialysis two days after being admitted and proceeding with investigation. A peripheral blood smear did not show schizocytes. C3 complement level was decreased (52 mg/dL). C4 and antistreptolysin were normal. Screening for antinuclear antibody, antineutrophil cytoplasmic antibody, anti-glomerular basement membrane antibody, cryoglobulins, and antiphospholipid antibody and VDRL test were negative. After an inconclusive Doppler renal ultrasound, a contrast enhanced computed tomography angiography was performed four days after admission and showed no abnormalities. A transthoracic echocardiogram was done and illustrated normal sized left chambers without intracardiac thrombus. After 3 sessions of hemodialysis a normal aPTT was accomplished and due to persistent oliguria a biopsy was performed.

Five glomeruli appeared normal. The tubulointerstitium had large intratubular RBC casts, extensive tubular necrosis, and interstitial hemorrhage (Figures 1 and 2). By immunofluorescence there were mesangial deposits of IgA (++), C3 (++), K, and λ chains on 3 glomeruli (Figure 3).

So the diagnosis of IgA nephropathy, anticoagulant nephropathy with acute tubular necrosis, and interstitial hemorrhage was made. Following the kidney biopsy there were perirenal haematoma and hypotension. Three units of RBC were provided and resolution was achieved under tight follow-up. After intravenous fluid reposition she restored diuresis (hematuria). Two weeks later, renal function improved, urine cleared, and patient was discharged. Creatinine was 1.9 mg/dL in the last clinical evaluation.

3. Discussion

Anticoagulant-related nephropathy (ARN) is a form of acute kidney injury caused by excessive anticoagulation first described with warfarin, and because of that it is called

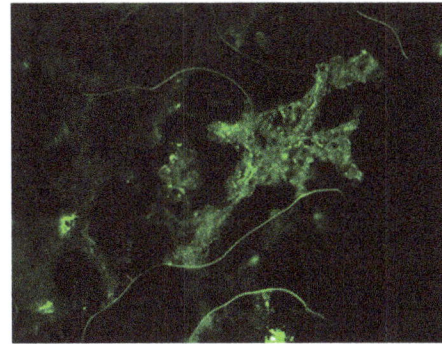

FIGURE 3: Direct immunofluorescence showing granular mesangial staining for IgA in the expanded mesangium of the biopsy, magnification 400x.

warfarin-related nephropathy (WRN) [1]. Diagnosis should be suspected among patients who present with unexplained acute renal injury defined as a serum creatinine increase greater than 0.3 mg/dL within one week of an INR measurement greater than 3 in a patient treated with warfarin, excluding other causes of AKI and bleeding [1, 2]. Recent evidence suggests that WRN-like syndromes are not confined to anticoagulation with warfarin but may occur with other anticoagulants, such as acenocoumarol [3] and dabigatran [2].

In WRN AKI occurs through glomerular hematuria with subsequent widespread tubular obstruction [4]. Biopsy studies showed RBCs in tubules and occlusive RBCs casts predominantly in distal nephron segments [4, 5]. Several pathogenic mechanisms were proposed. The combination of even mild glomerular disease and warfarin-induced coagulopathy seems to be the key point [4]. This leads to glomerular hematuria and to a significant accumulation of RBCs within nephrons that form occlusive casts, especially when urinary flow is diminished [4, 6]. Although glomerular hematuria is essential, it seems that interstitial hemorrhage may also have an important role [3]. So the dominant mechanism of AKI in WRN is probably tubular obstruction by RBC casts, which, associated with interstitial hemorrhage, leads to increased oxidative stress in the kidney [7, 8].

There are many underlying risk factors for WRN, such as age, CKD, due to higher risk of supratherapeutic INR, diabetes and diabetic nephropathy, hypertension, and heart failure [5].

Dabigatran is an anticoagulant used for stroke prevention in atrial fibrillation [9]. Recent evidence suggests that dabigatran has many hemorrhagic complications. However, in what concerns kidney involvement, information is scarce [10]. Dabigatran has 80% renal elimination and is not recommended for patients with creatinine clearance less than 15 mL/min or on dialysis, needing a dose adjustment in patients with creatinine clearance between 15 and 30 mL/min, in order to reduce hemorrhagic complications [11].

Evidence from animal studies revealed that dabigatran may cause AKI by two major pathogenic mechanisms: first, tubular obstruction by RBCs and, second, a mechanism possibly involving protease-activated receptor 1 (PAR-1) [1]. PAR-1 is a G protein-coupled receptor that participates in the regulation of the endothelial functions, vascular permeability, leukocyte migration, and adhesion and is the major effector of thrombin signaling [3]. Either vitamin K antagonists or direct thrombin inhibitors decrease thrombin activity. By acting on thrombomodulin, thrombin activates protein C and modulates the anticoagulation cascade. The same happens with PAR-1. In the aforementioned study the authors proposed that thrombin plays an important role in the glomerular filtration barrier function, and its decreased activity (secondary to anticoagulation) results in glomerular filtration barrier abnormalities. Indeed, treatment with selective PAR-1 inhibitor results in increased creatinine, hematuria, and tubular RBC casts, findings similar to those in animals with WRN or treated with dabigatran. These effects are similar to WRN. However in contrast to WRN, where kidney injury was seen only in animals with CKD, the effects of dabigatran were prominent in control rats as well. These findings suggest that the kidney risk with dabigatran may be greater than that of warfarin [3].

To the best of our knowledge, only two cases of dabigatran-induced AKI have been reported [12, 13]. In both cases patients presented with hematuria and had histologic evidence of hemorrhage into renal tubules. In the Moeckel et al. clinical report the patient had previously mild undiagnosed IgA nephropathy [13], as presented in our case. This raises the question if IgA nephropathy is a risk factor or a predisposing condition in anticoagulated patients with dabigatran as was described in WRN. The main clinical feature of IgA nephropathy is hematuria, which can be micro- or macroscopic, both unnoticed by our patient, and it is plausible to think that an entity, which, by nature, already predisposes hematuria, may be related or may be a risk factor to ARN. Fundamental WRN pathological lesions as described above were also observed in our patient, which suggests that the physiopathological mechanisms that induce AKI may have a common way, particularly with regard to tubular obstruction and interstitial hemorrhage. In our patient's case we propose that the combination of IgA nephropathy which associated with the age, CKD, and the medical history of hypertension possibly leads to the perfect background.

Concerning treatment, restoring the aPTT into a therapeutic range while doing supportive renal treatment is primordial [1]. In what concerns dabigatran-related AKI

hemodialysis seems to be effective [9, 13, 14]. About the prognosis, there seem to be discrepancies between WRN and dabigatran-related AKI. The clinical outcome in a WRN study was unfavorable: 66% of patients did not recover baseline function [4]. With regard to the two reported cases of dabigatran-induced AKI, in both renal function improved [12, 13]. In our case, there seems to be a recovery of renal function and we think that the absence of histological markers of poor prognosis of IgA nephropathy, such as the lack of interstitial fibrosis, tubular atrophy, glomerular sclerosis, or endocapillary hypercellularity, may possibly have contributed to this good outcome. The short period of administration and the lower dose of dabigatran may also have had influence. However, since there are so few published cases of dabigatran-related nephropathy, it is impossible to compare outcomes of these two entities.

This raises the note of caution about oral anticoagulation in patients with kidney disease. They are at a higher risk of overanticoagulation, gross hematuria, and AKI [15]. So physicians involved in the clinical management of anticoagulated patients should be aware of the ARN, either by warfarin or other anticoagulants like dabigatran. A correct coagulation and kidney function monitoring is required and, if needed, anticoagulants should be stopped or decreased [15].

Consent

The patient described in the case report had given informed consent for the case report to be published.

Conflict of Interests

The authors declare that there is no conflict of interests regarding the publication of this paper.

References

[1] M. Ryan, K. Ware, Z. Qamri et al., "Warfarin-related nephropathy is the tip of the iceberg: direct thrombin inhibitor dabigatran induces glomerular hemorrhage with acute kidney injury in rats," *Nephrology Dialysis Transplantation*, vol. 29, no. 12, pp. 2228–2234, 2014.

[2] D. V. Rizk and D. G. Warnock, "Warfarin-related nephropathy: another newly recognized complication of an old drug," *Kidney International*, vol. 80, no. 2, pp. 131–133, 2011.

[3] C. M. Cleary, J. A. Moreno, B. Fernández et al., "Glomerular haematuria, renal interstitial haemorrhage and acute kidney injury," *Nephrology Dialysis Transplantation*, vol. 25, no. 12, pp. 4103–4106, 2010.

[4] S. V. Brodsky, A. Satoskar, J. Chen et al., "Acute kidney injury during warfarin therapy associated with obstructive tubular red blood cell casts: a report of 9 cases," *The American Journal of Kidney Diseases*, vol. 54, no. 6, pp. 1121–1126, 2009.

[5] S. V. Brodsky, T. Nadasdy, B. H. Rovin et al., "Warfarin-related nephropathy occurs in patients with and without chronic kidney disease and is associated with an increased mortality rate," *Kidney International*, vol. 80, no. 2, pp. 181–189, 2011.

[6] D. Wheeler and J. Rangaswami, *Anticoagulation-Related Nephropathy: The Clot Thickens*, 2014, http://www.acc.org/.

[7] K. Ware, Z. Qamri, A. Ozcan et al., "N-acetylcysteine ameliorates acute kidney injury but not glomerular hemorrhage in an animal model of warfarin-related nephropathy," *The American Journal of Physiology—Renal Physiology*, vol. 304, no. 12, pp. F1421–F1427, 2013.

[8] M. J. Tracz, J. Alam, and K. A. Nath, "Physiology and pathophysiology of heme: implications for kidney disease," *Journal of the American Society of Nephrology*, vol. 18, no. 2, pp. 414–420, 2007.

[9] A. Majeed, H.-G. Hwang, S. J. Connolly et al., "Management and outcomes of major bleeding during treatment with dabigatran or warfarin," *Circulation*, vol. 128, no. 21, pp. 2325–2332, 2013.

[10] G. J. Hankey and J. W. Eikelboom, "Dabigatran etexilate: a new oral thrombin inhibitor," *Circulation*, vol. 123, no. 13, pp. 1436–1450, 2011.

[11] Z. Hijazi, S. H. Hohnloser, J. Oldgren et al., "Efficacy and safety of dabigatran compared with warfarin in relation to baseline renal function in patients with atrial fibrillation: a RE-LY (randomized evaluation of long-term anticoagulation therapy) trial analysis," *Circulation*, vol. 129, no. 9, pp. 961–970, 2014.

[12] D. Kadiyala, U. C. Brewster, and G. W. Moeckel, "Dabigatran induced acute kidney injury," in *Proceedings of the American Society of Nephrology Annual Meeting*, 2012.

[13] G. W. Moeckel, R. L. Luciano, and U. C. Brewster, "Warfarin-related nephropathy in a patient with mild IgA nephropathy on dabigatran and aspirin," *Clinical Kidney Journal*, vol. 6, no. 5, pp. 507–509, 2013.

[14] F. Knauf, C. M. Chaknos, J. S. Berns, and M. A. Perazella, "Dabigatran and kidney disease: a bad combination," *Clinical Journal of the American Society of Nephrology*, vol. 8, no. 9, pp. 1591–1597, 2013.

[15] C. Santos, A. M. Gomes, A. Ventura, C. Almeida, and J. Seabra, "An unusual cause of glomerular hematuria and acute kidney injury in a chronic kidney disease patient during warfarin therapy," *Nefrologia*, vol. 33, no. 3, pp. 400–403, 2013.

9

Spontaneous Forniceal Rupture in Pregnancy

Roshni Upputalla,[1] Robert M. Moore,[2] and Belinda Jim[1]

[1]*Department of Nephrology/Medicine, Jacobi Medical Center, Albert Einstein College of Medicine, Bronx, NY 10461, USA*
[2]*Department of Obstetrics and Gynecology, Jacobi Medical Center, Albert Einstein College of Medicine, Bronx, NY 10461, USA*

Correspondence should be addressed to Belinda Jim; belindajim286@gmail.com

Academic Editor: Yoshihide Fujigaki

Forniceal rupture is a rare event in pregnancy. We report a case of a 26-year-old primigravid woman who experienced a forniceal rupture at 23 weeks of gestation with no inciting cause except for pregnancy. Pregnancy is associated with ureteral compression due to increase in pelvic vasculature with the right ureter more dilated due to anatomic reasons. Hormones such as prostaglandins and progesterone render the ureter more distensible to allow for pressure build-up and an obstructive picture at the collecting system. We will discuss physiologic changes in pregnancies that predispose to this uncommon phenomenon and the most up-to-date management strategies.

1. Introduction

Forniceal rupture of the kidney in pregnancy is an uncommon entity. Pregnancy induced physiological changes predispose to this condition. Due to its relative rarity, management and treatment of this condition is often unclear.

2. Case Presentation

We present a case of a 26-year-old pregnant female (G_1P_0) who presents at 23 weeks of gestation complaining of acute right sided flank pain for one day with no other associated symptoms such as fever or dysuria. Her physical exam was remarkable for right costovertebral angle tenderness. The patient's chemistry and hematologic laboratory values remained normal (Table 1). She was admitted with an impression of pyelonephritis and was started on antibiotics. Imaging studies including renal ultrasound, CT (Figure 1), and MRI were performed which revealed a right forniceal rupture with no evidence of nephrolithiasis. The initial aspiration of the fluid returned a sterile culture. She improved symptomatically with conservative therapy and was discharged home. However, four days later, she returned to a different hospital with similar complaints of right flank pain. A repeat CT scan revealed a urinoma measuring 17.5 cm. The urinoma

was subsequently drained followed by the placement of a nephrostomy tube. The patient improved symptomatically and was discharged home. She was to follow up in outpatient urology, renal, and obstetric clinics. The patient continued to be symptom-free for the rest of the pregnancy and delivered at 37 weeks via a spontaneous vaginal delivery. The nephrostomy tube remained in through the remainder of the pregnancy with careful monitoring for infection; it was removed successfully two weeks postpartum.

3. Discussion

To qualify as a spontaneous forniceal rupture, the following criteria must be met: the absences of recent ureteric instrumentation, surgery, external trauma, a destructive kidney lesion, kidney stones, or external compression [1]. In a retrospective review of 108 cases of forniceal rupture diagnosed by CT scan, the causes were ureteric stones in 80 cases (74.1%), malignant extrinsic ureteric compression in nine cases (8.3%), benign extrinsic ureteric compression in two cases (1.9%), pelvic-ureteric junction obstruction in two cases (1.9%), vesicoureteric junction obstruction in one case (0.9%), bladder outlet obstruction in one case (0.9%), and iatrogenic causes in four cases (3.7%) [2]. In fact, no definitive cause was found in nine cases (8.3%). Pregnancy has been

TABLE 1: Admission laboratory values.

Laboratory values	Admission
Sodium (mmol/L)	142
Potassium (mmol/L)	4.2
Chloride (mmol/L)	108
Bicarbonate (mmol/L)	24.4
BUN (mmol/L)	3.21
Serum creatinine (μmol/L)	44.2
WBC (/nL)	10.1
Hemoglobin (g/dL)	11.6
Hematocrit (%)	33.7
Platelets (/nL)	164

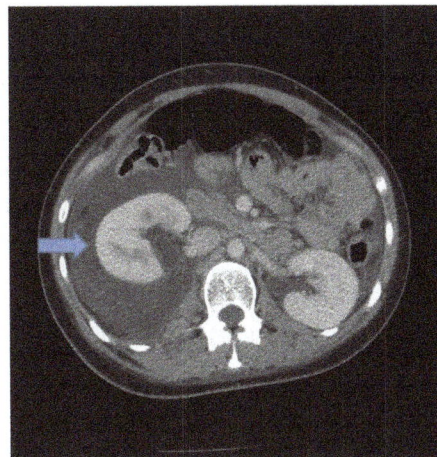

FIGURE 1: CT scan of abdomen on admission. Blue arrow indicates presence of urinoma.

described as a much more rare cause of forniceal rupture [3]. Pregnancy with a solitary kidney, however, has also been reported to result in forniceal rupture [4].

It is surmised that forniceal rupture is a safety valve for alleviation of increased intrapelvic pressure. According to Laplace's law (Tension = Pressure × Radius) the tensile stress that accumulates within a dilated collecting system would increase with size, thereby causing earlier forniceal rupture in a more dilated system [2]. A pressure that exceeds the tensile strength of forniceal tissues leads to rupture and extravasation of urine. Ultimately, this phenomenon is meant to be renoprotective by decreasing pressure in the collecting system [5].

The state of pregnancy results in physiologic hormonal and hemodynamic changes of kidney size, structure, and function. Both kidneys increase in size by 1–1.5 cm due to the increase in the renal vascular volume, hence increasing the glomerular filtrate rate by 50% [6]. The ureters are retroperitoneal structures that go from the renal pelvis to the bladder. They are around 25 to 30 cm in length from the renal pelvis to the trigone of the bladder. They are divided by the pelvic brim into abdominal and pelvic segments, each of which is around 12 to 15 cm in length. That physiologic hydronephrosis and hydroureters that occur in pregnancy have been well-described for more than 200 years. Both Morgagni in 1761 and Rayer in 1839 discerned from postmortem examination that the uterus compressing the ureters produced retention of urine in the kidneys. This then causes dilatation of structures such as ureters, pelvis, and calyces, which results in a delay in the excretion of urine [7]. With increase in the pelvic vasculature in pregnancy, ureteral compression occurs, more on the right because of anatomic relationship of right ureter to less distensible right iliac artery and right ovarian blood vessels. The ureters and renal pelvis dilate more so on the right than left (up to 80%) [7]. The dilatation involves only the renal pelvis and the abdominal ureter and is evident by the third trimester of pregnancy in almost 90% of pregnant patients. This effect usually resolves in half of the females within two days of delivery.

Apart from mechanical reasons, endocrine factors also contribute to ureteropelvic distension. Hormones such as progesterone and prostaglandins can cause diminished tone and peristalsis of the ureter. This allows for small increments of extraluminal pressure to produce substantial reductions in urine flow and distension of the collecting system proximal to a point of obstruction. Interestingly, high-dose hormonal therapy failed to produce ureteropelvic dilatation reliably, suggesting that hormonal causes alone are not enough to explain the structural alterations [8].

With all the above features, there is progressive dilatation of the renal pelvis and the risk of forniceal rupture. The incidence for rupture will be highest at points where there is scarring and infection due to decreased structural integrity. In the absence of these factors, the site of rupture is unclear but may be traced to the calyx or pelvis where a collection of urine may be found.

The clinical presentation of a forniceal rupture in pregnancy may be confused with many abdominal processes, including but not limited to cholecystitis, hepatitis, appendicitis, pyelonephritis, uterine rupture, abruption placentae, and more. Laboratory testing is usually not very helpful in delineating the exact etiology, though normal liver function tests may help to rule out liver pathologies. Imaging of the collecting system, initially with an ultrasound, usually followed with a CT or MRI scan, would be more definitive. A limited excretory urogram is not commonly performed during pregnancy but may help to delineate the site and nature of the rupture or obstruction, the amount of extravasation, and the function of the kidneys.

Management is individualized and depends on the location and type of extravasation. Hwang et al. report the use of serial ultrasonography to detect, monitor, and manage the rupture [9]. On ultrasound, the presence of perinephric fluid may be difficult to distinguish between a urinoma and a hematoma, with helpful hints from the presence of internal echoes or septations indicating the latter. However, oftentimes, an MRI is necessarily performed to view the characteristic high-intensity signals of acute hematoma on T1-images [10]. If the rupture occurred through the renal parenchyma, then surgical exploration is necessary because of the associated hemorrhage. A partial or total nephrectomy may be necessary to control the bleeding [11]. In cases where the collecting system is ruptured, the goal is to alleviate the outflow obstruction. For the patient with a gravid uterus that compresses the ureter, placement of a double J ureteral stent [4] or a nephrostomy tube should relieve the pressure [10]. Appropriate antibiotic coverage and close follow-up are required until definitive treatment is possible, that is, the delivery of the child. It is recommended to change ureteral stents and nephrostomy tubes every 4–6 weeks during pregnancy [12]. Ureteral stents, in particular, have a high risk of encrustation. Why this phenomenon is increased during pregnancy is not completely clear but may be related to the hypercalciuric and hyperuricosuric states that are associated with pregnancy [13]. Frequent urinary tract infections or asymptomatic bacteriuria may exacerbate this as well. Prolonged nephrostomies are associated with increased risk of infection. Since radiation exposure is a concern, it is possible to perform ultrasound-guided ureteral stent placement with local anesthesia and intravenous sedation [14]. However, if this expertise is not available, placement under pulsed fluoroscopy will help to minimize radiation exposure. Oesterling et al. reported one case report of a spontaneous forniceal rupture during pregnancy that was managed only with the temporary insertion of a ureteral catheter for 72 hours [11]. A retrograde pyelogram conducted after removal of the catheter showed no further extravasation and the patient remained asymptomatic for the remainder of her pregnancy. The authors recommend that a short trial of ureteral catheter placement of 48 to 72 hours may be tried; if recurrence is noted, a self-retaining indwelling catheter should be inserted for the duration of the pregnancy. Hwang et al. performed a retrograde ureteral catheterization and were able to relieve the patient's flank pain and rapidly resorb the perinephric urinoma, which suggested that there was an open communication between the site of rupture and the urinoma [9]. Conservative management is usually adequate; however, should the patient demonstrate clinical deterioration in the form of decreasing hemoglobin or increasing in the size of collection, nephrectomy may be necessary to control the hemorrhage provided the other kidney is normal [4].

In conclusion, though ureteral dilatation is common in pregnancy, forniceal rupture is not. Management of this condition ranges from temporary insertion of a ureteral catheter to total nephrectomy depending on the site and severity of rupture. There have not been reports on whether the rupture recurs in subsequent pregnancies, though, given the anatomic damage, the risk should be higher. Careful postpartum follow-up with nephrology and urology would be crucial.

Conflict of Interests

The authors declare that there is no conflict of interests regarding the publication of this paper.

References

[1] A. Schwartz, M. Caine, G. Hermann, and W. Bittermann, "Spontaneous renal extravasation during intravenous urography," *The American Journal of Roentgenology, Radium Therapy, and Nuclear Medicine*, vol. 98, no. 1, pp. 27–40, 1966.

[2] B. Gershman, N. Kulkarni, D. V. Sahani, and B. H. Eisner, "Causes of renal forniceal rupture," *BJU International*, vol. 108, no. 11, pp. 1909–1912, 2011.

[3] J. T. van Winter, P. L. Ogburn Jr., D. E. Engen, and M. J. Webb, "Spontaneous renal rupture during pregnancy," *Mayo Clinic Proceedings*, vol. 66, no. 2, pp. 179–182, 1991.

[4] G. Nabi, D. Sundeep, and P. N. Dogra, "Spontaneous rupture of hydronephrotic solitary functioning kidney during pregnancy," *International Urology and Nephrology*, vol. 33, no. 3, pp. 453–456, 2001.

[5] M. Georgieva, M. Thieme, W. Pernice, and R.-B. Tröbs, "Urinary ascites and perirenal urinoma—a renoprotective 'Complication' of posterior urethral valves," *Aktuelle Urologie*, vol. 34, no. 6, pp. 410–412, 2003.

[6] R. R. Bailey and G. L. Rolleston, "Kidney length and ureteric dilatation in the puerperium," *Journal of Obstetrics and Gynaecology of the British Commonwealth*, vol. 78, no. 1, pp. 55–61, 1971.

[7] P. E. Rasmussen and F. R. Nielsen, "Hydronephrosis during pregnancy: a literature survey," *European Journal of Obstetrics Gynecology and Reproductive Biology*, vol. 27, no. 3, pp. 249–259, 1988.

[8] P. Klarskov, T. Gerstenberg, D. Ramirez, P. Christensen, and T. Hald, "Prostaglandin type E activity dominates in urinary tract smooth muscle in vitro," *The Journal of Urology*, vol. 129, no. 5, pp. 1071–1074, 1983.

[9] S. S. Hwang, Y. H. Park, C. B. Lee et al., "Spontaneous rupture of hydronephrotic kidney during pregnancy: value of serial sonography," *Journal of Clinical Ultrasound*, vol. 28, no. 7, pp. 358–360, 2000.

[10] A. W. Middleton Jr., G. W. Middleton, and L. K. Dean, "Spontaneous renal rupture in pregnancy," *Urology*, vol. 15, no. 1, pp. 60–63, 1980.

[11] J. E. Oesterling, R. E. Besinger, and C. B. Brendler, "Spontaneous rupture of the renal collecting system during pregnancy: successful management with a temporary ureteral catheter," *Journal of Urology*, vol. 140, no. 3, pp. 588–590, 1988.

[12] C. M. Cormier, B. J. Canzoneri, D. F. Lewis, C. Briery, L. Knoepp, and J. B. Mailhes, "Urolithiasis in pregnancy: current diagnosis, treatment, and pregnancy complications," *Obstetrical and Gynecological Survey*, vol. 61, no. 11, pp. 733–741, 2006.

[13] R. A. Goldfarb, G. J. Neerhut, and E. Lederer, "Management of acute hydronephrosis of pregnancy by ureteral stenting: risk of stone formation," *Journal of Urology*, vol. 141, no. 4 I, pp. 921–922, 1989.

[14] D. J. Jarrard, G. S. Gerber, and E. S. Lyon, "Management of acute ureteral obstruction in pregnancy utilizing ultrasound-guided placement of ureteral stents," *Urology*, vol. 42, no. 3, pp. 263–268, 1993.

10

Rhabdomyolysis and Acute Kidney Injury Requiring Dialysis as a Result of Concomitant Use of Atypical Neuroleptics and Synthetic Cannabinoids

Aiyu Zhao, Maybel Tan, Aung Maung, Moro Salifu, and Mary Mallappallil

State University of New York Downstate Medical Center, 450 Clarkson Avenue, Brooklyn, NY 11203, USA

Correspondence should be addressed to Aiyu Zhao; aiyuzhao@gmail.com

Academic Editor: Neil Boudville

The use of synthetic cannabinoids (SCBs) is associated with many severe adverse effects that are not observed with marijuana use. We report a unique case of a patient who developed rhabdomyolysis and acute kidney injury (AKI) requiring dialysis after use of SCBs combined with quetiapine. Causes for the different adverse effects profile between SCBs and marijuana are not defined yet. Cases reported in literature with SCBs use have been associated with reversible AKI characterized by acute tubular necrosis and interstitial nephritis. Recent studies have showed the involvement of cytochromes P450s (CYPs) in biotransformation of SCBs. The use of quetiapine which is a substrate of the CYP3A4 and is excreted (73%) as urine metabolites may worsen the side effect profiles of both quetiapine and K2. SCBs use should be included in the differential diagnosis of AKI and serum Creatinine Phosphokinase (CPK) level should be monitored. Further research is needed to identify the mechanism of SCBs nephrotoxicity.

1. Introduction

AKI is the abrupt loss of kidney function, resulting in the retention of urea and other nitrogenous waste products and in the dysregulation of volume and electrolytes [1]. Rhabdomyolysis is characterized by muscle necrosis and the leakage of muscle-cell contents like electrolytes, myoglobin, and sarcoplasmic proteins (CPK, aldolase, lactate dehydrogenase, alanine aminotransferase, and aspartate aminotransferase) into the circulation [2]. AKI is a complication of severe rhabdomyolysis and is seen in about 7–10% of all cases of AKI in the United States. The causes of rhabdomyolysis may be classified as traumatic, nontraumatic exertional, and nontraumatic nonexertional causes [2, 3].

Cannabis is the most commonly used illegal substance in the world [4]. It contains over 400 compounds, including more than 60 cannabinoids. The primary psychoactive cannabinoid is delta-9-tetrahydrocannabinol (THC) [5].

SCBs have multiple brand names most commonly "Spice" or "K2" and many street names such as "Fake Pot" [5]. They are a heterogeneous group of compounds developed to probe the endogenous cannabinoid system (ECS) [4, 5]. SCBs can be divided into 7 major structural groups: naphthoylindoles (JWH-018 and JWH-073), naphthylmethylindoles, naphthoylpyrroles, naphthylmethylindenes, phenylacetylindoles (JWH-250), cyclohexylphenols (CP-47,497), and classical cannabinoids (HU-210). There are no structural similarities in SCBs with THC [5, 6].

Recreational use of SCBs was noticed initially in the early 2000s in Europe. After European and Russian authorities banned SCBs in 2010, the K2 epidemic emerged in the United States [5]. Previously they were referred to as "legal highs" or "herbal highs"; these compounds are now classified as Class I controlled substances by the United States Drug Enforcement Administration [7]. Illicit use remains significant and reports of illness are increasing. In March 2012, 16 cases of AKI after SCBs use were reported in six states [8]. Four cases of oliguric AKI associated with use of SCBs were reported in 2013 [9]. However, rhabdomyolysis was not reported in the above cases. To our knowledge, there is only case report of rhabdomyolysis associated with SCB use in the USA [10].

We are reporting a unique case of a patient with history of Cannabis dependence and paranoid schizophrenia who developed severe rhabdomyolysis and AKI requiring dialysis after use of K2 combined with quetiapine.

TABLE 1: Daily laboratory values.

	CK (IU/L)	Potassium (mmol/L)	BUN (mg/dL)	Creatinine (mg/dL)	AST (IU/L)	ALT (IU/L)	Urine output (mL)	Note
Day 1	>22,000	6.9	68	6.09	3167	964	10	IVF
Day 2	148,643	6.5	83	7.56	2307	724	20	IVF
Day 3	>22,000	6.8	92	9.39	1520	597	0	HD
Day 4	81,620	5.2	84	9.15	973	530	0	HD
Day 5	>22,000	5.6	87	9.69	610	442	0	HD
Day 6	51,030	4.8	75	8.36	523	406	0	HD
Day 7	28,060	4.9	76	8.77	315	331	0	HD
Day 8	16,339	4.4	62	7.79	222	237	50	No HD
Day 9	10,701	5	75	9.7	188	218	100	HD
Day 10	6242	4.4	63	8.87	128	200	150	HD
Day 11	4230	4.8	58	8.75	91	161	200	HD
Day 12	2719	4.9	58	8.61	65	123	300	No HD
Day 13	2199	4.6	64	9.38	57	112	900	HD
Day 14	1835	4.4	57	8.69	51	109	1200	HD

CK: Creatine Kinase, BUN: Blood Urea Nitrogen, AST: Aspartate Transaminase, and ALT: Alanine Transaminase.

2. Case Presentation

A 39-year-old African American man from a supervised living facility, with history of paranoid schizophrenia and Cannabis dependence, presented with generalized bodyache, back pain, and weakness. He had been smoking one joint of K2 daily purchased from the street for several years, with increased use in the one week prior to admission. The day prior to admission he took 10 tablets of quetiapine from his roommate with the intention of suicide. Subsequently he felt nauseated and vomited. He noticed that his urine "was darker." He had a history of paranoid schizophrenia with many failed antipsychotic regimens. In the last 2 years, he had been receiving monthly intramuscular haloperidol decanoate 250 mg and the last injection was 3 weeks prior to admission. He denied history of trauma or injury and denied chest pain, shortness of breath or dizziness or other medications, and supplement or other illicit drugs' use. There was no similar episode in the past.

On examination, he was afebrile, initial blood pressure was 136/87 mmHg with pulse of 111 per minute, and respiratory rate was 18 per minute. There was no orthostatic hypotension. Oxygenation saturation was 100% in room air. He was lethargic but oriented to person, place, and date. His pupils were equal and reactive to light and measured about 3 mm in size. His lungs were clear to auscultation; heart rate was regular with no murmurs; abdomen was soft and there is no tenderness or organomegaly. There was 2+ pitting edema in bilateral lower extremities up to the knees; there was diffuse tenderness upon palpation. Foley catheter was inserted with 50 milliliters of tea color urine returned.

Table 1 shows the daily laboratory values. His creatinine was 1 mg/dL (88.4 μmol/L) in November 2013. Urine microscopy showed muddy brown casts of acute tubular necrosis. Urine myoglobin was strongly positive, FeNa (the fractional excretion of sodium) was 1.8%. Urine toxicity

screen for barbiturate, benzodiazepines, cocaine, methadone, and opiates was negative. Urine for cannabinoid was negative as expected with SCBs use. Alcohol and salicylate level was undetectable. HIV (the human immunodeficiency virus), HBV (hepatitis B virus), HCV (hepatitis C virus), EBV (Epstein-Barr virus), anti-DNase B, ANA (antinuclear antibody), P-ANCA (Perinuclear Anti-Neutrophil Cytoplasmic Antibodies), C-ANCA (Cytoplasmic Anti-Neutrophil Cytoplasmic Antibodies), and anti-glomerular basement membrane (anti-GBM) antibody were all negative; complements were within normal limits. ABG revealed pH of 7.29, PCO_2 of 30.6 mmHg, PO_2 of 178 mmHg, and bicarbonate of 16 mmol/L, which was consistent with high anion gap metabolic acidosis with respiratory compensation. High anion metabolic acidosis is likely due to AKI, as there was no evidence of lactic acidosis, ketoacidosis, toxic alcohol, acetaminophen, or salicylate ingestion.

Electrocardiogram showed normal sinus rhythm with no PT prolongation. There was no hydronephrosis in renal sonogram.

A diagnosis of AKI secondary to rhabdomyolysis and K2 use was made. His FeNa was more than 1 which is different from typical rhabdomyolysis-induced AKI when FeNa may frequently be less than 1%. The workup for AKI has been unrevealing except for positive urine myoglobin. The additional K2 nephrotoxicity might have explained this finding [11, 12]. The etiology of rhabdomyolysis was thought to be secondary to use of K2 combined with quetiapine. Neuroleptic malignant syndrome was in the differential diagnosis, however, thought to be less likely as the patient had never been febrile with no rigidity and no tremor or signs of autonomic dysfunction.

He was started on aggressive intravenous hydration with normal saline at 200 mL/hr. After 12 hours, no increase in urine output was noticed. The IV fluid rate increased to

500 mL/hour; he remained oliguric with persistent hyperkalemia. Hemodialysis was started on Day 3 of the hospitalization. He was dialyzed for 10 sessions. Urine output started to improve on Day 13 when his 24 hours' urine output was 900 mL. His last dialysis was on Day 14 of hospitalization after which creatinine and CK continued to decrease without dialysis. After 26 days of hospitalization he was discharged back to the supervised living facility; upon discharge, his creatinine was 2.25 mg/dL and CK was 299 IU/L.

With the resolution of oliguria in AKI which is the commonest marker for improvement in renal function, we noted a decrease in serum CPK and decrease in the number of muddy brown casts on sequential urine microscopy [11].

3. Discussion

Unlike many other "traditional" drugs of abuse, SCBs appear to have variable and unknown toxicities, including many not seen with marijuana use like tachycardia, hypertension, nausea, vomiting, convulsions, agitation, hallucinations, and psychosis [4, 5]. More recently, separate reports of rhabdomyolysis and kidney failure after SCBs use have been published [4, 5, 7–10, 13]. SCBs use has also been implicated in cases of acute myocardial infarction in three otherwise healthy teenagers. Dependence and withdrawal symptoms associated with chronic use have also been reported [6].

SCBs interact with cannabinoid receptors (CBRs) and elicit cannabimimetic effects similar to THC [6, 14, 15]. The endogenous cannabinoid system (ECS) is widely dispersed through the body. To date, two endogenous cannabinoid receptors, CBR1 and CBR2, are well characterized [6, 14, 15]. CBR1 and CBR2 are G protein-coupled receptors (GPCRs). CBR1 is mainly expressed in the brain and mediates the CNS effects of THC and other cannabinoids. CBR1 also is expressed peripherally in adipocytes and skeletal muscle. Recent studies have showed that ECS affects skeletal muscle oxidation [6]. CBR2 is located primarily on the T cells, B cells, and macrophages and in hematopoietic cells and is involved in regulating immune function. In general, CBR2 activation is immunosuppressive, inhibits production of proinflammatory cytokines, enhances production of anti-inflammatory cytokines, induces apoptosis of immune cells, and suppresses macrophage chemotaxis. Activation of CBR2 is thought to underlie the anti-inflammatory and immunosuppressive effects of marijuana [6, 16].

Causes for the different adverse effects profile between SCBs and marijuana are not defined yet. Four possible mechanisms are postulated [6]. The first two mechanisms are potential differences in pharmacodynamics. First, these effects are probably mediated by actions of SCBs at non-cannabinoid receptors. Second, as most SCBs examined to date possess higher potency and efficacy than THC at CBRs it is possible that SCBs, especially taken in the various combinations found in SCB products, achieve levels of CBR1 and CBR2 activation high enough to produce severe, clinically observable physiological and psychological disturbances.

Third, the active components of marijuana and SCBs are likely metabolized differently and thus have distinct pharmacokinetic profiles. Some active metabolites of SBCs

likely contribute to the effects by activating CBRs. THC is metabolized by CYP2C9 to a predominant single biologically active metabolite, 11-hydroxy-D9-THC, which then inactivated carboxylation and glucuronidated prior to excretion. In contrast, several major metabolites of SCBs exhibit greater CBR1 affinity, potency, and efficacy than THC, both in vitro and in vivo. And these metabolites also retain in vitro pharmacological activity at CBR2s with greater potency.

The fourth mechanism is that drug-drug interactions, such as synergy, may increase risk of adverse effects as multiple drug use is common with SCBs abuse.

According to a study by Ginsburg et al. in 2012, adverse effects following consumption of SCBs are unlikely due to impurities or residue from the manufacturing process [17]. However, different content of nonpsychoactive substances in the marijuana plant versus SCB products might play a role in the adverse symptoms.

Neuroleptics can cause acute rhabdomyolysis as part of a neuroleptic malignant syndrome (NMS) or via direct toxic effect on myocytes. One suggested mechanism of rhabdomyolysis in the absence of NMS is an increase of skeletal muscle-cell membrane permeability [2, 3]. It is unknown whether rhabdomyolysis is dose or duration dependent when neuroleptics are involved [13]. There has been evidence that endocannabinoid has effect on the skeletal muscle oxidation [18]. But the complete endocannabinoid action on skeletal muscle metabolism is still to be elucidated. If both SCBs and quetiapine have effect on skeletal muscle, the combination of them might have made the injury more severe.

SCB causing AKI is thought to be via acute tubular necrosis which does not present with rhabdomyolysis. Cases reported in literature with K2 use and AKI have been associated with reversible acute kidney injury characterized by acute tubular necrosis and interstitial nephritis [9]. THC is initially metabolized via oxidation by CYP2C9 and CYP3A4 [19, 20]. Recent in vitro metabolism studies, using recombinant CYPs, identified CYP2C9 and CYP1A2 as the primary hepatic P450 isoforms involved in the oxidation of JWH-018 [19, 21]. Other structural groups of SCBs might have involved CYP3A4. In this case the combination with quetiapine which is a substrates of the CYP3A4 system and which is excreted mostly (73%) in the urine as metabolites may worsen the side effect profiles of both quetiapine and K2.

4. Conclusion

Complete pharmacological knowledge of synthetic cannabinoids is lacking. The confirmation of SCBs use was hindered by lack of known biomarkers. It is important for the clinician to always take a thorough history and have a complete list of medications the patients are exposed to. SCBs use should be included in the differential diagnosis of AKI and CK level should be monitored. Further research is needed to identify the mechanism of SCBs nephrotoxicity.

Conflict of Interests

The authors declare that there is no conflict of interests regarding the publication of this paper.

References

[1] R. L. Mehta and G. M. Chertow, "Acute renal failure definitions and classification: time for change?" *Journal of the American Society of Nephrology*, vol. 14, no. 8, pp. 2178–2187, 2003.

[2] X. Bosch, E. Poch, and J. M. Grau, "Rhabdomyolysis and acute kidney injury," *The New England Journal of Medicine*, vol. 361, no. 1, pp. 62–72, 2009.

[3] R. Vanholder, M. S. Sever, E. Erek, and N. Lameire, "Rhabdomyolysis," *Journal of the American Society of Nephrology*, vol. 11, no. 8, pp. 1553–1561, 2000.

[4] T. Leggett, "A review of the world cannabis situation," *Bulletin on Narcotics*, vol. 58, no. 1-2, pp. 1–155, 2006.

[5] L. Lindsay and M. L. White, "Herbal marijuana alternatives and bath salts—'barely legal' toxic highs," *Clinical Pediatric Emergency Medicine*, vol. 13, no. 4, pp. 283–291, 2012.

[6] L. K. Brents and P. L. Prather, "The K2/Spice phenomenon: emergence, identification, legislation and metabolic characterization of synthetic cannabinoids in herbal incense products," *Drug Metabolism Reviews*, vol. 46, no. 1, pp. 72–85, 2014.

[7] US Drug Enforcement Administration, "Chemicals used in 'Spice' and 'K2' type products now under federal control and regulation," 2011, http://www.dea.gov/pubs/pressrel/pr030111.html.

[8] Centers for Disease Control and Prevention (CDC), "Acute kidney injury associated with synthetic cannabinoid use—multiple states, 2012," *Morbidity and Mortality Weekly Report*, vol. 62, no. 6, pp. 93–98, 2013.

[9] G. K. Bhanushali, G. Jain, H. Fatima, L. J. Leisch, and D. Thornley-Brown, "AKI associated with synthetic cannabinoids: a case series," *Clinical Journal of the American Society of Nephrology*, vol. 8, no. 4, pp. 523–526, 2013.

[10] D. Durand, L. L. Delgado, D. M. de la Parra-Pellot, and D. Nichols-Vinueza, "Psychosis and severe rhabdomyolysis associated with synthetic cannabinoid use," *Clinical Schizophrenia & Related Psychoses*, vol. 8, no. 4, pp. 205–208, 2015.

[11] M. C. Mallappallil, R. Mehta, E. Yoshiuchi, G. Briefel, E. Lerma, and M. Salifu, "Parameters used to discontinue dialysis in acute kidney injury recovery: a survey of United States Nephrologists," *Nephron*, vol. 130, no. 1, pp. 41–47, 2015.

[12] H. L. Corwin, M. J. Schreiber, and L. S. T. Fang, "Low fractional excretion of sodium. Occurrence with hemoglobinuric- and myoglobinuric-induced acute renal failure," *Archives of Internal Medicine*, vol. 144, no. 5, pp. 981–982, 1984.

[13] R. Aggarwal, N. Guanci, K. Marambage, and J. P. Caplan, "A patient with multiple episodes of rhabdomyolysis induced by different neuroleptics," *Psychosomatics*, vol. 55, no. 4, pp. 404–408, 2014.

[14] M. S. Castaneto, D. A. Gorelick, N. A. Desrosiers, R. L. Hartman, S. Pirard, and M. A. Huestis, "Synthetic cannabinoids: epidemiology, pharmacodynamics, and clinical implications," *Drug and Alcohol Dependence*, vol. 144, pp. 12–41, 2014.

[15] C. R. Harris and A. Brown, "Synthetic cannabinoid intoxication: a case series and review," *The Journal of Emergency Medicine*, vol. 44, no. 2, pp. 360–366, 2013.

[16] S. Steffens and P. Pacher, "Targeting cannabinoid receptor CB_2 in cardiovascular disorders: promises and controversies," *British Journal of Pharmacology*, vol. 167, no. 2, pp. 313–323, 2012.

[17] B. C. Ginsburg, L. R. McMahon, J. J. Sanchez, and M. A. Javors, "Purity of synthetic cannabinoids sold online for recreational use," *Journal of Analytical Toxicology*, vol. 36, no. 1, Article ID bkr018, pp. 66–68, 2012.

[18] P. Cavuoto, A. J. McAinch, G. Hatzinikolas, D. Cameron-Smith, and G. A. Wittert, "Effects of cannabinoid receptors on skeletal muscle oxidative pathways," *Molecular and Cellular Endocrinology*, vol. 267, no. 1-2, pp. 63–69, 2007.

[19] W. E. Fantegrossi, J. H. Moran, A. Radominska-Pandya, and P. L. Prather, "Distinct pharmacology and metabolism of K2 synthetic cannabinoids compared to Δ^9-THC: mechanism underlying greater toxicity?" *Life Sciences*, vol. 97, no. 1, pp. 45–54, 2014.

[20] K. Watanabe, S. Yamaori, T. Funahashi, T. Kimura, and I. Yamamoto, "Cytochrome P450 enzymes involved in the metabolism of tetrahydrocannabinols and cannabinol by human hepatic microsomes," *Life Sciences*, vol. 80, no. 15, pp. 1415–1419, 2007.

[21] K. C. Chimalakonda, K. A. Seely, S. M. Bratton et al., "Cytochrome P450-mediated oxidative metabolism of abused synthetic cannabinoids found in K2/Spice: identification of novel cannabinoid receptor ligands," *Drug Metabolism and Disposition*, vol. 40, no. 11, pp. 2174–2184, 2012.

11

Pauci-Immune Necrotizing and Crescentic Glomerulonephritis with Membranous Lupus Nephritis, Fifteen Years after Initial Diagnosis of Secondary Membranous Nephropathy

Ryan Burkhart,[1] Nina Shah,[2] Michael Abel,[3] James D. Oliver III,[4] and Matthew Lewin[5]

[1]Department of Internal Medicine, William Beaumont Army Medical Center, 5005 N. Piedras Street, El Paso, TX 79920, USA
[2]Department of Nephrology, William Beaumont Army Medical Center, 5005 N. Piedras Street, El Paso, TX 79920, USA
[3]Department of Rheumatology, William Beaumont Army Medical Center, 5005 N. Piedras Street, El Paso, TX 79920, USA
[4]Nephrology Service, Walter Reed National Military Medical Center, 8901 Rockville Pike, Bethesda, MD 20889, USA
[5]ProPath Services, LLP, 1355 River Bend Drive, Dallas, TX 75247, USA

Correspondence should be addressed to Ryan Burkhart; ryan.v.burkhart.mil@mail.mil

Academic Editor: Kouichi Hirayama

Renal involvement in systemic lupus erythematosus (SLE) is usually immune complex mediated and may have multiple different presentations. Pauci-immune necrotizing and crescentic glomerulonephritis (NCGN) refers to extensive glomerular inflammation with few or no immune deposits that may result in rapid decline in renal function. We report a case of a 79-year-old Hispanic male with a history of secondary membranous nephropathy (diagnosed by renal biopsy 15 years previously) who was admitted with acute kidney injury and active urinary sediment. P-ANCA titers and anti-myeloperoxidase antibodies were positive. The renal biopsy was diagnostic for NCGN superimposed on a secondary membranous nephropathy. A previous diagnosis of SLE based on American College of Rheumatology criteria was discovered via Veteran's Administration records review after the completion of treatment for pauci-immune NCGN. ANCAs are detected in 20–31% of patients with SLE. There may be an association between SLE and ANCA seropositivity. In patients with lupus nephritis and biopsy findings of necrotizing and crescentic glomerulonephritis, without significant immune complex deposition, ANCA testing should be performed. In patients with secondary membranous nephropathy SLE should be excluded.

1. Introduction

Pauci-immune necrotizing and crescentic glomerulonephritis (NCGN) refers to extensive glomerular inflammation with few or no immune deposits that may result in rapid decline in renal function if left untreated. Lupus nephritis (LN) can present with a NCGN. This often presents as a clinical syndrome of type 2 rapidly progressive glomerulonephritis (RPGN), pathologically consistent with class IV lupus nephritis and is immune complex mediated [1]. Often those patients have evidence of clinically or immunologically active lupus [2–5]. The first two cases of biopsy proven antineutrophil cytoplasmic antibody (ANCA) associated NCGN superimposed on a patient with class V LN were published in 1997 [5]. Since then this has remained a rare occurrence with three additional cases reported [3, 6, 7].

We describe a rare case of a patient with inactive SLE who presented with ANCA associated NCGN superimposed on class V LN fifteen years after his initial diagnosis of secondary membranous nephropathy.

2. Case Presentation

A 79-year-old Hispanic male presented to the emergency room with complaints of increased fatigue and decreased appetite. Fifteen years prior, he had presented with nephrotic range proteinuria (7.5 g/day on 24-hour collection) and underwent a renal biopsy showing secondary membranous glomerulopathy of unspecified etiology. Since the biopsy, his renal function was preserved and he was noted to have spontaneous remission of his proteinuria on prednisone without cytotoxic therapy. His other past medical history included mild dementia, hypertension, hypothyroidism, hyperlipidemia, gout, cerebral vascular disease, fatty liver, and alcohol abuse. Twelve years prior to his current presentation, his ANCA antibodies were negative. Six months prior, his serum creatinine was 114.92 μmol/L (1.3 mg/dL). His medications were levothyroxine, allopurinol, sertraline, metoprolol tartrate, aspirin, galantamine, calcium/vitamin D, loratadine, vitamin E, and multivitamin. On presentation the blood pressure was 225/90 mmHg. The exam was significant for bilateral crackles on pulmonary exam and absence of lower extremity edema. Labs were significant for BUN of 32.84 mmol/L (92 mg/dL) and serum creatinine was 813.28 μmol/L (9.2 mg/dL). Urinalysis was notable for 3+ proteinuria, 3+ blood, and specific gravity of 1.009. Urine sediment demonstrated 0–2 granular casts/hpf, 0-1 broad granular cast/lpf, and sheets of RBCs with >30% dysmorphic RBCs/hpf. Proteinuria was noted to be 3 g/day on a 24-hour collection. Serologies for HIV, hepatitis B, hepatitis C, and RPR were negative. Complement levels were normal. CRP was 2120.99 nmol/L (22.27 mg/dL), and ESR was 96 mm/hr. ANA was equivocal and anti-dsDNA antibodies were negative. Anti-Smith antibodies were negative. C-ANCA and anti-proteinase 3 antibodies were negative, as were anti-glomerular basement membrane (anti-GBM) antibodies. P-ANCA antibodies were positive with a 1 : 640 titer and anti-MPO antibodies were positive at 657 AU/mL (positive, >120 AU/mL). Chest X-ray showed small pleural effusions and patchy opacities bilaterally. Renal ultrasound noted normal parenchyma and no evidence of hydronephrosis or renal vein thrombosis.

Echocardiogram noted a preserved ejection fraction, moderate mitral stenosis, and elevated pulmonary artery pressures in the setting of a low normal central venous pressure. CT chest was consistent with chronic interstitial lung disease. Interstitial lung disease in combination with his mitral stenosis was likely contributing to his elevated pulmonary arterial pressures and pulmonary crackles on physical exam findings.

His blood pressure was treated with hydralazine and labetalol, and dialysis was initiated. A renal biopsy was performed and 39 glomeruli were obtained. Twelve out of 39 glomeruli were obsolescent, and 15 had cellular or fibrocellular crescents (Figure 1). Fibrinoid necrosis was present. There was mild increase in mesangial matrix but minimal hypercellularity and no endocapillary proliferation. The capillary walls were thickened, deposits were visible on Masson trichrome stain, and spikes were seen on Jones silver stain, consistent with a membranous glomerulopathy. The tubulointerstitium had inflammation with occasional eosinophils and mild interstitial fibrosis and tubular atrophy. No vasculitis was present in the vessels.

Immunofluorescence was positive for IgG (3+), IgM (trace), C3 (3+), kappa (2+), and lambda (3+) in the mesangium and glomerular capillary wall. C1q was negative. There was segmental staining for fibrinogen (3+) in Bowman's

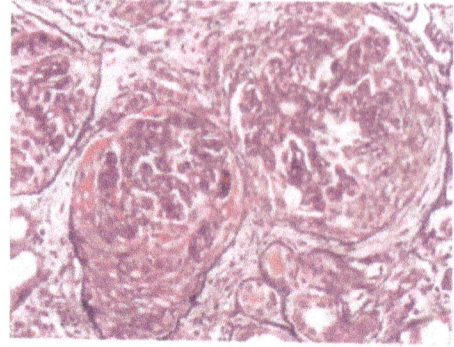

FIGURE 1: Light micrograph of crescentic glomerulonephritis with fibrinoid necrosis, showing mild mesangial expansion and minimal increase in cellularity without endocapillary proliferation. Subepithelial spikes were noted on the silver stain.

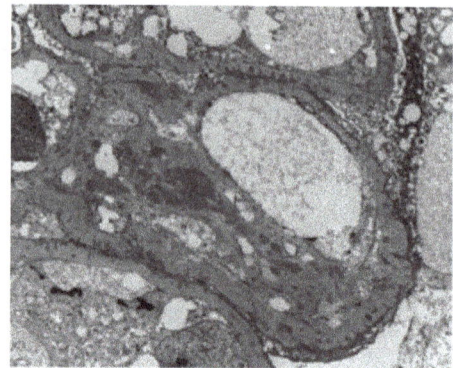

FIGURE 2: Electron microscopy showing extensive foot process effacement, numerous subepithelial deposits with GBM reaction-spike formation, and occasional enveloping of deposits. There are occasional mesangial deposits. Fibrin deposition was noted within Bowman's capsule.

capsule. Electron microscopy showed extensive foot process effacement and numerous subepithelial deposits with spike formation and occasional enveloping of deposits consistent with stage 3 membranous nephropathy (Figure 2). There were occasional mesangial deposits but no tubuloreticular inclusions or tubular basement membrane deposits.

Glomerular basement membrane immunofluorescent histology evaluation for IgG subclasses 1–4 was positive only for IgG2 which was strongly suggestive of secondary membranous nephropathy. Staining for anti-phospholipase A2 receptor (anti-PLA2R) antibodies was negative.

Treatment was initiated for renal-limited NCGN with corticosteroids (1 gram of methylprednisolone, 1 gm intravenously daily for three days, followed by prednisone 60 mg orally daily with gradual taper), plasmapheresis (seven treatments, one plasma volume every other day), and rituximab (375 mg/m^2 once weekly for four doses). Despite therapy, renal recovery was insufficient to withdraw dialysis. On clinical followup at sixteen months the patient remained dialysis dependent but free of systemic manifestations of vasculitis.

A diagnosis of SLE from fifteen years ago based on American College of Rheumatology (ACR) and Systemic Lupus International Collaborating Clinics (SLICC) criteria was discovered via Veteran's Administration records review after the completion of treatment for pauci-immune NCGN.

3. Discussion

The patient had a history of secondary membranous nephropathy of unspecified etiology since 1998. Prior work-up at that time was negative for viral hepatitis and negative for RPR, with no known history of drug induced membranous nephropathy or malignancy. ANCA antibodies were negative three years after the initial renal biopsy but were not checked at the time of the initial diagnosis of secondary membranous nephropathy. In the fifteen years prior to his presentation, the proteinuria had resolved spontaneously without cytotoxic therapy.

A diagnosis of SLE was discovered via Veteran's Administration records review after the completion of treatment for pauci-immune NCGN. ANA titer with speckled pattern of 1 : 2560 was noted in 2001. There is prior dermatologist documentation of photosensitivity and skin biopsy report consistent with cutaneous lupus. He also had prior nephrotic range proteinuria documented with secondary membranous nephropathy of unspecified etiology. He met 4 of the 11 criteria diagnostic for systemic lupus erythematosus based on the prior ACR criteria. Subsequent discussion with the pathologist in conjunction with the above history confirmed that the patient's secondary membranous nephropathy would be consistent with International Society of Nephrology (ISN) Class V lupus nephritis. He would therefore also meet criteria for the diagnosis of SLE based on the Systemic Lupus International Collaborating Clinics (SLICC) criteria. We suspect that at some point in time he likely developed synovitis, probably from his underlying SLE, and given his positive low titer rheumatoid factor, was given the diagnosis of rheumatoid arthritis. His overall picture would fit better with SLE as well given his lack of erosive joint disease. It is well described that about a third of patients with SLE will have positive rheumatoid factor.

He was conjectured to have either renal limited vasculitis or early microscopic polyangiitis as he had no other systemic involvement. Given the severity of his disease, initial decision was to treat him with pulse methylprednisolone of 1 gram for three days followed by prednisone (1 mg/kg) with gradual taper and oral cyclophosphamide. Rituximab has shown evidence of noninferiority in randomized controlled trials [8, 9] and possibly reduces relapse among patient with renal vasculitis. KDOQI guidelines also note that rituximab may be used as an alternative [10]. Notably one critique for the use of rituximab is that it has not been well studied in patients with severely elevated creatinine ($>354\,\mu$mol/L [>4.0 mg/dL]) as they were excluded from the RAVE trial. Our patient presented with a serum creatinine of 813.28 μmol/L (9.2 mg/dL); however, there was concern for the increased risk of adverse effects, particularly leukopenia and infection with cyclophosphamide, given the patient's age, baseline comorbidities, transition to oliguric state, and

anemia. Rituximab was therefore used as the induction agent utilizing the RAVE trial protocol [9]. Prior data has suggested that the treatment of severe renal vasculitis with the use of plasma exchange [11, 12] may be of benefit to decrease the progression to ESRD. Plasma exchange was used as an adjunctive therapy prior to rituximab. Seven sessions of plasma exchange were performed every other day for the first two weeks as assigned in the MEPEX trial [12]. Given that the patient showed no evidence of renal recovery on followup nor manifestations of systemic vasculitis, his prednisone was tapered and no further immunologic agents were started.

The patient did not regain sufficient renal function to become dialysis independent. This was not all together unexpected given the patient's serum creatinine of 813.28 μmol/L (9.2 mg/dL) on presentation, the mild interstitial fibrosis, and the fact that 12 of 39 glomeruli were obsolescent on renal biopsy. Serum creatinine at time of biopsy is an important predictor of progression to ESRD [13]. On clinical follow-up at sixteen months, the patient had not displayed evidence of systemic vasculitis despite remaining persistently anti-MPO antibody positive. Notably, since the patient's hospitalization, additional follow-up data has been published from the RAVE study at 18 months which noted sustained benefit from single course of induction therapy with rituximab [14], though our patient (who was anti-MPO antibody positive) may be at lower risk for relapse given that C-ANCA and anti-proteinase 3 antibody positivity is at higher risk for relapse [15].

When crescents and necrosis are noted superimposed on membranous nephropathy, the possibility of a mixed ISN/RPS class V LN with class III or IV LN may be considered. The renal biopsy noted minimal hypercellularity which would indicate that the necrotic lesions were "pauci-immune" in nature. In addition, the cellularity was limited to the mesangial areas without significant endocapillary proliferation and the degree of crescents and necrosis was out of proportion to the proliferative changes and the amount of immune complex deposits.

ANCA associated NCGN has been described to occur superimposed on primary [13, 16] and secondary membranous nephropathy [17] and has been reported with multiple classes of LN (at least classes II–V) [2–4] with different manifestations of systemic vasculitis. Since the first two cases of ANCA associated NCGN superimposed on class V LN in 1997 only three additional cases have been reported [3, 6, 7]. While there appears to be an association between SLE and ANCA positivity, it is unclear if there is a pathophysiologic mechanism for class V LN nephropathy resulting in NCGN. Our patient had documented negative ANCA antibodies twelve years prior and it is uncertain when the ANCA antibodies actually became positive, or if they were drug induced (i.e., allopurinol). Anti-MPO antibodies can be also be induced with hydralazine which was used for inpatient management of his hypertension. It would be unlikely to develop after two doses of hydralazine. Additionally he was in renal failure prior to the initial administration of the hydralazine.

Review of the literature has noted two case reports of NCGN that manifested or "transformed" years after a diagnosis of idiopathic membranous nephropathy. James et al. in 1995 [18] described a 67-year-old male with idiopathic membranous nephropathy diagnosed fifteen years prior to his presentation with anasarca and AKI in setting of recent CABG, TURP, and urinary tract infection. Repeat renal biopsy showed crescentic GN and allergic interstitial nephritis.

Kwan et al. in 1991 [19] described a 31-year-old male idiopathic membranous nephropathy with persistent nephrotic range proteinuria despite treatment with steroids. Seven years later he presented clinically with rapidly progressive glomerulonephritis with biopsy noting crescentic GN. Both of these patients were ANCA and anti-GBM negative. Our patient presented with P-ANCA associated NCGN superimposed on class V LN, fifteen years after the initial diagnosis of secondary membranous nephropathy, which to the best of our knowledge has not yet been described.

4. Conclusion

There appears to be an association between SLE and ANCA seropositivity [20, 21]; however, the number of cases reported with class V LN and ANCA associated GN is small. In patients with lupus nephritis and biopsy findings of necrotizing and crescentic glomerulonephritis, without significant subendothelial immune complex deposition, endocapillary proliferation, or immunologic evidence of active SLE, ANCA testing should be considered. In patients with membranous nephropathy and renal biopsy suggestive of a secondary process, work-up must include the exclusion of underlying SLE.

Disclaimer

The views expressed in this document are those of the authors and do not reflect the official policy of William Beaumont Army Medical Center, Walter Reed National Military Medical Center, the Department of the Army, or the United States Government.

Consent

Verbal and written consent was obtained from both the patient and the patient's guardian for the publication of this paper.

Conflict of Interests

The authors declare that there is no conflict of interests regarding the publication of this paper.

References

[1] F. Yu, Y. Tan, G. Liu, S.-X. Wang, W.-Z. Zou, and M.-H. Zhao, "Clinicopathological characteristics and outcomes of patients with crescentic lupus nephritis," Kidney International, vol. 76, no. 3, pp. 307–317, 2009.

[2] B. Hervier, M. Hamidou, J. Haroche, C. Durant, A. Mathian, and Z. Amoura, "Systemic lupus erythematosus associated with ANCA-associated vasculitis: an overlapping syndrome?" Rheumatology International, vol. 32, no. 10, pp. 3285–3290, 2012.

[3] S. H. Nasr, V. D. D'Agati, H.-R. Park et al., "Necrotizing and crescentic lupus nephritis with antineutrophil cytoplasmic antibody seropositivity," Clinical Journal of the American Society of Nephrology, vol. 3, no. 3, pp. 682–690, 2008.

[4] N. N. Masani, L. J. Imbriano, V. D. D'Agati, and G. S. Markowitz, "SLE and rapidly progressive glomerulonephritis," American Journal of Kidney Diseases, vol. 45, no. 5, pp. 950–955, 2005.

[5] S. Marshall, R. Dressier, and V. D'Agati, "Membranous lupus nephritis with antineutrophil cytoplasmic antibody-associated segmental necrotizing and crescentic glomerulonephritis," American Journal of Kidney Diseases, vol. 29, no. 1, pp. 119–124, 1997.

[6] R. Lekkham, E. Bloom, and R. Rasib, "Membranous lupus nephritis with ANCA-associated crescentic glomerulonephritis in non-specific interstitial pneumonia [NKF abstract 173]," American Journal of Kidney Diseases, vol. 61, no. 4, p. B59, 2013.

[7] A. Chang, O. Aneziokoro, S. M. Meehan, and R. J. Quigg, "Membranous and crescentic glomerulonephritis in a patient with anti-nuclear and anti-neutrophil cytoplasmic antibodies," Kidney International, vol. 71, no. 4, pp. 360–365, 2007.

[8] J. H. Stone, P. A. Merkel, R. Spiera et al., "Rituximab versus cyclophosphamide for ANCA-associated vasculitis," The New England Journal of Medicine, vol. 363, no. 3, pp. 221–232, 2010.

[9] R. B. Jones, J. W. C. Tervaert, T. Hauser et al., "Rituximab versus cyclophosphamide in ANCA-associated renal vasculitis," The New England Journal of Medicine, vol. 363, no. 3, pp. 211–220, 2010.

[10] L. Beck, A. S. Bomback, M. J. Choi et al., "KDOQI US commentary on the 2012 KDIGO clinical practice guideline for glomerulonephritis," American Journal of Kidney Diseases, vol. 62, no. 3, pp. 403–441, 2013.

[11] M. Walsh, F. Catapano, W. Szpirt et al., "Plasma exchange for renal vasculitis and idiopathic rapidly progressive glomerulonephritis: a meta-analysis," American Journal of Kidney Diseases, vol. 57, no. 4, pp. 566–574, 2011.

[12] D. R. W. Jayne, G. Gaskin, N. Rasmussen et al., "Randomized trial of plasma exchange or high-dosage methylprednisolone as adjunctive therapy for severe renal vasculitis," Journal of the American Society of Nephrology, vol. 18, no. 7, pp. 2180–2188, 2007.

[13] S. H. Nasr, S. M. Said, A. M. Valeri et al., "Membranous glomerulonephritis with ANCA-associated necrotizing and crescentic glomerulonephritis," Clinical Journal of the American Society of Nephrology, vol. 4, no. 2, pp. 299–308, 2009.

[14] U. Specks, P. A. Merkel, P. Seo et al., "Efficacy of remission-induction regimens for ANCA-associated vasculitis," The New England Journal of Medicine, vol. 369, no. 5, pp. 417–427, 2013.

[15] S. P. McAdoo and C. D. Pusey, "Should rituximab be used to prevent relapse in patients with ANCA-associated vasculitis?" Clinical Journal of the American Society of Nephrology, vol. 9, no. 4, pp. 641–644, 2014.

[16] H. Fatima, E. D. Siew, J. P. Dwyer, and P. Paueksakon, "Membranous glomerulopathy with superimposed pauci-immune necrotizing crescentic glomerulonephritis," Clinical Kidney Journal, vol. 5, no. 6, pp. 587–590, 2012.

[17] M. Shimada, T. Fujita, N. Nakamura et al., "A case of myeloperoxidase anti-neutrophil cytoplasmic antibody (MPO-ANCA)-associated glomerulonephritis and concurrent membranous nephropathy," BMC Nephrology, vol. 14, article 73, 2013.

[18] S. H. James, Y.-H. H. Lien, S. J. Ruffenach, and G. E. Wilcox, "Acute renal failure in membranous glomerulonephropathy: a

result of superimposed crescentic glomerulonephritis," *Journal of the American Society of Nephrology*, vol. 6, no. 6, pp. 1541–1546, 1995.

[19] J. T. C. Kwan, R. H. Moore, S. M. Dodd, and J. Cunningham, "Crescentic transformation in primary membranous glomerulonephritis," *Postgraduate Medical Journal*, vol. 67, no. 788, pp. 574–576, 1991.

[20] D. Sen and D. A. Isenberg, "Antineutrophil cytoplasmic autoantibodies in systemic lupus erythematosus," *Lupus*, vol. 12, no. 9, pp. 651–658, 2003.

[21] P. A. Merkel, R. P. Polisson, Y. Chang, S. J. Skates, and J. L. Niles, "Prevalence of antineutrophil cytoplasmic antibodies in a large inception cohort of patients with connective tissue disease," *Annals of Internal Medicine*, vol. 126, no. 11, pp. 866–873, 1997.

12

A Rare Cause of Reversible Renal Hemosiderosis

Rima Abou Arkoub,[1] Don Wang,[2] and Deborah Zimmerman[3]

[1]*Division of nephrology, The Ottawa Hospital, Ottawa, ON, Canada K1H 7W9*
[2]*Division of Anatomical Pathology, Department of Pathology and Laboratory Medicine, The Ottawa Hospital and
  Kidney Research Centre of the Ottawa Hospital Research Institute, University of Ottawa, Ottawa, ON, Canada K1H 7W9*
[3]*Division of Nephrology, The Ottawa Hospital and University of Ottawa, Ottawa, ON, Canada K1H 7W9*

Correspondence should be addressed to Deborah Zimmerman; dzimmerman@toh.on.ca

Academic Editor: Anja Haase-Fielitz

Kidney failure secondary to renal hemosiderosis has been reported in diseases with intravascular hemolysis, like paroxysmal nocturnal hemoglobinuria, and valvular heart diseases. We present here a case of hemosiderin induced acute tubular necrosis secondary to intravascular hemolysis from Clostridium difficile infection with possible role of supratherapeutic INR. We discuss the pathophysiology, causes, and prognosis of acute tubular injury from hemosiderosis.

1. Case Report Presentation

A 54-year-old Caucasian man presented to his infectious disease physician in October 2014 with fatigue, nausea, and anorexia for the last 5 days that had been preceded by several episodes of bloody diarrhea of 10 days' duration. He denied abdominal pain, diminished urine output, or macroscopic hematuria. His past medical history was significant for HIV infection for 10 years with the most recent CD4 count of 180; current treatment consisted of Atazanavir, Emtricitabine, Tenofovir, and Ritonavir. He also had a history of chronic hepatitis C infection. He had a previous history of injection drug use that had been complicated by 2 episodes of infective endocarditis requiring a mechanical mitral valve replacement in 1997. Since that time, he had been treated with warfarin anticoagulation, INR 2.5–3.5. He admitted taking additional doses of warfarin when he had migraine headaches as he thought this would improve blood flow. On physical examination, he was afebrile with a supine blood pressure (BP) of 109/65 mmHg but with postural drop to 95/55 mmHg. His JVP was flat with no evidence of lower extremity edema. He did not have a skin rash or detectable heart murmur. The remainder of his examination was otherwise unremarkable.

His laboratory data on admission are outlined in Table 1. His urinalysis was significant for 5–30 RBC/HPF and hyaline casts; no heme granular or red blood cell casts were seen. His urine albumin : creatinine ratio was 217 g/mol Cr. His creatinine which was 1.4 mg/dL in July 2014 had increased to 19.9 mg/dL. Abdominal ultrasonography showed normal-sized kidneys with slightly increased right renal parenchymal echogenicity.

After fluid resuscitation failed to improve his acute kidney injury (AKI), he underwent hemodialysis for metabolic acidosis. Other investigations included (1) anemia work-up for a declining hemoglobin [11.1 g/dL to 6.6 g/dL after fluid resuscitation without evidence of bleeding or falling platelet count (137 × 10^9/L)] included blood film review which showed polychromasia without schistocytes, LDH 153 (N: 100–205 units), haptoglobin < 0.08 (N: 0.3–2.0 units), total bilirubin of 43 (N: 3–17 units), direct bilirubin of 6 (N: 2–9 units), iron percent saturation 86 (N: 20–50), and ferritin 314 (N: 24–336), making TTP and HUS unlikely with the stable platelet count and absence of schistocytes on blood smear. Further investigations showed (1) a positive random urine for hemosiderin and (2) renal biopsy that showed severe acute tubular necrosis (ATN) caused by extensive renal hemosiderosis with extensive iron depositions in the tubules; the glomeruli were spared from deposition and damage (Figures 1 and 2). There was focal interstitial

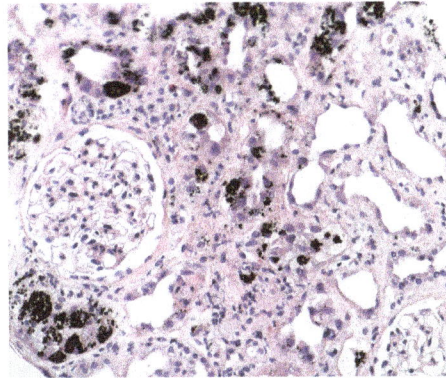

FIGURE 1: H&E stain showing extensive iron deposits in the tubules and glomerulus spared from deposition (H&E, ×300).

TABLE 1: Basic laboratory data on admission.

Creatinine	19.9	mg/dL
Urea	95.2	mg/dL
Potassium	3.7	mEq/L
Sodium	124	mEq/L
CO_2	10	mEq/L
Chloride	95	mEq/L
INR	5.9	
Hemoglobin	11.1	g/dL
WBC	7.8	$\times 10^9$/L
MCV	97	fL
Platelets	164	$\times 10^9$/L

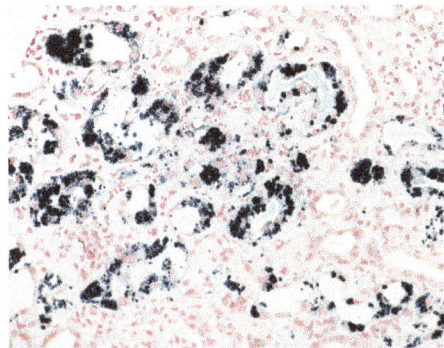

FIGURE 3: Prussian blue stain showing strong diffuse positivity in the tubules as coarse blue granules (Prussian blue, ×300).

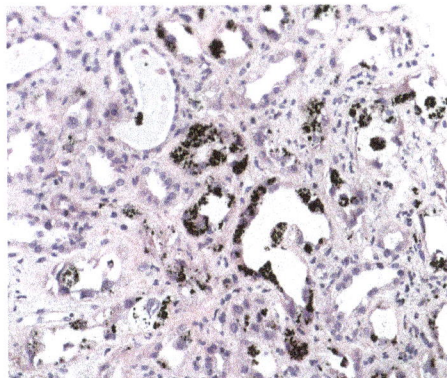

FIGURE 2: H&E stain showing severe acute tubular necrosis (ATN) caused by extensive iron depositions in the tubules (H&E, ×300).

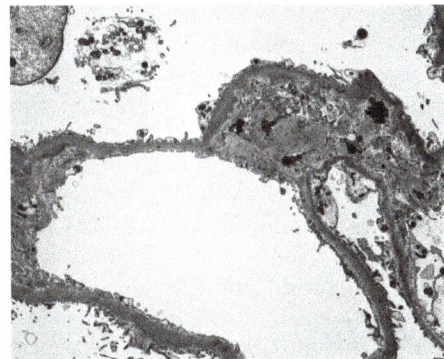

FIGURE 4: Electron microscopy shows segmental effacement of foot process with iron deposits (dark granules) (electron microscopy magnification ×8000).

chronic inflammation, mild interstitial fibrosis, mild tubular atrophy, and mild-to-moderate arterial atherosclerosis. Immunofluorescent staining: IgG: Negative, IgA: negative, IgM: equivocal, complement (C3): equivocal, C1q: negative, albumin: negative, and Kappa/Lambda: negative. Special stains for iron show strong diffuse positivity in the tubules (Figure 3). Electron microscopy showed segmental effacement of foot process with no evidence of electron dense deposits (Figure 4).

(3) Clostridium difficile toxin B was detected by PCR, (4) normal genetic testing for HFE (human hemochromatosis protein gene) mutation excluding hemochromatosis, negative flow cytometry for PNH (paroxysmal nocturnal hemoglobinuria), a normal glucose-6-phosphate dehydrogenase screen (excluding hemolysis secondary to G6PD deficiency anemia), and (5) transesophageal echocardiogram which showed that the prosthetic mitral valve is functioning well without evidence of paravalvular leak or mitral valve regurgitation

The patient stabilized in hospital with treatment of his AKI and Clostridium difficile infection. He remained on 3-times-per-week hemodialysis for ten weeks when his AKI recovered and his central venous catheter was removed.

2. Discussion

We report a case of acute hemolysis and nonoliguric AKI secondary to hemosiderin induced tubular necrosis. Upon hemolysis of red blood cells, hemoglobin alpha-beta dimers are released that, if unbound to haptoglobin, are filtered by the glomerulus and appear in the urine as hemoglobinuria. The hemoglobin dimers are taken up by renal proximal tubular cells and degraded and the free chelatable iron is stored as hemosiderin in the lysosomes [1, 2]. Under normal conditions, modest hemosiderin deposition is only mildly toxic to the kidney. However, with hemolysis in the presence of concentrated urine secondary to extracellular fluid volume depletion, hemosiderin can induce hemoglobinuria-associated acute renal failure [1]. Cytotoxic effects of large amounts of heme result from its lipophilic, oxidant, proinflammatory, and apoptotic effects.

Studies in an experimental model of heme protein-induced kidney injury show that mitochondria in particular are vulnerable to heme-mediated damage [3].

Hemosiderin deposition in kidney tubular cells has been reported in different types of hemolytic anemia including autoimmune hemolytic anemia and PNH [1, 4, 5] and sickle cell anemia [6, 7] and after cardiac valve replacement with residual valvular regurgitation or perivalvular leak [8]. In hemochromatosis, hemosiderin accumulation in tubular epithelial cells has also been reported [9]. ATN secondary to highly active antiretroviral therapy (HAART) including Tenofovir has been reported in HIV-infected patients. Moreover approximately 70% of the published cases of Tenofovir-induced nephrotoxic effects are observed with concomitant use of low-dose Ritonavir, the combination used by our patient [10]. However iron deposition in tubular cells causing ATN has not been reported with these medications making this an unlikely cause of this patient's renal failure.

All of these possibilities were considered in our differential diagnosis but all of them were subsequently excluded. Other potential etiologies included hemolysis secondary to Clostridium difficile infection or overanticoagulation with warfarin.

Several infections have also been associated with hemolysis and hemosiderin in the urine. Since 1990, 50 patients with Clostridium perfringens septicemia with hemolysis have been reported [11]; renal failure was reported in some but there was no mention of biopsy proven renal hemosiderosis. There are also case reports of hemolysis and severe jaundice in G-6-PD-deficient neonates with Clostridium difficile infection [12]. However, renal involvement and acute kidney injury did not appear to be part of the presentation in infants.

With respect to the potential role of warfarin and the supratherapeutic INR in our patient, Brodsky et al. examined renal biopsy specimens from 9 patients with AKI and an abnormal international normalized ratio (mean 4.4 + 0.7 IU). There was evidence of acute tubular injury and glomerular

hemorrhage: red blood cells in Bowman space with numerous occlusive RBC casts in the tubules, none with hemosiderin deposition [13]. However in one other case report, a kidney biopsy from a patient with IgA nephropathy, macroscopic hematuria, AKI, and INR of 6.2 IU showed extensive interstitial and intratubular red blood cell extravasation and interstitial hemosiderin deposits [14].

In summary, our patient appears to have developed AKI secondary to hemosiderin induced acute tubular necrosis perhaps from a combination of extracellular fluid volume depletion, elevated INR, and Clostridium difficile infection.

Conflict of Interests

The authors declare that there is no conflict of interests regarding the publication of this paper.

References

[1] K. Qi, X.-G. Zhang, S.-W. Liu, Z. Yin, X.-M. Chen, and D. Wu, "Reversible acute kidney injury caused by paroxysmal nocturnal hemoglobinuria," *American Journal of the Medical Sciences*, vol. 341, no. 1, pp. 68–70, 2011.

[2] H. Wang, K. Nishiya, H. Ito, T. Hosokawa, K. Hashimoto, and T. Moriki, "Iron deposition in renal biopsy specimens from patients with kidney diseases," *American Journal of Kidney Diseases*, vol. 38, no. 5, pp. 1038–1044, 2001.

[3] K. A. Nath, J. P. Grande, A. J. Croatt, S. Likely, R. P. Hebbel, and H. Enright, "Intracellular targets in heme protein-induced renal injury," *Kidney International*, vol. 53, no. 1, pp. 100–111, 1998.

[4] P. Leonardi and A. Ruol, "Renal hemosiderosis in the hemolytic anemias: diagnosis by means of needle biopsy," *Blood*, vol. 16, pp. 1029–1038, 1960.

[5] S. Hussain, A. Qureshi, and J. Kazi, "Renal involvement in paroxysmal nocturnal hemoglobinuria," *Nephron: Clinical Practice*, vol. 123, no. 1-2, pp. 28–35, 2013.

[6] A. Schein, C. Enriquez, T. D. Coates, and J. C. Wood, "Magnetic resonance detection of kidney iron deposition in sickle cell disease: a marker of chronic hemolysis," *Journal of Magnetic Resonance Imaging*, vol. 28, no. 3, pp. 698–704, 2008.

[7] L. M. Calazans, R. F. D. S. Santos, M. D. S. Gonçalves, W. L. C. Dos-Santos, and P. N. Rocha, "Renal hemosiderosis complicating sickle cell anemia," *Kidney International*, vol. 81, no. 7, p. 709, 2012.

[8] B. Concepcion, S. M. Korbet, and M. M. Schwartz, "Intravascular hemolysis and acute renal failure after mitral and aortic valve repair," *American Journal of Kidney Diseases*, vol. 52, no. 5, pp. 1010–1015, 2008.

[9] S. Ozkurt, M. F. Acikalin, G. Temiz, O. M. Akay, and M. Soydan, "Renal hemosiderosis and rapidly progressive glomerulonephritis associated with primary hemochromatosis," *Renal Failure*, vol. 36, no. 5, pp. 814–816, 2014.

[10] R. Kalyesubula and M. A. Perazella, "Nephrotoxicity of HAART," *AIDS Research and Treatment*, vol. 2011, Article ID 562790, 11 pages, 2011.

[11] T. G. Simon, J. Bradley, A. Jones, and G. Carino, "Massive intravascular hemolysis from clostridium perfringens septicemia: a review," *Journal of Intensive Care Medicine*, vol. 29, no. 6, pp. 327–333, 2014.

[12] A. Lodha, M. S. Kamaluddeen, E. Kelly, and H. Amin, "*Clostridium difficile* infection precipitating hemolysis in glucose-6-phosphate dehydrogenase-deficient preterm twins causing severe neonatal jaundice," *Journal of Perinatology*, vol. 28, no. 1, pp. 77–78, 2008.

[13] S. V. Brodsky, A. Satoskar, J. Chen et al., "Acute kidney injury during warfarin therapy associated with obstructive tubular red blood cell casts: a report of 9 cases," *American Journal of Kidney Diseases*, vol. 54, no. 6, pp. 1121–1126, 2009.

[14] C. M. Cleary, J. A. Moreno, B. Fernández et al., "Glomerular haematuria, renal interstitial haemorrhage and acute kidney injury," *Nephrology Dialysis Transplantation*, vol. 25, no. 12, pp. 4103–4106, 2010.

13

The Impact of Intensified Hemodialysis on Pruritus in an End Stage Renal Disease Patient with Biliary Ductopenia

Sandra Chomicki[1] and Omar Dahmani[2]

[1]Service de Néphrologie, Centre Hospitalier Louis Pasteur, 4 rue Claude Bernard, 28 630 Le Coudray, France
[2]Service de Néphrologie, Centre Hospitalier Louis Jaillon, 2 rue Hôpital, 39 206 Saint-Claude, France

Correspondence should be addressed to Sandra Chomicki; sandrachomicki@hotmail.com

Academic Editor: Władysław Sułowicz

We report a unique observation characterized by the coexistence of idiopathic adulthood ductopenia (IAD), a rare cholestatic disease, and end stage renal failure treated by conventional hemodialysis in a patient awaiting double renal and liver transplantation. As pruritus gradually worsened, we hypothesized that intensified dialysis could alleviate the symptoms. Conventional hemodialysis following 3 hours/3 times a week regimen was initiated in December 2013. Due to increasing pruritus not responding to standard medical therapy, intensified hemodialysis following 2.5 hours/5 times a week regimen was started in May 2014. During two weeks, a temporary decrease in bilirubin levels was observed. No major changes on other liver function tests and inflammatory markers occurred. Nevertheless, a persistent improvement on pruritus and general wellbeing was obtained during the four weeks' study period. The pathogenesis of itch encompasses multiple factors, and, in our case, both uremic and cholestatic pruritus are involved, although the latter is likely to account for a greater proportion. By improving itch intensity, through better clearance of uremic and cholestatic toxins which we detail further, intensive dialysis appears to be an acceptable short-term method for patients with hepatic cholestasis and moderate pruritus not responding to conventional therapy. Additional studies are needed to assess and differentiate precisely factors contributing to pruritus of both origins.

1. Introduction

Idiopathic adulthood ductopenia (IAD) is a rare cholestatic liver disease of unknown etiology first described by Ludwig et al. in 1988 [1]. To date, less than a hundred cases have been described in the literature. It is characterized by adult onset, biochemical evidence of cholestatic liver disease, negative antibodies, absence of bowel inflammatory disease, normal cholangiography, and loss of interlobular bile ducts on liver biopsy. The diagnosis requires exclusion of other conditions of chronic cholestasis. Interestingly, Li et al. [2] found an excellent correlation between the histologic classification and the clinical diagnosis. The course of the disease varies, severe IAD types typically progressing to end stage liver disease and requiring transplantation [3–5].

2. Case Presentation

We report the case of a 55-year-old patient presenting with a typical idiopathic adulthood ductopenia diagnosed earlier in the course of chronic renal failure requiring hemodialysis, awaiting double liver and renal transplantation. She was referred in 2008 to our clinic for impaired renal function and a biological cholestatic profile. Medical history included moderate hypertension and hysterectomy for fibroids causing metrorrhagia. There had been no family history of renal or liver disease and no personal history of recurrent urinary tract infection, medication treatments, illicit drug, or alcohol use. Physical examination showed moderate hypertension, mild jaundice, and mild pruritus. No clinical or biological signs of liver failure or encephalopathy were present. Laboratory tests revealed serum creatinine levels of 204 μmol/L, hemoglobin 13.1 g/dL, calcium 2.48 mmol/L, phosphorus 1.07 mmol/L, elevation of transaminases three times the upper limit (AST 156 UI/L and ALT 182 UI/L), gamma-glutamyl transferase (GGT) 1000 UI/L, and ALP 1029 UI/L. Bilirubin levels were normal. Thyroid-stimulating hormone levels, urinary electrolytes, iron studies, serum immunoglobulins, and protein electrophoresis were normal.

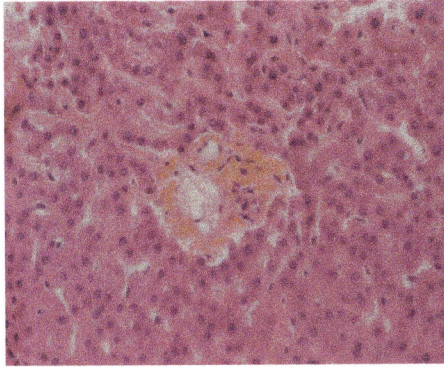

FIGURE 1: The liver biopsy specimen (H&E, ×200) shows branches of the hepatic artery and portal vein, but absence of interlobular bile duct. Lymphocyte infiltrate, cholangiolar proliferation, and fibrosis are absent.

Hepatitis and autoimmune antibodies were negative. Proteinuria was 0.24 g/24 h. Renal ultrasound showed bilateral small kidneys (7 and 8 cm) with no signs of obstruction; abdominal ultrasound showed a normal liver size (10.5 cm), smooth contours, and no signs of biliary dilation. Renal biopsy was not performed due to kidneys' small size and a chronic renal failure profile. The diagnosis of IAD was obtained on a second liver biopsy in 2012, showing loss of interlobular bile ducts, no lymphocyte inflammatory infiltrate, no fibrosis, and no cholangiolar proliferation (Figure 1). Biological follow-up showed development of secondary hyperparathyroidism (parathyroid hormone (PTH) 539 pg/mL, calcium 1.82 mmol/L, and phosphorus 2.35 mmol/L in December 2013), stabilisation of transaminase levels around three times the upper fold, a decrease of GGT levels (226 UI/L in December 2013), and a steady increase of bilirubin levels (total bilirubin 144 μmol/L, conjugated bilirubin 129 μmol/L in December 2013). Along with emollients, pruritus was treated first with cholestyramine and second with ursodeoxycholic acid; however neither showed a significant improvement. Conventional dialysis was started in December 2013, five years after the initial diagnosis of chronic renal failure. The patient was registered for double renal and liver transplantation shortly after. As the liver disease progressed, with jaundice and pruritus gradually worsening, we decided in May 2014 to perform intensified dialysis in order to assess whether this regimen could alleviate the symptoms.

Conventional hemodialysis following a 3 hours/3 times a week regimen was initiated in December 2013, switched on May 27, 2014, for intensified hemodialysis following 2.5 hours/5 times a week regimen. Both were performed as high-flux hemodialysis and did not differ in terms of ultrapure water quality, dialysis machine (5008, Fresenius Medical Care), heparin use, vascular access (jugular dialysis catheter), high-flux dialysis filter (FX 80), surface (1.8 m^2), blood flow (300 mL/min), and dialysate flow (500 mL/min). Mean Kt/V did not differ much ranging between 1.3 and 1.4. MARS and SPAD were not available at our centre and as for plasmapheresis, reports in these situations are anecdotal. At commencement of this regimen, no symptoms and signs of hepatic encephalopathy or liver failure were present with TP being 74% and serum albumin being 31.7 g/L.

Initially, during an approximate two-week period, a decrease in bilirubin levels was observed (conjugated bilirubin levels were 238 μmol/L on May 27, 186 μmol/L on June 7), however followed by a continuous increase later on (261 μmol/L on June 24). There were no major changes on other liver enzymes including ASP, ALT, GGT, and ALP and inflammatory markers including CRP and ferritin. PTH levels did not decrease after implementation of this regimen (560 pg/mL on July 8 versus 358 pg/mL in April 2014) and predialysis calcemia and phosphorus levels remained overall stable after intensified dialysis (resp., 1.92 mmol/L and 3.08 mmol/L on June 24 versus 1.94 mmol/L and 2.67 mmol/L on May 27). Taking a glance at the bilirubin curve, intensified dialysis did not change its increasing course (Figure 2). Nevertheless, a persistent improvement on pruritus was obtained over the four-week period we applied this regimen, with itch intensity being reduced by half. As this study was performed on one patient, a numeric assessment such as the visual analogue scale was not used as considered too subjective. Another weighty point in favor of this scheme is the pruritus rising on nondialysis days, thus showing a degree of effectiveness from hemodialysis on this symptom. Therefore we decided to continue this regimen until transplantation, as the improvement on pruritus and general wellbeing outweighed the inconvenience caused by daily travels.

3. Discussion

Pruritus is a common symptom in cholestatic disorders, occurring in about 30 to 70% patients with cholestatic liver disease according to available data. The pathogenesis of cholestatic pruritus is not clear. Some studies suggest that the accumulation of bile salts in the plasma and tissues of patients with cholestatic disease leads to pruritus, while some others propose that endogenous opioids play a key role in the development of pruritus [6, 7]. The latest studies have however focused on lysophosphatidic acid (LPA, monoacylglycerol-3-phosphate, <3 kDalton, and $t_{1/2}$ = a few minutes) a water soluble phospholipid that could possibly act as a neuronal activator. In recent studies by Kremer et al. [8, 9], LPA acted as a major Ca^{2+} agonist in pruritic sera and its concentration was increased in patients with cholestatic pruritus. The presence of autotaxin (ATX, >100 kDalton), the enzyme that converts lysophosphatidylcholine into LPA, was also increased in these patients. Its activity was associated with cholestatic pruritus and correlated with the intensity of pruritus, which was not the case for serum bile salts, histamine, tryptase, substance P, or μ opioids. Additionally, Rifampicin, MARS treatment, and nasobiliary drainage all markedly reduced ATX serum levels, whereas ATX protein was neither directly drained into bile nor removed in albumin dialysate (MARS membrane pores having a molecular weight cutoff of 50 kDalton). The authors hypothesized that a factor capable of increasing ATX expression (or reducing its clearance) was removed by these treatments. Moreover, Beuers et al. [10] suggested that some inflammatory cytokines could contribute to increasing ATX levels during cholestasis. In light of these recent results, we

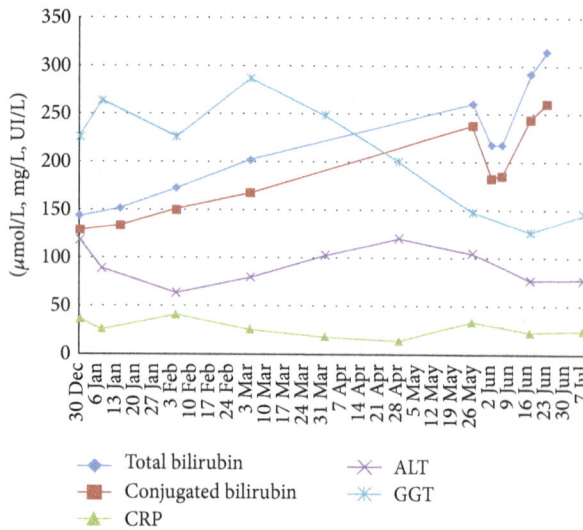

FIGURE 2: The graph shows a temporary drop in conjugated bilirubin levels after the initiation of intensified dialysis (May 27, 2014), followed by a consistent increase. No other changes of Liver Function Tests or CRP were observed.

could imagine that some small to medium molecular weight toxins responsible for pruritus could be partially removed by hemodialysis.

It would be very tempting to assume that the renal dysfunction in our patient was secondary to the liver condition. Recently, van Slambrouck et al. [11] carried out a remarkable study on bile cast nephropathy, a histologic entity observed in the spectrum of cholestatic pruritus. Following their results, a good correlation was observed between patients with hepatorenal syndrome and the presence of bile casts (85%) but poor in patients whose initial condition was cholestatic/obstructive jaundice (43%). Moreover, the presence of bile cast nephropathy is correlated with high bilirubin levels, while, on presentation, our patient's bilirubin levels were normal. Therefore, we cannot conclude here on a clear link between these two conditions.

Concerning intensified dialysis, this method has been the subject of growing interest for the past few years as conventional regimens (usually 4-hour sessions 3 times a week) did not offer optimal physiological replacement of renal function. Increasing dialysis time and/or allowing a more physiological renal replacement through daily sessions could offer better results. Intensified dialysis usually consists in short daily sessions, lasting 2 or 3 hours, or nocturnal 6- to 8-hour intermittent sessions 3 to 7 times a week. Intensified dialysis has shown in several previous studies improved outcomes on various measures, including arterial blood pressure, left ventricular hypertrophy, uremia associated variables, erythropoiesis parameters, and necessity of dietary restriction compared to conventional dialysis [12, 13]. A positive impact on inflammation has been suggested, as CRP tended to decline, although this has not been the case in our study.

We aimed to assess whether intensified hemodialysis could relieve cholestatic pruritus not responding to standard medical therapy. It is now generally accepted that liver dialysis

devices such as molecular adsorbents recirculation system (MARS) and single pass albumin dialysis (SPAD) are effective in the management of intractable cholestatic pruritus as they remove a number of toxins including ammonia, albumin-bound bilirubin, bile acids, and phenols. Their use is currently a new emerging indication for severe pruritus [14–16].

However, these devices are not available everywhere and paramedical staff is not always trained. Moreover, our patient expressed moderate pruritus and no signs of liver failure or encephalopathy were present.

From our experience, intensified dialysis appears to be an acceptable short-term method (in our case, until transplantation) for moderate pruritus in patients affected with end stage renal disease and hepatic cholestasis not responding to conventional therapy. The pathogenesis of pruritus involves multiple factors. In our observation, cholestatic pruritus is likely to account for a greater proportion than uremic pruritus, as itch slowly but constantly increased over months, which correlates well with the natural course of the liver disease. Moreover, little benefit was achieved on parameters such as phosphorus, PTH, and calcium, thus suggesting a less important influence of uremic pruritus on itch [17]. Unfortunately, we did not measure autotaxin activity, which could have been a potential marker to differentiate its origin. Our case report also supports the hypothesis that other molecules, for instance, inflammatory cytokines, could play a role in the generation of cholestatic pruritus [10], as improving their clearance through intensive dialysis decreases itch intensity.

In this regard, studies including hemodiafiltration methods could shed light on the benefits of improved clearance of medium and high molecular weight solutes compared to hemodialysis. In any case, further studies are needed to assess and differentiate precisely factors contributing to pruritus of both origins.

Conflict of Interests

The authors declare that there is no conflict of interests regarding this paper.

Acknowledgments

Special thanks go to (i) Dr. André Pruna, Dr. Catherine Albert, Dr. Catherine Godart, Dr. Virginie Chaigne, and Dr. Charlotte Jouzel, Service de Néphrologie, Centre Hospitalier Louis Pasteur, Le Coudray, France; (ii) Dr. Léandre Mackaya, Service de Néphrologie, Centre Hospitalier Louis Jaillon, Saint-Claude, France; (iii) Dr. Alexander Chen, Monash Health, Melbourne, Australia; (iv) Dr. Jean-Frédéric Bruch, Service d'Anatomopathologie, Centre Hospitalier Louis Pasteur, Le Coudray, France; (v) Dr. Antoine Brault, Service de Radiologie, Centre Hospitalier Régional d'Orléans, Orléans, France, for histopathological examination and expertise on idiopathic adulthood ductopenia.

References

[1] J. Ludwig, R. H. Wiesner, and N. F. LaRusso, "Idiopathic adulthood ductopenia: a cause of chronic cholestatic liver

disease and biliary cirrhosis," *Journal of Hepatology*, vol. 7, no. 2, pp. 193–199, 1988.

[2] Y. Li, G. Ayata, S. P. Baker, and B. F. Banner, "Cholangitis: a histologic classification based on patterns of injury in liver biopsies," *Pathology Research and Practice*, vol. 201, no. 8-9, pp. 565–572, 2005.

[3] J. Ludwig, "Idiopathic adulthood ductopenia: an update," *Mayo Clinic Proceedings*, vol. 73, no. 3, pp. 285–291, 1998.

[4] B. C. Park, S. M. Park, E. Y. Choi et al., "A case of idiopathic adulthood ductopenia," *Korean Journal of Internal Medicine*, vol. 24, no. 3, pp. 270–273, 2009.

[5] A. Kaung, V. Sundaram, D. Dhall, and T. T. Tran, "A case of mild idiopathic adulthood ductopenia and brief review of literature," *Gastroenterology Report*, 2014.

[6] C. Levy, "Management of pruritus in patients with cholestatic liver disease," *Gastroenterology and Hepatology*, vol. 7, no. 9, pp. 615–617, 2011.

[7] R. P. Oude Elferink, A. E. Kremer, and U. Beuers, "Mediators of pruritus during cholestasis," *Current Opinion in Gastroenterology*, vol. 27, no. 3, pp. 289–293, 2011.

[8] A. E. Kremer, J. J. W. W. Martens, W. Kulik et al., "Lysophosphatidic acid is a potential mediator of cholestatic pruritus," *Gastroenterology*, vol. 139, no. 3, pp. 1008–1018, 2010.

[9] A. E. Kremer, R. van Dijk, P. Leckie et al., "Serum autotaxin is increased in pruritus of cholestasis, but not of other origin, and responds to therapeutic interventions," *Hepatology*, vol. 56, no. 4, pp. 1391–1400, 2012.

[10] U. Beuers, A. E. Kremer, R. Bolier, and R. P. J. O. Elferink, "Pruritus in cholestasis: facts and fiction," *Hepatology*, vol. 60, pp. 399–407, 2014.

[11] C. M. van Slambrouck, F. Salem, S. M. Meehan, and A. Chang, "Bile cast nephropathy is a common pathologic finding for kidney injury associated with severe liver dysfunction," *Kidney International*, vol. 84, no. 1, pp. 192–197, 2013.

[12] S. P. Curran and C. T. Chan, "Intensive hemodialysis: normalizing the 'Unphysiology' of conventional hemodialysis?" *Seminars in Dialysis*, vol. 24, no. 6, pp. 607–613, 2011.

[13] J. Thumfart, W. Pommer, U. Querfeld, and D. Müller, "Intensified hemodialysis in adults, and in children and adolescents," *Deutsches Arzteblatt International*, vol. 111, no. 14, pp. 237–243, 2014.

[14] S. Sen, R. Williams, and R. Jalan, "Emerging indications for albumin dialysis," *The American Journal of Gastroenterology*, vol. 100, no. 2, pp. 468–475, 2005.

[15] I. M. Sauer, M. Goetz, I. Steffen et al., "In vitro comparison of the molecular adsorbent recirculation system (MARS) and single-pass albumin dialysis (SPAD)," *Hepatology*, vol. 39, no. 5, pp. 1408–1414, 2004.

[16] P. Leckie, G. Tritto, R. Mookerjee, N. Davies, D. Jones, and R. Jalan, "'Out-patient' albumin dialysis for cholestatic patients with intractable pruritus," *Alimentary Pharmacology and Therapeutics*, vol. 35, no. 6, pp. 696–704, 2012.

[17] I. Narita, B. Alchi, K. Omori et al., "Etiology and prognostic significance of severe uremic pruritus in chronic hemodialysis patients," *Kidney International*, vol. 69, no. 9, pp. 1626–1632, 2006.

14

Membranoproliferative Glomerulonephritis in Patients with Chronic Venous Catheters: A Case Report and Literature Review

John Sy,[1] Cynthia C. Nast,[2] Phuong-Thu T. Pham,[3] and Phuong-Chi T. Pham[1]

[1] Division of Nephrology and Hypertension, Department of Internal Medicine, UCLA-Olive View Medical Center,
14445 Olive View Drive, 2B-182, Sylmar, CA 91342, USA
[2] Cedars Sinai Medical Center, Department of Pathology, Los Angeles, CA 90048, USA
[3] David Geffen School of Medicine at UCLA, Kidney and Pancreas Transplant Program, Los Angeles, CA 90095, USA

Correspondence should be addressed to Phuong-Chi T. Pham; pctp@ucla.edu

Academic Editors: Y. Fujigaki, K. Hirayama, A. K. Saxena, and W. Sułowicz

Chronic indwelling catheters have been reported to be associated with membranoproliferative glomerulonephritis (MPGN) *via* the activation of the classical complement pathway in association with bacterial infections such as coagulase negative staphylococcus. We herein provide supporting evidence for the direct causal relationship between chronic catheter infections and MPGN *via* a case of recurrent MPGN associated with recurrent catheter infections used for total parenteral nutrition (TPN) in a man with short gut syndrome. We also present a literature review of similar cases and identify common clinical manifestations that may serve to aid clinicians in the early identification of MPGN associated with infected central venous catheterization or *vice versa*. The importance of routine monitoring of kidney function and urinalysis among patients with chronic central venous catheterization is highlighted as kidney injury may *herald* or coincide with overtly infected chronic indwelling central venous catheters.

1. Introduction

Membranoproliferative glomerulonephritis (MPGN) is a pattern of disease characterized by the deposition of immunoglobulins, complement factors, or both along capillary walls and within the glomerular mesangium. The classic finding of lobular accentuation of glomerular tufts on light microscopy is attributed to mesangial hypercellularity, endocapillary proliferation, and capillary wall remodeling resulting in the formation of "double contours." Depositions of the third component of complement (C3) with or without immunoglobulins may be observed on immunofluorescent studies [1]. The underlying etiologies of MPGN comprise a spectrum of conditions including infection, monoclonal gammopathy, autoimmune or rheumatologic disease, and dysregulation of the alternative complement pathway. It is well known that chronic infection from indwelling ventriculosystemic shunts can cause "shunt nephritis", an entity first reported in 1965 by Black et al. after the placement of a ventriculoatrial shunt

for the relief of hydrocephalus in two pediatric patients [2, 3]. Further experiments in animal studies have similarly shown a relation between chronic infections associated with indwelling catheters and MPGN [4, 5]. Although uncommon, there have been few reports of MPGN associated with central venous catheters placed for total parenteral nutrition (TPN) [6]. We herein report a case of recurrent MPGN in association with recurrent coagulase negative *Staphylococcus epidermidis* Hickman catheter infection, and review the literature for common clinical presentations of MPGN in patients requiring chronic central venous catheter placement.

2. Case Report

2.1. Clinical History and Initial Laboratory Data. A 23-year-old male with prior multiple gunshot wounds to the abdomen requiring complete small bowel resection and chronic TPN support *via* a Hickman catheter since the age of 17 presented with anasarca and low grade fevers in June 1996. Basic urine

(a)

(b)

(c)

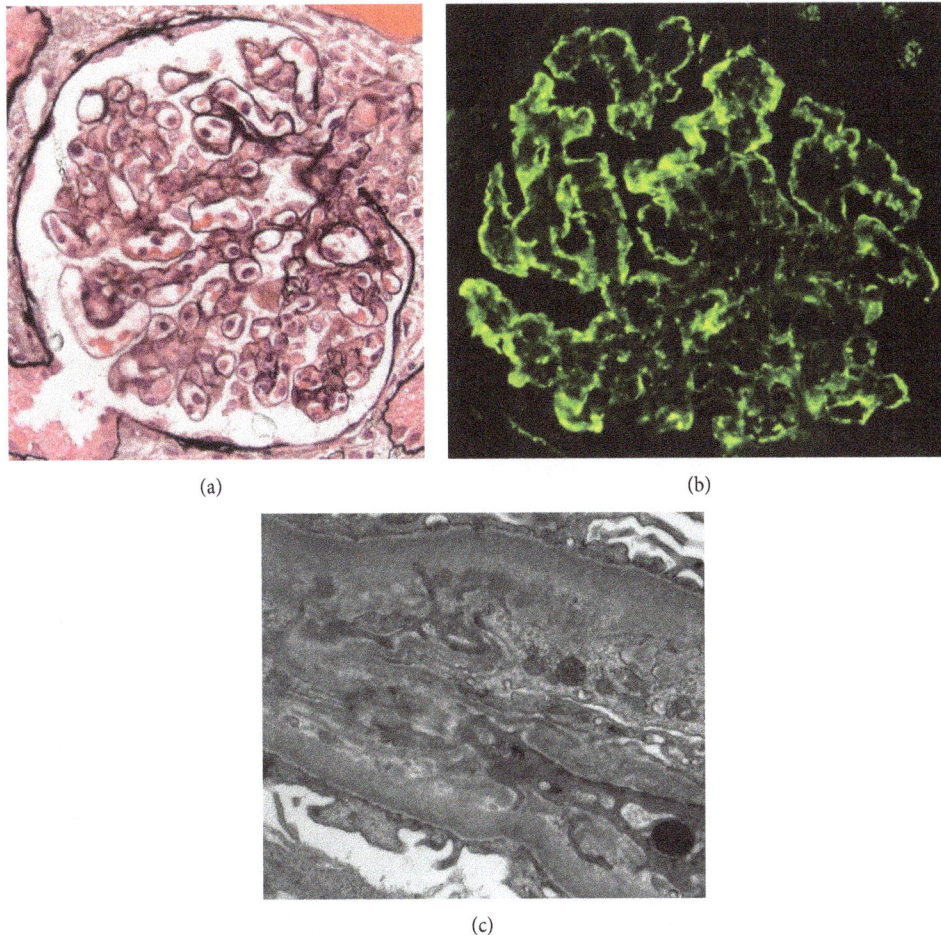

FIGURE 1: Glomerular renal biopsy findings. (a) Mesangial and endocapillary hypercellularity with a lobular pattern and segmental capillary double contours (periodic acid methenamine silver ×400). (b) Peripheral granular staining for C3 (×400). (c) Capillary wall subendothelial electron dense deposits with peripheral mesangial migration and new subendothelial basement membrane material forming a double contour (×19,000).

evaluations revealed 2+ blood without evidence of casts and 2.0 g proteinuria from a 24-hour collection. A serum chemistry panel revealed creatinine of 1.9 mg/dL (estimated glomerular filtration rate of 50 mL/min/1.73 m²), blood urea nitrogen (BUN) of 37 mg/dL, and albumin of 2 gm/dL. His baseline creatinine levels were unknown. Routine serology evaluation including human immunodeficiency virus (HIV), rapid plasma reagin (RPR), antinuclear antibody (ANA), and hepatitis B and C screen were all negative. Complement studies revealed C3 of 68 mg/dL (reference range, 90–180 mg/dL), fourth component of complement (C4) of 19 mg/dL (reference range 16–47 mg/dL), and total complement levels (CH50) of <28 mg/dL (reference range 60–90 mg/dL). Echocardiogram showed no vegetations. Blood cultures were positive for coagulase negative *staphylococcus*. Kidney ultrasound revealed right kidney measuring 10.6 cm and left kidney measuring 10.8 cm without structural abnormalities or evidence of obstruction. A kidney biopsy was performed.

2.2. Kidney Biopsy (June 1996).

Light microscopy revealed 15 glomeruli showing a lobular pattern with mesangial hypercellularity, a moderate number of capillary wall double contours,

and leukocytes within capillary lumina. Three glomeruli had segmental crescents. There were interstitial inflammation and edema, associated with acute tubular cell injury. Immunofluorescence microscopy disclosed five glomeruli staining for IgM (3+), C3 (3+), and kappa (trace to 1+) and lambda (trace) light chains along capillary walls in a granular pattern and peripheral distribution. Mesangial regions were stained for IgM (1 to 2+), C1q (trace), C3 (1+), and kappa (trace) and lambda (trace) light chains in a granular pattern. Electron microscopy of three glomeruli revealed small subendothelial and few mesangial electron dense deposits. There were no tubuloreticular structures in the cytoplasm of any cells (Figure 1).

Diagnoses of membranoproliferative glomerulonephritis type I and acute tubulointerstitial nephritis were rendered.

2.3. Clinical Follow-Up.

The patient received vancomycin and underwent Hickman catheter replacement with subsequent rapid and complete resolution of his acute kidney injury (serum creatinine improved to 1.3 mg/dL), proteinuria, and anasarca. Due to the temporal association of treatment and

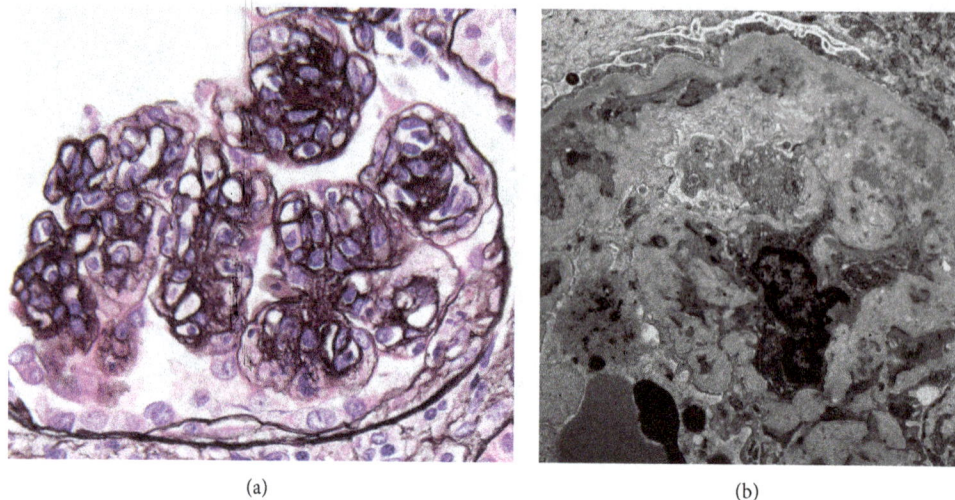

(a)   (b)

FIGURE 2: Glomerular features of second renal biopsy. (a) Lobular hypercellular glomerulus with capillary wall double contours (periodic acid methenamine silver ×600). (b) Capillary wall with subendothelial deposits and peripheral mesangial migration and interposition producing a double contour (×7200).

renal disease resolution, the MPGN was presumed to be secondary to *staphylococcal* bacteremia.

He was lost to follow-up for several years until February 2010 when he presented with upper extremity edema and chills. On admission he had anemia, reduced kidney function, and hypoalbuminemia. Again, he was found to be infected with coagulase negative staphylococcus bacteremia (*S. epidermidis*). His spot urine protein to creatinine ratio at presentation was 2.4 g/g creatinine but increased to 5.8 g/g over several days without associated blood pressure changes. Routine laboratory investigations revealed creatinine of 2.2 mg/dL, BUN 19 mg/dL, WBC 4,400/mm^3, and hemoglobin 5.9 g/dL. Urinalysis revealed 300 mg/dL protein, large blood, large leukocyte esterase, 196 WBC/high power field (HPF), 224 RBC/HPF, 33 hyaline casts, few WBC clumps, 14 granular casts, and 24 cellular casts. He was treated with vancomycin pending repeat evaluation of the underlying nephrotic syndrome. Of interest, the patient commented that "every time I swell up, they give me antibiotics and the swelling goes away." Further evaluation of his renal disease was again pursued as all his previous medical records were lost in a hospital fire. Serum protein electrophoresis (SPEP), urine protein electrophoresis (UPEP), serum protein immunofixation (SPIF), urine protein immunofixation (UPIF), antineutrophil cytoplasmic antibody (ANCA), RPR, ANA, and HIV were all negative. C3 was low at 71 mg/dL with normal C4 of 23 mg/dL. A kidney ultrasound revealed normal sized kidneys (right 11.0 cm and left 11.7 cm) without structural abnormalities. Evaluation for subacute bacterial endocarditis was negative. His Hickman catheter was replaced and subsequent blood cultures confirmed resolution of his bacteremia. His proteinuria improved markedly (greater than 50% reduction) within a few days of antibiotic therapy initiation. Serial creatinine measurements documented improvement in his creatinine to 1.75 mg/dL within 20 days of presentation. A repeat kidney biopsy performed in June 2010 confirmed MPGN type I (Figure 2), with acute tubulointerstitial nephritis and mild-to-moderate chronic renal parenchymal injury.

In July 2010, he presented for the third time with anasarca, fevers, and acute kidney injury (creatinine of 3.29 mg/dL, elevated from baseline level 1.7–2.0 mg/dL). Initial urinalysis showed 100 mg/dL protein, large blood, 215 WBC/HPF, 252 RBC/HPF, and 42 hyaline casts. Complement levels revealed C3 of 45 mg/dL, C4 of 18 mg/dL, and CH50 < 13 mg/dL. Blood cultures revealed coagulase negative staphylococcus bacteremia (*S. epidermidis*) and spot urine protein-creatinine ratios rapidly rose from 5.1 g/g to a peak of 9.5 g/g within 2 days without accompanying blood pressure changes. Treatment with vancomycin and Hickman line replacement led to rapid reduction in proteinuria and anasarca with creatinine improving to his recent baseline of 1.7 mg/dL by October 2010. As the two previous kidney biopsies demonstrated MPGN type I, this third episode of acute kidney injury accompanied by hematuria and nephrotic range proteinuria was attributed to a recurrence of MPGN secondary to recurrent Hickman catheter infection.

3. Discussion

The pathophysiology of MPGN caused by chronic indwelling central catheters has been previously described [4, 6, 8]. The production of immunoglobulins against an infectious agent and the subsequent binding of two or more of these immunoglobulins result in activation of C1, which then cleaves C4 and C2 to generate C4b and C2a to form C4b2a, the classical pathway convertase, leading to the activation of C3 convertase and generation of the terminal complement complex. Glomerular involvement is instigated by deposition of immune-complexes and complement factors of the classical and terminal pathway in the subendothelial region of capillary walls [6]. The injury phase of MPGN is characterized by the influx of leukocytes with associated cytokine and protease release, inducing capillary wall damage and ensuing

TABLE 1: Clinical manifestations of reported cases and current case.

References	Medical history	Initial presentation	Baseline creatinine (mg/dL.)	Presenting creatinine (mg/dL.)	Urinalysis	Complements (mg/dL.)	Renal Biopsy	Blood cultures	Number of catheter changes
Yared et al. [7]	66-year-old male with mesenteric ischemia and bowel resection with parenteral nutrition for hyperalimentation	Worsening kidney function and new skin rash	1.5	3.2	>25 RBC/HPF, proteinuria, 4–10 granular casts	"Normal" complements (values not reported)	MPGN	S. epidermidis and C. jeikeium	6
Yared et al. [7]	45-year-old female TAH/BSO complicated by ischemic bowel requiring resection, required parenteral nutrition for hyperalimentation	Worsening kidney function, new skin rash, and severe anemia	1.8	7.7	Proteinuria and hematuria with RBC and mixed-cell casts	Initially normal complements, then C3 and C4 levels slightly depressed	MPGN	Unknown	5
Ohara et al. [6]	13-year-old male midgut volvulus and resection of necrotic ileum, required parenteral nutrition for hyperalimentation	Hematuria and proteinuria on routine urinary screening	Unknown	0.6	Many RBCs, 10–15 WBC, 1–2 granular casts/HPF	C3 30 (low), C4 8 (low), CH50 <10 (low)	MPGN	S. epidermidis	7
Current case report	23-year-old male multiple gunshot wounds to abdomen at age 17, required parenteral nutrition for hyperalimentation	First episode July 1996: proteinuria, hematuria, and renal insufficiency on routine testing	Unknown	1.9	2+ blood, >100 RBC, no cellular casts	C3 69 (low), C4 19 (low-normal), CH50 < 28 (low)	MPGN	S. epidermidis	Unknown
		Second episode February 2010 at age 37: fevers, anasarca, and renal insufficiency	1.3–1.5	2.2	Protein 300 mg/dL, large blood, WBC 196, RBC 224, +hyaline, granular, and cellular casts/HPF	C3 71 (low), C4 23 (low-normal), CH50 < 13 (low)	MPGN (biopsy done June 2010)	S. epidermidis	>2
		Third episode July 2010: anasarca and fatigue	1.7–2.0	3.3	Protein 100 mg/dL, large blood, WBC 215, RBC 252, 42 hyaline casts/HPF	C3 45 (low), C4 18 (low-normal), CH50 < 13 (low)	No biopsy*	S. epidermidis	>2

Abbreviations: TAH/BSO: total abdominal hysterectomy and bilateral salpingooopherectomies; S. epidermidis: Staphylococcus epidermidis; C. jeikeium: Clostridium jeikeium; RBC: red blood cells; WBC: white blood cells; HPF: high power field.
* Presumptive diagnosis of recurrent MPGN based on previous biopsy findings, clinical course, and response to appropriate therapy.

hematuria and proteinuria. In addition to *Staphylococcus*, other bacteria reported in association with MPGN include *Mycobacterium tuberculosis, streptococci, Propionibacterium acnes, Mycoplasma pneumoniae, brucella, Coxiella burnetii, nocardia,* and *Meningococcus* [8].

A literature search for biopsy proven MPGN associated with chronic central venous catheterization revealed only three cases [6, 7]. In these three reported cases, the central venous catheter was used for home parenteral nutrition for short bowel syndrome (Table 1). Of note, all patients had multiple (five to seven) episodes of infectious catheter complications prior to overt renal manifestations. Specific renal presentations ranged from incidental finding of microscopic hematuria, mild proteinuria (0.3 g/g creatinine), and granular casts in one patient to an insidious or relatively rapid rise in serum creatinine over 18 days to 2 months in the two other patients. Patients with increasing serum creatinine had concurrent significant proteinuria and an active urinary sediment including microscopic hematuria with or without cellular casts. Associated extrarenal clinical manifestations reported include edema/anasarca, fevers, and/or palpable purpura due to biopsy proven leukocytoclastic vasculitis. Complement levels varied from normal to significantly depressed. Blood and catheter tip cultures obtained in three out of four cases revealed *Staphylococcus epidermidis*. Following catheter replacement and appropriate antibiotic administration, all patients promptly and markedly improved in renal function, proteinuria, and/or hematuria. Of interest, signs of recovery such as reduction in proteinuria may be noted within a few days and fall in serum creatinine within 1-2 weeks of antibiotic therapy and catheter removal (8, present case). Complete recovery of renal function may occur within three to 10 months. Unfortunately, in our current case, only partial renal functional recovery and reduction in proteinuria were observed following the third documented episode of infection with glomerulonephritis. This likely was due to significant renal parenchymal scarring consequent to inadequate treatment of prior infectious insults in association with poor patient compliance and follow-up.

Recurrent biopsy proven MPGN in parallel with recurrent line infection/bacteremia, as observed in the current case, leaves little doubt regarding a direct causal relationship between chronic central line infections and MPGN. Subtle renal manifestations such as microscopic hematuria and slow rise in serum creatinine may herald overtly apparent manifestations of catheter infections; therefore, routine urinalysis and close monitoring of serum creatinine in patients with chronic central venous catheterization are indicated to allow early detection of catheter infection and prevention of progressive kidney injury. It should be noted that animal studies involving sheep and baboons have shown that renal parenchymal injury may occur even prior to overt renal manifestations [4, 5]. Nevertheless, some extent of disease reversal is expected with prompt intervention, including appropriate antimicrobial therapy and removal or replacement of the indwelling catheter, as reported [6, 7].

In summary, we have presented a case of recurrent MPGN associated with recurrent bacteremia from a chronically indwelling Hickman catheter in an adult. Given the repeated strong temporal correlations of MPGN with recurrent catheter infections, the latter is likely the key factor in the development of MPGN in this setting. In a patient with an infected catheter and concurrent evidence of kidney injury, with or without a prior biopsy-proven MPGN, short time allowance for antibiotic treatment and catheter replacement may be indicated prior to renal biopsy performance, particularly when the only abnormal serologic finding is a low C3 level. However, it should be emphasized that a kidney biopsy should be considered if renal function and/or proteinuria do not resolve within 2–4 weeks, or if serologic testing suggests the possibility of another disease entity.

In conclusion, patients with chronic indwelling central venous catheters should be given routine surveillance for both infections and markers of kidney injury including serum creatinine and urinalysis. Similarly, patients should be educated to recognize early signs and symptoms of infections as well as development of unusual urinary foaming and/or change in urine output and color.

Conflict of Interests

The authors declare that there is no conflict of interests regarding the publication of this paper.

References

[1] H. G. Rennke, "Secondary membranoproliferative glomerulonephritis," *Kidney International*, vol. 47, no. 2, pp. 643–656, 1995.

[2] E. Noiri, S. Kuwata, K. Nosaka et al., "Shunt nephritis: efficacy of an antibiotic trial for clinical diagnosis," *Internal Medicine*, vol. 32, no. 4, pp. 291–294, 1993.

[3] J. A. Black, D. N. Challacombe, and B. G. Ockenden, "Nephrotic syndrome associated with bacteraemia after shunt operations for hydrocephalus," *The Lancet*, vol. 286, no. 7419, pp. 921–924, 1965.

[4] V. P. Rao, T. Poutahidis, R. P. Marini, H. Holcombe, A. B. Rogers, and J. G. Fox, "Renal infarction and immune-mediated glomerulonephritis in sheep (*Ovis aries*) chronically implanted with indwelling catheters," *Journal of the American Association for Laboratory Animal Science*, vol. 45, no. 4, pp. 14–19, 2006.

[5] S. L. Leary, W. D. Sheffield, and J. D. Strandberg, "Immune complex glomerulonephritis in baboons (*Papio cynocephalus*) with indwelling intravascular catheters," *Laboratory Animal Science*, vol. 31, no. 4, pp. 416–420, 1981.

[6] S. Ohara, Y. Kawasaki, K. Takano et al., "Glomerulonephritis associated with chronic infection from long-term central venous catheterization," *Pediatric Nephrology*, vol. 21, no. 3, pp. 427–429, 2006.

[7] G. Yared, D. L. Seidner, E. Steiger, P. M. Hall, and J. V. Nally, "Tunneled right atrial catheter infection presenting as renal failure," *Journal of Parenteral and Enteral Nutrition*, vol. 23, no. 6, pp. 363–365, 1999.

[8] S. Sethi and F. C. Fervenza, "Membranoproliferative glomerulonephritis—a new look at an old entity," *The New England Journal of Medicine*, vol. 366, no. 12, pp. 1119–1131, 2012.

15

Hyperchloremic Metabolic Acidosis due to Cholestyramine: A Case Report and Literature Review

Fareed B. Kamar[1] **and Rory F. McQuillan**[2]

[1]*University of Calgary, Suite G15, 1403-29 Street NW, Calgary, AB, Canada T2N 2T9*
[2]*University of Toronto and University Health Network, Toronto General Hospital, Room 8N-842, 200 Elizabeth Street, Toronto, ON, Canada M5G 2C4*

Correspondence should be addressed to Fareed B. Kamar; fbkamar@ucalgary.ca

Academic Editor: Yoshihide Fujigaki

Cholestyramine is a bile acid sequestrant that has been used in the treatment of hypercholesterolemia, pruritus due to elevated bile acid levels, and diarrhea due to bile acid malabsorption. This medication can rarely cause hyperchloremic nonanion gap metabolic acidosis, a complication featured in this report of an adult male with concomitant acute kidney injury. This case emphasizes the caution that must be taken in prescribing cholestyramine to patients who may also be volume depleted, in renal failure, or taking spironolactone.

1. Introduction

The orally administered medication cholestyramine is a nonabsorbable anion exchange resin that serves as a bile acid sequestrant. It has been used in the treatment of hypercholesterolemia, pruritus due to biliary obstruction and elevated bile acid levels, and diarrhea due to bile acid malabsorption in the setting of ileal disease or resection [1]. Adverse effects are uncommon, though typical gastrointestinal reactions include constipation, nausea, and flatulence [1]. A handful of reports have described the rare complication of metabolic acidosis [1–11]. The following case adds to this literature in describing the occurrence of hyperchloremic nonanion gap metabolic acidosis in a 45-year-old male liver transplant patient on cholestyramine for pruritus who developed acute kidney injury.

2. Case Presentation

A 45-year-old Caucasian man was admitted to hospital for an elective biliary drain insertion for his recurrent bile duct stricture since a liver transplant seven years earlier. Because of the chronic cholestasis, he had been taking cholestyramine 4 g PO TID for his pruritus.

Days after the biliary drain insertion, the patient developed acute kidney injury (creatinine of 261 μmol/L), in the setting of an *Enterococcus faecium* bacteremia. At this time, the serum pH was 7.09 and serum electrolytes were as follows: sodium 140 mmol/L, potassium 3.9 mmol/L, chloride 118 mmol/L, and bicarbonate 12 mmol/L (anion gap 10 mmol/L). The urine pH was 5.5 and the urinalysis was positive for bilirubin, proteinuria (1.0 g/L), and heme-granular casts. The urine electrolytes were as follows: sodium 48 mmol/L, potassium 30 mmol/L, and chloride 57 mmol/L (urine anion gap 21 mmol/L). No phosphaturia or glycosuria was noted.

Having discontinued the cholestyramine, he was given intravenous sodium bicarbonate, and his hyperchloremic metabolic acidosis resolved.

3. Discussion

Cholestyramine is a resin that exchanges anions once orally administered by way of its ammonium groups. It swaps chloride anions for bile acids in the lumen of the small intestine, resulting in bile acid complexes that are excreted fecally instead of being reabsorbed in the ileum [10, 12].

TABLE 1: Summary of the literature describing cholestyramine-induced hyperchloremic metabolic acidosis.

Age	Sex (male (M), female (F))	Serum pH	Chloride (mmol/L)	Bicarbonate (mmol/L)	Precipitating factors	Case reference
1.5 days	M	7.15	125	9	Diarrhea	[6]
4 weeks	F	—	128	19	Diarrhea	[9]
5 weeks	M	6.83	130	5.4	Volume depletion, renal failure	[8]
13 weeks	M	7.28	145	15	Upper respiratory tract infection, diarrhea	[9]
6 months	M	6.88	112	—	Upper respiratory tract infection	[2]
10.5 years	F	7.18	114	9	Renal failure	[7]
45 years	M	7.09	118	12	Bacteremia, renal failure	Case presentation
45 years	M	7.12	127	8	Renal failure	[5]
51 years	F	—	115	8	Spironolactone	[10]
57 years	M	—	122	11	Diarrhea	[10]
70 years	F	7.15	128	5	Upper respiratory tract infection, renal failure, and spironolactone	[1]
70 years	F	7.34	119	14	Spironolactone	[4]

This exchange causes gastrointestinal secretion of bicarbonate and absorption of chloride, mediated by the duodenal brush border's apical chloride/bicarbonate antiporter [13]. The effect of this resin on chloride and bicarbonate in the gastrointestinal tract alone does not, however, lead to hyperchloremic metabolic acidosis, since the kidneys can compensate by increasing chloride excretion and bicarbonate retention. These compensatory mechanisms are impeded in states of impaired urinary acidification such as renal insufficiency and aldosterone antagonism [10, 14], which unmask cholestyramine-induced hyperchloremia and bicarbonate loss. In this report, the patient's impaired urinary acidification, as evidenced by a positive urine anion gap, was the result of renal insufficiency.

Other reported cases of cholestyramine-induced hyperchloremic metabolic acidosis have occurred in children with renal impairment [7, 8] and volume depletion (a probable cause of renal impairment) in the setting of infection [2, 9] and diarrhea ([6, 9], see Table 1). Adult cases of metabolic acidosis in the context of cholestyramine use have also been described in the setting of renal insufficiency [1, 5, 10] and spironolactone use ([1, 4, 10, 11], see Table 1).

This case and literature review highlight the complication of hyperchloremic metabolic acidosis that may occur with cholestyramine use in adult and pediatric patients. Patients taking this medication should have their electrolytes monitored, particularly in the setting a precipitating factor such as renal failure, volume depletion, and spironolactone use. If this complication occurs along with no other identified causes, then cholestyramine should be stopped, precipitants should be addressed, and sodium bicarbonate could be administered.

Conflict of Interests

The authors declare that there is no conflict of interests regarding the publication of this paper.

References

[1] E. R. Eaves and M. G. Korman, "Cholestyramine induced hyperchloremic metabolic acidosis," *Australian and New Zealand Journal of Medicine*, vol. 14, no. 5, pp. 670–672, 1984.

[2] B. Bernsten and S. Zoger, "Hyperchloremic metabolic acidosis with cholestyramine therapy for biliary cholestasis," *The American Journal of Diseases of Children*, vol. 132, no. 12, p. 1220, 1978.

[3] H. J. Blom and E. Monasch, "Metabolic acidosis in a patient with kidney dysfunction following administration of cholestyramine," *Nederlands Tijdschrift voor Geneeskunde*, vol. 127, no. 32, pp. 1446–1447, 1983.

[4] W. M. Clouston and H. M. Lloyd, "Cholestyramine induced hyperchloremic metabolic acidosis," *Australian and New Zealand Journal of Medicine*, vol. 15, no. 2, article 271, 1985.

[5] F. S. Y. Fan, K. M. Chow, C. C. Szeto, and P. K. T. Li, "Hyperchloraemic metabolic acidosis," *Emergency Medicine Journal*, vol. 25, no. 9, article 613, 2008.

[6] J. V. Hartline, "Hyperchloremia, metabolic acidosis, and cholestyramine," *The Journal of Pediatrics*, vol. 89, no. 1, p. 155, 1976.

[7] P. K. Kleinman, "Letter: cholestyramine and metabolic acidosis," *The New England Journal of Medicine*, vol. 290, no. 15, article 861, 1974.

[8] M. Pattison and S. M. Lee, "Life-threatening metabolic acidosis from cholestyramine in an infant with renal insufficiency," *The American Journal of Diseases of Children*, vol. 141, no. 5, pp. 479–480, 1987.

[9] W. A. Primack, L. M. Gartner, H. E. McGurk, and A. Spitzer, "Hypernatremia associated with cholestyramine therapy," *The Journal of Pediatrics*, vol. 90, no. 6, pp. 1024–1025, 1977.

[10] P. J. Scheel Jr., A. Whelton, K. Rossiter, and A. Watson, "Cholestyramine-induced hyperchloremic metabolic acidosis," *Journal of Clinical Pharmacology*, vol. 32, no. 6, pp. 536–538, 1992.

[11] P. Zapater and D. Alba, "Acidosis and extreme hyperkalemia associated with cholestyramine and spironolactone," *Annals of Pharmacotherapy*, vol. 29, no. 2, pp. 199–200, 1995.

[12] W. G. Thompson, "Cholestyramine," *Canadian Medical Association journal*, vol. 104, no. 4, pp. 305–309, 1971.

[13] Z. Wang, S. Petrovic, E. Mann, and M. Soleimani, "Identification of an apical Cl^-/HCO_3^- exchanger in the small intestine," *American Journal of Physiology—Gastrointestinal and Liver Physiology*, vol. 282, no. 3, pp. G573–G579, 2002.

[14] M. A. Manuel, G. J. Beirne, J. P. Wagnild, and M. W. Weiner, "An effect of spironolactone on urinary acidification in normal man," *Archives of Internal Medicine*, vol. 134, no. 3, pp. 472–474, 1974.

16

A Rare Case of Acute Renal Failure Secondary to Rhabdomyolysis Probably Induced by Donepezil

Osman Zikrullah Sahin,[1] Teslime Ayaz,[2] Suleyman Yuce,[2] Fatih Sumer,[2] and Serap Baydur Sahin[3]

[1] Department of Nephrology, Recep Tayyip Erdogan University Medical School, 53100 Rize, Turkey
[2] Department of Internal Medicine, Recep Tayyip Erdogan University Medical School, 53100 Rize, Turkey
[3] Department of Endocrinology and Metabolic Disease, Recep Tayyip Erdogan University Medical School, 53100 Rize, Turkey

Correspondence should be addressed to Osman Zikrullah Sahin; drosahin@yahoo.com

Academic Editor: Ricardo Enríquez

Introduction. Acute renal failure (ARF) develops in 33% of the patients with rhabdomyolysis. The main etiologic factors are alcoholism, trauma, exercise overexertion, and drugs. In this report we present a rare case of ARF secondary to probably donepezil-induced rhabdomyolysis. *Case Presentation.* An 84-year-old male patient was admitted to the emergency department with a complaint of generalized weakness and reduced consciousness for two days. He had a history of Alzheimer's disease for one year and he had taken donepezil 5 mg daily for two months. The patient's physical examination revealed apathy, loss of cooperation, and decreased muscle strength. Laboratory studies revealed the following: urea: 128 mg/dL; Creatinine 6.06 mg/dL; creatine kinase: 3613 mg/dL. Donepezil was discontinued and the patient's renal function tests improved gradually. *Conclusion.* Rhabdomyolysis-induced acute renal failure may develop secondary to donepezil therapy.

1. Introduction

Rhabdomyolysis is defined as a clinical condition in which damaged skeletal muscle breaks down rapidly, releasing toxic substances such as creatine kinase (CK) and myoglobin into the bloodstream [1]. The severity of symptoms depends upon the extent of muscle damage and development of renal failure [2, 3]. It may be asymptomatic or have symptoms including muscle pains, vomiting, and confusion. Some patients may develop severe hypovolemia, shock, arrhythmia, and acute renal failure (ARF) [4, 5].

ARF develops in 33% of the patients with rhabdomyolysis [6]. The main etiologic factors are alcoholism, trauma, exercise overexertion, sunstroke, heat intolerance, hypophosphatemia, convulsions, infections, ischemia, and drug use or overdose [3, 7, 8]. Drugs reported to induce rhabdomyolysis include cocaine, amphetamines, statins, fenofibrate, heroin, corticosteroids, and colchicine [3, 7, 8].

In this report we present a rare case of ARF secondary to rhabdomyolysis probably induced by donepezil.

2. Case Report

An 84-year-old male patient was admitted to the emergency department with a complaint of generalized weakness and reduced consciousness for two days. He had a history of Alzheimer's disease for one year and he had taken donepezil 5 mg daily for two months. He had no other diseases and he had not taken any other medications. He had no history of trauma, convulsion, previous fall, or alcohol intake.

The patient's physical examination revealed apathy, loss of cooperation, and decreased muscle strength. His temperature was 36.8°C, blood pressure 140/90 mm/Hg, and pulse rate 88 bpm. He had bilateral moderate pretibial edema.

Laboratory studies revealed the following: urea: 128 mg/dL; creatinine: 6.06 mg/dL; aspartate aminotransferase: 93 U/L; CK: 3613; calcium: 8.1 mg/dL; phosphorous: 4.9 mg/dL; sodium: 149 mmol/L; potassium: 4,3 mmol/L; albumin: 3.7 g/dL; lactate dehydrogenase: 349 U/L; hemoglobin: 14.2 g/dL; fT3: 3.5 (N: 1.71–3.71 pg/mL); fT4: 1.35 (N: 0.7 1.18 ng/dL); TSH: 2.04 (N: 0.35–4.94 uIU/mL). Urinary dipstick analysis was 1+ positive for protein and 3+ positive in the Haem test. Urinary sediment showed a few red blood cells and 2-3 leukocytes per high-power field. Arterial blood gases analysis was PH: 7.44, PCO_2: 23 mmHg, PO_2: 151 mmHg, SO_2: 99.5%, and HCO_3: 19 mmol/L.

The patient's renal function tests were performed by other health centers before two months and they were completely normal. His renal ultrasound evaluation was normal. The patient was evaluated by a neurologist and there was no neurologic pathology other than Alzheimer's disease. Echocardiography was performed and ejection fraction was 60%, left ventricle was concentric hypertrophic, and a minimal pericardial effusion was reported. The patient was admitted to the nephrology ward with a diagnosis of ARF. Donepezil was discontinued. There was no indication for emergent hemodialysis. Intravenous hydration therapy was given. The patient's renal function tests improved gradually and were normal after 12 days of the treatment. He was discharged with complete recovery.

3. Discussion

We have reported a rare case of rhabdomyolysis associated with donepezil treatment that had progressed to ARF. In literature there was only one case report of rhabdomyolysis related to donepezil treatment in a 76-year-old man with type 2 diabetes mellitus and pulmonary emphysema who had been diagnosed with Alzheimer's and recovered shortly after discontinuing the drug [9]. The patient in our case had no history of trauma, convulsion, exercise, or alcohol intake and he had not taken any other medications such as statin or colchicine that may induce rhabdomyolysis.

Donepezil is a centrally acting reversible acetylcholinesterase inhibitor (ChE) [10]. It is used in palliative treatment of mild to moderate Alzheimer's disease [11]. The safety of donepezil has been demonstrated in many studies ranging from 12-week to 5-year duration [12–15]. Renal function is known to be decreased with increasing age [16]. Donepezil has been found also to be safely administered to patients with moderate to severely impaired renal function [17].

In our case ARF was a result of rhabdomyolysis probably induced by donepezil and not a direct nephrotoxic effect of the drug. It is not known how donepezil can cause rhabdomyolysis. Further studies may be needed to clarify this effect. The routine control measurement of CK may be suggested after administration of donepezil or other drugs that may have rhabdomyolysis effect in elderly patients. Clinicians should be alert for rhabdomyolysis in patients with generalized body weakness and muscle pain. Early management in these patients is vital in protecting the renal functions and preventing morbidity and mortality.

In conclusion, rhabdomyolysis may be associated with many medications. So drugs should be given carefully to the patients particularly the aged or those with chronic diseases and patients should be warned of possible side effects.

Conflict of Interests

The authors declare that there is no conflict of interests regarding the publication of this paper.

References

[1] R. Vanholder, M. S. Sever, E. Erek, and N. Lameire, "Rhabdomyolysis," *Journal of the American Society of Nephrology*, vol. 11, no. 8, pp. 1553–1561, 2000.

[2] J. Farmer, "Rhabdomyolysis," in *In Critical Care*, J. Civetta, R. Taylor, and R. Kirby, Eds., pp. 1785–1791, Lippincott, Philadelphia, Pa, USA, 2nd edition, 1997.

[3] J. D. Warren, P. C. Blumbergs, and P. D. Thompson, "Rhabdomyolysis: a review," *Muscle and Nerve*, vol. 25, no. 3, pp. 332–347, 2002.

[4] G. Melli, V. Chaudhry, and D. R. Cornblath, "Rhabdomyolysis: an evaluation of 475 hospitalized patients," *Medicine*, vol. 84, no. 6, pp. 377–385, 2005.

[5] D. J. Graham, J. A. Staffa, D. Shatin et al., "Incidence of hospitalized rhabdomyolysis in patients treated with lipid-lowering drugs," *Journal of the American Medical Association*, vol. 292, no. 21, pp. 2585–2590, 2004.

[6] F. Y. Khan, "Rhabdomyolysis: a review of the literature," *Netherlands Journal of Medicine*, vol. 67, no. 9, pp. 272–283, 2009.

[7] A. L. Huerta-Alardín, J. Varon, and P. E. Marik, "Bench-to-bedside review: rhabdomyolysis—an overview for clinicians," *Critical Care*, vol. 9, no. 2, pp. 158–169, 2005.

[8] X. Bosch, E. Poch, and J. M. Grau, "Rhabdomyolysis and acute kidney injury," *The New England Journal of Medicine*, vol. 361, no. 1, pp. 62–72, 2009.

[9] K. - Yanagisawa, S. Nagai, Y. Kimura et al., "A case of rhabdomyolysis by donepezil hydrochloride in an elder type 2 diabetes mellitus," *Acta Medica Nosocomi Sapporo*, vol. 65, pp. 21–25, 2005.

[10] J. Birks and R. J. Harvey, "Donepezil for dementia due to Alzheimer's disease," *Cochrane Database of Systematic Reviews*, no. 1, Article ID CD001190, 2006.

[11] "'Aricept' The American Society of Health-System Pharmacists," 2011.

[12] S. Rogers, L. T. Friedhoff, J. T. Apter et al., "The efficacy and safety of donepezil in patients with Alzheimer's disease: results of a US multicentre, randomized, double-blind, placebo-controlled trial," *Dementia*, vol. 7, no. 6, pp. 293–303, 1996.

[13] S. L. Rogers, M. R. Farlow, R. S. Doody, R. Mohs, and L. T. Friedhoff, "A 24-week, double-blind, placebo-controlled trial of donepezil in patients with Alzheimer's disease," *Neurology*, vol. 50, no. 1, pp. 136–145, 1998.

[14] S. L. Rogers, R. S. Doody, R. C. Mohs, and L. T. Friedhoff, "Donepezil improves cognition and global function in Alzheimer disease: a 15-week, double-blind, placebo-controlled study," *Archives of Internal Medicine*, vol. 158, no. 9, pp. 1021–1031, 1998.

[15] S. L. Rogers, R. S. Doody, R. D. Pratt, and J. R. Ieni, "Long-term efficacy and safety of donepezil in the treatment of Alzheimer's disease: final analysis of a US multicentre open-label study," *European Neuropsychopharmacology*, vol. 10, no. 3, pp. 195–203, 2000.

[16] M. M. Lubran, "Renal function in the elderly," *Annals of Clinical and Laboratory Science*, vol. 25, no. 2, pp. 122–133, 1995.

[17] P. J. Tiseo, K. Foley, and L. T. Friedhoff, "An evaluation of the pharmacokinetics of donepezil HCl in patients with moderately to severely impaired venal function," *British Journal of Clinical Pharmacology, Supplement*, vol. 46, no. 1, pp. 56–60, 1998.

17

Nephrotic Syndrome Secondary to Proliferative Glomerulonephritis with Monoclonal Immunoglobulin Deposits of Lambda Light Chain

Seongseok Yun,[1,2] Beth L. Braunhut,[3] Courtney N. Walker,[1] Waheed Bhati,[1] Amy N. Sussman,[1] and Faiz Anwer[4]

[1] Department of Medicine, University of Arizona, Tucson, AZ 85721, USA

[2] Department of Medicine, Arizona Health Sciences Center, 6th Floor, Room 6336, 1501 N. Campbell Avenue, Tucson, AZ 85719, USA

[3] Division of Pathology, University of Arizona, Tucson, AZ 85721, USA

[4] Division of Hematology, Oncology, Blood & Marrow Transplantation, Department of Medicine, University of Arizona, Tucson, AZ 86721, USA

Correspondence should be addressed to Seongseok Yun; namaska97@gmail.com

Academic Editor: Ricardo Enríquez

We describe a rare case of a 46-year-old woman with history of refractory nephrotic syndrome and hypertension who presented with worsening proteinuria and kidney function. Work-up for both autoimmune and infectious diseases and hematologic malignancies including multiple myeloma were negative. Kidney biopsy demonstrated glomerular sclerotic change with lambda light chain deposits in the subendothelial space, which is consistent with proliferative glomerulonephritis with monoclonal immunoglobulin deposit (PGNMID). The patient was treated with bortezomib and dexamethasone without clinical improvement and eventually became hemodialysis dependent.

1. Introduction

PGNMID is a recently described as a rare disorder that belongs to the class of disorders known as monoclonal gammopathy of renal significance (MGRS) [1]. PGNMID has been shown to be associated with various underlying diseases including myeloma, chronic lymphocytic leukemia (CLL), and parvovirus infection [1–5], and the most common clinical manifestation is renal involvement. PGNMID has unique histological and pathophysiological features, which distinguish it from other entities of MGRS or malignant monoclonal diseases. The renal deposit in PGNMID is composed of monoclonal immunoglobulin (Ig). Microscopic findings typically show a nonfibrillar or nonmicrotubular pattern of Ig deposit without any organized structure. Although histologic features have been well described and the clinical course of PGNMID is known to be poor, the underlying mechanisms of PGNMID remain elusive. Based on the evidence of other clonal disorders, bortezomib, cyclophosphamide, and high dose of chemotherapy followed by stem cell transplant are the current recommended treatments, although with variable response.

2. Case Presentation

A 46-year-old woman with history of nephrotic syndrome was referred from an outside hospital for further evaluation and management of recurrent and progressively worsening nephrotic syndrome with stage III chronic kidney disease (CKD). Kidney biopsy and immunofluorescence (IF) staining one year ago had shown focal segmental proliferative glomerulonephritis and the patient had been treated with 16 weeks of cyclosporine followed by prednisone. Unfortunately, one year later, she presented with recurrent nephrotic symptoms including elevated serum creatinine, hypoalbuminemia, and significant proteinuria (Figure 1).

Vital signs revealed blood pressure of 155/83 mmHg, heart rate of 81 beats per minute, respiratory rate of 14/minute,

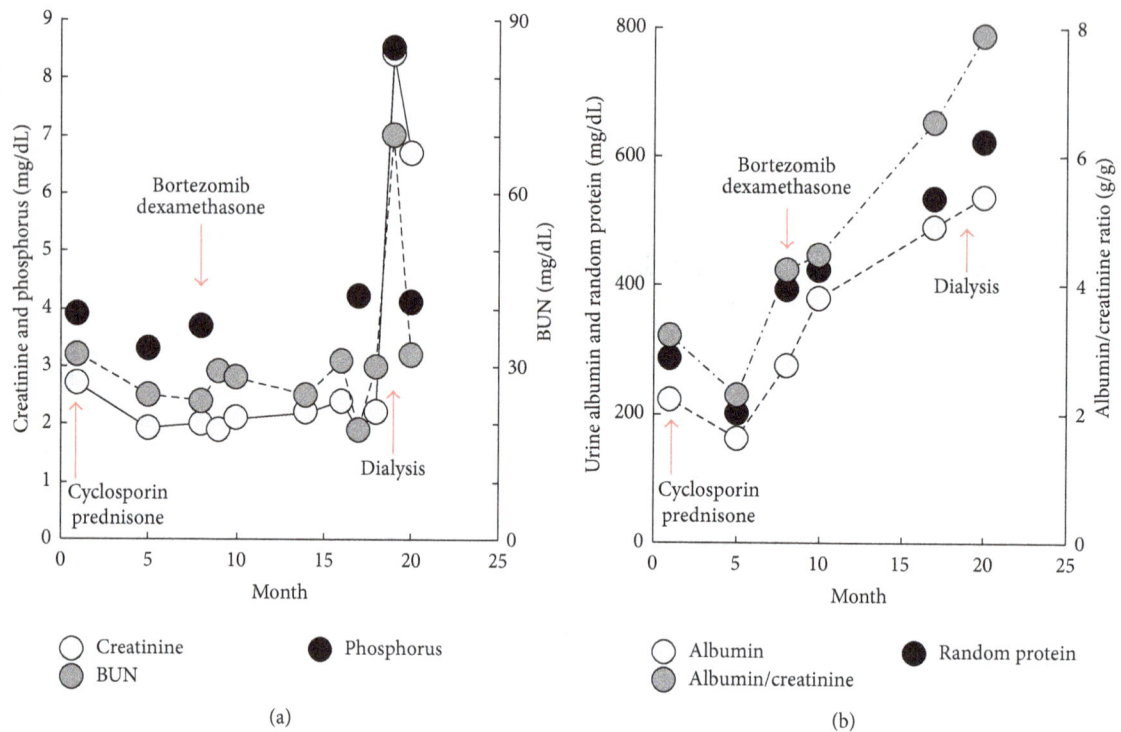

FIGURE 1: Laboratory values during the chemotherapy. 16-week treatment with cyclosporine followed by prednisone failed to prevent disease progression. Patient received a total of 4 cycles of bortezomib and dexamethasone, however, with no clinical or laboratory improvement. Disease progressed and patient eventually became hemodialysis dependent.

and temperature of 37.6°C. Lung and heart exams were normal and there was no palpable cervical, supraclavicular, axillary, or inguinal lymphadenopathy. Bilateral, one plus pitting lower extremity edema was present. Laboratory exam showed serum creatinine of 1.92 (normal 0.67–1.17 mg/dL) (Figure 1), IgG of 1333 (normal 552–1631 mg/dL), elevated kappa chain of 3.67 (normal 0.33–1.94 mg/dL), and lambda chain of 2.29 (normal 0.57–2.63 mg/dL) with normal ratio of 1.62. A 24-hour urine protein excretion was 8 g (normal 80 mg), and urine and serum immunofixation demonstrated positive monoclonal-free lambda light chain. Serum IgA (201 mg/dL), IgM (102 mg/dL), C3 (152 mg/dL), and C4 (32 mg/dL) levels were within normal range. Additional rheumatologic work-up included anti-SSA, anti-SSB, anti-nuclear antibodies (ANA), anti-neutrophil cytoplasmic antibody (ANCA), serum cryoglobulin, hepatitis panel, and serum protein electrophoresis (SPEP), which were all negative. Renal biopsy with light microscopic examination revealed multiple globally sclerosed glomeruli and occasional glomeruli with segmental sclerosis. The glomerular capillary loops showed patchy endocapillary proliferation and mononuclear inflammatory cell infiltration. A patchy mononuclear cell infiltrate was observed with associated tubulitis (Figures 2(a) and 2(b)). Immunofluorescence (IF) examination revealed mesangial staining for IgG (trace) and IgM (trace) and glomerular capillary loops were stained positive for C3 (1 to 2+) and lambda light chain (2+) (Figures 3(a)–3(d)). Subsequent electron microscopic ultrastructural examination demonstrated scattered electron dense

immune-type deposits within mesangial areas and focally within the subendothelial space. The complexes did not show any organized substructural features, and the glomerular basement membrane had markedly irregular thickness in areas involved with deposits and/or endocapillary proliferation (Figures 4(a) and 4(b)). Further work-up for multiple myeloma, including skeletal survey and bone marrow biopsy, was normal with only 5% plasma cells on bone marrow immunohistochemistry and only 0.6% CD20+ B cells on flow cytometry. Additional fluorescence in situ hybridization (FISH) analysis included 1q21 (CKS1B), 9q34 (ASS1), 11q13 (CCND1), 14q32 (IGH), 15q22 (PML), and 17p13 (TP53), which were all negative. Although the IF staining for IgG is weaker than that of previous case reports, suggesting either early stage of disease or suboptimal staining condition, the microscopic findings and laboratory results confirmed the diagnosis of proliferative glomerulonephritis with monoclonal immunoglobulin deposit (PGNMID) with monoclonal lambda light chain.

The patient completed three cycles of weekly bortezomib along with dexamethasone without complication. Unfortunately, her disease progressed and she became hemodialysis dependent (Figure 1).

3. Discussion

PGNMID is a rare disease (incidence of 0.17%) with most published data extrapolated from case reports [1]. Proposed criteria to diagnosis PGNMID include (1) the presence of Ig

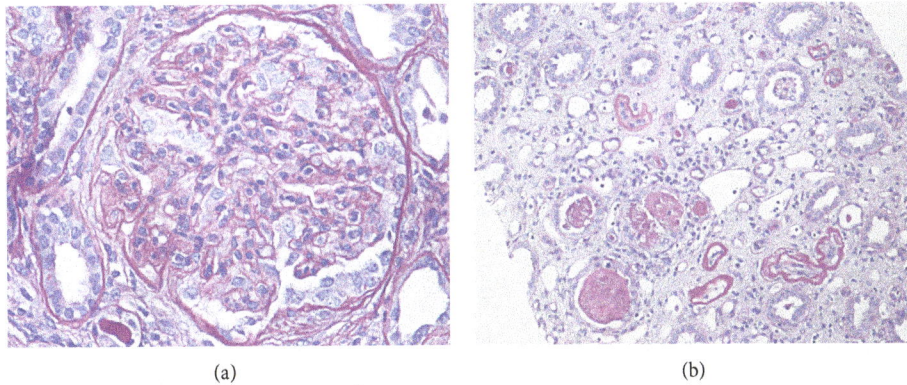

(a)

(b)

FIGURE 2: Light microscopic finding of kidney biopsy. PAS at 400x shows glomerulus with globally increased mesangial matrix and cellularity and segmental attachment to Bowman's capsule (a). The glomerular capillary loops show patchy endocapillary proliferation and focal mononuclear cell infiltration. No necrosis or crescents are seen in glomeruli, and the interstitium shows extensive fibrosis and patchy tubular atrophy. PAS at 200x demonstrates tubules containing intraluminal casts with smooth borders and flattening and sloughing of tubular epithelial cells (b).

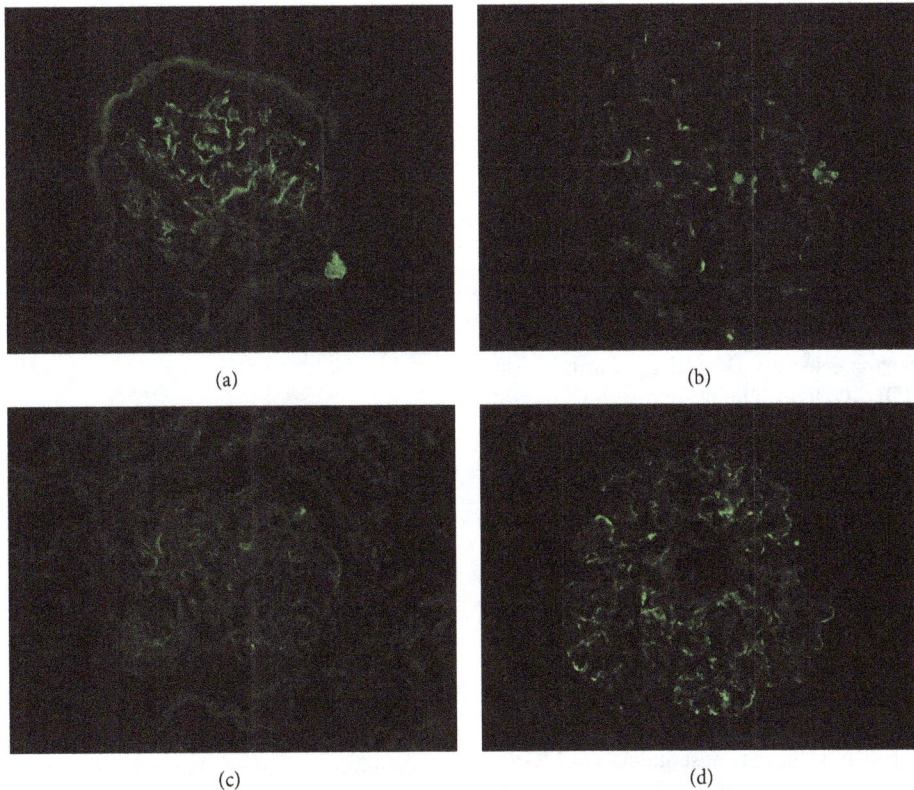

(a)

(b)

(c)

(d)

FIGURE 3: Immunofluorescence staining of kidney biopsy. Immunofluorescence staining shows trace mesangial staining for IgG (a), IgM (b), and kappa light chain (c) but 2+ mesangial and granular capillary loop staining for lambda light chain (d), confirming the diagnosis of PGNMID with monoclonal lambda light chain.

deposit with a single IgG subclass and a single light chain isotype, (2) granular pattern of deposit under microscopy, and (3) no evidence of cryoglobulinemia [6]. PGNMID belongs to the disease spectrum known as monoclonal gammopathy of renal significance (MGRS) that includes amyloidosis (AL), type I cryoglobulinemia, immunotactoid glomerulopathy (ITG), and Randall-type monoclonal immunoglobulin deposition disease (MIDD) [7]. AL is one of the most frequent diseases in MGRS and is associated with plasma cell clones [6]. The deposit is composed of monoclonal light chain or its fragments. Although 70–80% of AL patients have renal involvement, the mortality largely depends on cardiac

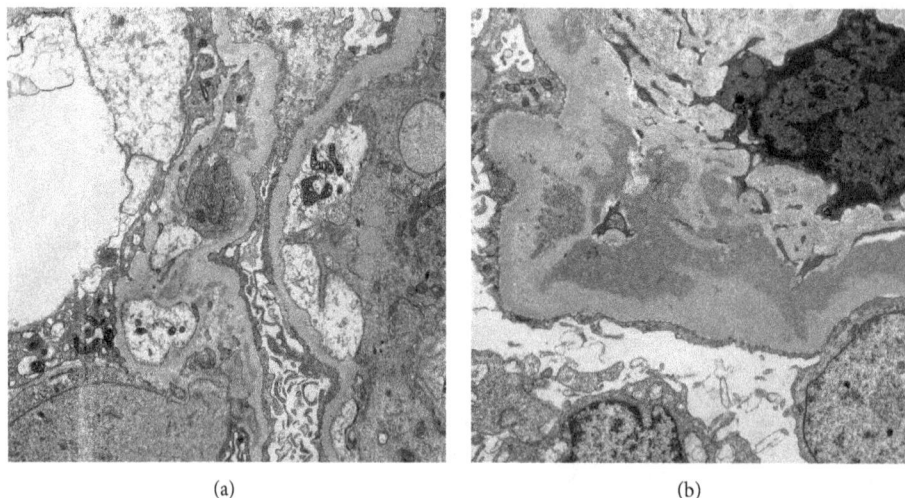

(a)   (b)

FIGURE 4: Electron microscopic finding of kidney biopsy. Electron microscopy demonstrates diffuse podocyte foot process effacement, proliferation in the capillary loop, and remodeling of the glomerular basement membrane with cellular interposition (a). The glomerular basement membrane is markedly irregular in thickness, and dense deposits are located in the mesangial areas and focally within subendothelial space without any organized substructural features (b). In loops without these abnormalities, the glomerular basement membrane is of normal thickness and has normal architecture.

involvement. Type I cryoglobulinemia is another monoclonal disease with single monoclonal Ig deposit [6]. IgG type is the most common type and is precipitated by cold temperature. Raynaud's phenomenon, glomerular disease of membranoproliferative glomerulonephritis (MPGN), hypertension, and articular involvement are common clinical manifestations (Table 1). Randal-type MIDD is frequently associated with multiple myeloma with more than 10% of bone marrow involvement with plasma cells [6]. The most common form of Randal-type MIDD is light chain deposition disease (LCDD). Light heavy chain deposition disease (LHCDD) and heavy chain deposition disease (HCDD) are relatively rare. Glomerular deposits with nodular glomerulosclerosis and linear amorphous deposits in the tubular basement membranes are common histologic findings. Majority of the patients present with renal involvement including proteinuria, hematuria, and renal insufficiency. Renal biopsy and pathologic review are mandatory for the differential diagnosis of MGRS.

B-cell clones that do not meet criteria for lymphoma or multiple myeloma are known to be responsible for MGRS. Most of the pathological and clinical consequences of MGRS arise from the deposition of monoclonal Ig in the organ rather than the proliferation of abnormal B-cell clones [8]. Moreover, PGNMID has a distinct microscopic appearance compared to other entities of MGRS, including a granular nonlinear pattern without deposits in glomerular or tubular basement membranes [1, 2, 6] and diffuse endocapillary proliferative glomerulonephritis (DPGN) or membranoproliferative glomerulonephritis (MPGN) pattern.

Patients with PGNMID most commonly present with proteinuria, renal insufficiency, and hematuria without clinical evidence of multiple myeloma or B-cell lymphoproliferative disorders such as lymphadenopathy, hepatosplenomegaly, or skeletal involvement, and extrarenal

TABLE 1: Clinical manifestations of PGNMID [1].

Pathologic findings	Clinical findings	Laboratory findings
Membranoproliferative GN	Peripheral edema	Proteinuria
Endocapillary proliferative GN	Hematuria	Hypoalbuminemia
Mesangial proliferative GN		Renal insufficiency
Membranous GN		Serum and urine paraprotein
Focal interstitial inflammation		Low C3 and C4
Tubular atrophy and interstitial fibrosis		

manifestations of PGNMID are extremely rare (Table 2). Additionally, the renal Ig deposits are not a consequence of glomerular damage secondary to autoimmune, infectious, or systemic disorders that can cause antigenic stimulation. Overall, the pathogenesis of PGNMID is poorly understood. Only one-third of patients showed a positive monoclonal spike in either SPEP or UPEP, and the plasma cells found in the bone marrow are usually less than 10% [1]. In our patient, serum kappa light chain was slightly elevated and lambda chain was normal with normal ratio of 1.62. However, monoclonal renal deposits indicate the presence of circulating monoclonal plasma cells and an underlying B-cell disorder as shown in our patient, and this has been the rationale for using chemotherapy targeting B-cells in PGNMID [9].

To date, there is no treatment that inhibits the process of Ig accumulation or removes already formed immune deposits. Currently, most therapies for PGNMID target

TABLE 2: Treatment recommendation for PGNMID [9].

CKD stage I and II Proteinuria (<1 g/day) No evidence of progressive disease	CKD stage I and II with high grade proteinuria (>1 g/day) Progressive disease CKD stage III and IV	CKD stage V

(1) Symptomatic measures only
(2) Careful surveillance
	(1) Chemotherapy,
	   cyclophosphamide, and
	   bortezomib
	(2) HDM/ASCT
	(3) Rituximab
		(1) Kidney transplantation
		(2) HDM/ASCT

the underlying B-cell disorder using chemotherapeutic or immune-modulatory agents, although evidence is lacking. There are several case reports of PGNMID patients treated with chlorambucil, mycophenolate mofetil, prednisone, thalidomide, and rituximab, but the outcomes are disappointing with low remission rates [1, 4, 10]. The International Kidney and Monoclonal Gammopathy Research Group recommends treatment according to the severity of renal disease (Table 2) [9]. Symptomatic management is recommended for CKD stage I or II with proteinuria less than 1 g/day and no evidence of disease progression. Chemotherapy with bortezomib or cyclophosphamide is recommended for CKD stage I or II with proteinuria greater than 1 g/day and progressive disease. High dose melphalan followed by autologous stem cell transplant (HDM/ASCT) is an alternative option for patients less than 65 years of age. However, the efficacy of these chemotherapy targeting plasma cells is unknown especially in a setting of less than 10% plasma cells in PGNMID warranting further clinical investigation. Accordingly, rituximab targeting CD20+ B cell clones is excluded from current recommendations due to its limited efficacy and delayed complications [11], although it has been shown to be effective in several PGNMID cases [4]. Lastly, kidney transplantation with or without pretransplant chemotherapy or HDM/ASCT is the best suggested option for patients with CKD stage V.

Following the recommendation of the International Kidney and Monoclonal Gammopathy Research Group, our patient was treated with bortezomib and dexamethasone, although without improvement. Rituximab was not considered for this patient due to lack of CD20+ population in flow cytometry in bone marrow cells. Eventually, the patient's renal disease progressed to hemodialysis dependence. Alternative treatment options are now HDM/ASCT or kidney transplant.

As described in this case, there are several limitations in the current treatment guidelines. First of all, therapies are not based on prospective, randomized controlled clinical trials but on a limited number of case studies. Secondly, treatment simply depends on CKD staging without an understanding of the underlying pathophysiology of monoclonal production and deposition. Thirdly, no prognostic factor or prognostic system has been investigated or developed yet. Finally, more clinical studies are necessary to better understand PGNMID and improve clinical outcomes of this rare disease.

4. Conclusion

PGNMID is a very rare disease of the MGRS spectrum. The pathologic abnormalities are limited to the renal system, and common clinical manifestations include proteinuria, hypoalbuminemia, and renal insufficiency. The underlying mechanisms of PGNMID remain elusive. However, the presence of monoclonal deposits in the kidney suggests an underlying plasma cell and B-cell disorder. Depending on the stage of CKD, the current therapeutic options are bortezomib, cyclophosphamide, hemodialysis, or stem cell transplant, although evidence is lacking.

Conflict of Interests

The authors declare that there is no conflict of interests regarding the publishing of this paper.

References

[1] S. H. Nasr, A. Satoskar, G. S. Markowitz et al., "Proliferative glomerulonephritis with monoclonal IgG deposits," *Journal of the American Society of Nephrology*, vol. 20, no. 9, pp. 2055–2064, 2009.

[2] E. Guiard, A. Karras, E. Plaisier et al., "Patterns of noncryoglobulinemic glomerulonephritis with monoclonal Ig deposits: correlation with IgG subclass and response to rituximab," *Clinical Journal of the American Society of Nephrology*, vol. 6, no. 7, pp. 1609–1616, 2011.

[3] M. D. Redondo-Pachón, R. Enríquez, A. E. Sirvent et al., "Proliferative glomerulonephritis with monoclonal IgG deposits in multiple myeloma," *Nefrologia*, vol. 32, no. 6, pp. 846–848, 2012.

[4] S. J. Barbour, M. C. Beaulieu, N. Y. Zalunardo, and A. B. Magil, "Proliferative glomerulonephritis with monoclonal IgG deposits secondary to chronic lymphocytic leukemia. Report of two cases," *Nephrology Dialysis Transplantation*, vol. 26, no. 8, pp. 2712–2714, 2011.

[5] E. Fujita, A. Shimizu, T. Kaneko et al., "Proliferative glomerulonephritis with monoclonal immunoglobulin G3κ deposits in association with parvovirus B19 infection," *Human Pathology*, vol. 43, no. 12, pp. 2326–2333, 2012.

[6] S. H. Nasr, G. S. Markowitz, M. B. Stokes et al., "Proliferative glomerulonephritis with monoclonal IgG deposits: a distinct entity mimicking immune-complex glomerulonephritis," *Kidney International*, vol. 65, no. 1, pp. 85–96, 2004.

[7] N. Leung, F. Bridoux, C. A. Hutchison et al., "Monoclonal gammopathy of renal significance: when MGUS is no longer

undetermined or insignificant," *Blood*, vol. 120, no. 22, pp. 4292–4295, 2012.

[8] G. Merlini and M. J. Stone, "Dangerous small B-cell clones," *Blood*, vol. 108, no. 8, pp. 2520–2530, 2006.

[9] J. P. Fermand, F. Bridoux, R. A. Kyle et al., "How I treat monoclonal gammopathy of renal significance (MGRS)," *Blood*, vol. 122, pp. 3583–3590, 2013.

[10] A. Ranghino, M. Tamagnone, M. Messina et al., "A case of recurrent proliferative glomerulonephritis with monoclonal IgG deposits after kidney transplant treated with plasmapheresis," *Case Reports in Nephrology and Urology*, vol. 2, no. 1, pp. 46–52, 2012.

[11] C. Tarella, R. Passera, M. Magni et al., "Risk factors for the development of secondary malignancy after high-dose chemotherapy and autograft, with or without rituximab: a 20-year retrospective follow-up study in patients with lymphoma," *Journal of Clinical Oncology*, vol. 29, no. 7, pp. 814–824, 2011.

18

Palliative Care for a Mentally Incompetent End Stage Renal Failure Patient: Why Is It Important?

Kwok-Ying Chan,[1] Terence Yip,[2] Mau-Kwong Sham,[1] Benjamin Hon-Wai Cheng,[1] Cho-Wing Li,[1] Yim-Chi Wong,[1] and Vikki Wai-Kee Lau[1]

[1]*Palliative Medical Unit, Grantham Hospital, Wong Chuk Hang, Hong Kong*
[2]*Renal Unit, Department of Medicine, Tung Wah Hospital, Sheung Wan, Hong Kong*

Correspondence should be addressed to Kwok-Ying Chan; cky842@yahoo.com.hk

Academic Editor: Władysław Sułowicz

People with intellectual disabilities are among the most disadvantaged groups in society. Here we report a mentally incompetent end stage renal failure (ESRF) patient with frequent emergency visits who made a significant improvement in symptoms control and reduction in casualty visits after introduction of renal palliative care service. Multidisciplinary approach would be useful in this case.

1. Introduction

As the risk of life-limiting diseases such as end stage renal disease (ESRD), it could be speculated that more people with intellectual disabilities now suffer such disease and may require palliative care if they are chosen for conservative therapy without dialysis [1]. Here we report a mentally incompetent ESRD patient with frequent emergency visits who made a significant improvement in symptoms control and reduction in casualty visits after introduction of renal palliative care service.

2. Case Report

Mr. K was a 53-year-old gentleman with history of diabetes mellitus and hypertension since his teenage years. His diabetic control had never been satisfactory and he suffered from end stage kidney disease since his 50s.

He was mildly mental incapacitated and received special education since 3 years old. Besides, his mother had moderate to severe dementia who requires regular medication and constant attention. His father died when he was young and his elder sister suffered from Parkinsonism at her 40s. Since his mother was a landlady, there was no financial difficulty for this family. He received formal assessment by nephrology team but was found to be difficult in hemodialysis (HD) due to the patient being unable to keep still during therapy. In addition, due to his complicated social history and lack of support, peritoneal dialysis (PD) could not be managed by the family. After a thorough discussion with his family, it was decided that his ESRF should be managed conservatively without dialysis.

His drug and fluid compliance was all along poor. Besides, he had attention seeking behavior related to his mental incompetence. Prior to the introduction of renal palliative care, he had frequent emergency department (ED) visits due to various reasons, including gouty attack (plasma urate = 6.5 mg/dL), dizziness, edema, pruritus, fatigue, and severe hyperkalemia (K = 7.3 mmol/L). Some of the episodes were of minor complaints and he could be discharged home without requiring ward admission. Family members and domestic helper mentioned that this had caused significant stress to them.

His baseline laboratory results revealed the following: hemoglobin level (Hb) 8.1 g/dL; plasma creatinine level 9.5 mg/dL; phosphate 5.8 mg/dL, calcium 8.5 mg/dL; PTH 23 pmol/L; and eGFR 9 mL/min/1.73 m^2. His blood gas showed pH 7.39, HCO3$^-$ 26.1 mmol/L and base excess 1 mmol/L.

After ruling out vitamins and iron deficiency, continuous erythropoietin receptor activator (CERA) which was a long acting erythropoietin stimulating agent (ESA) was started in the palliative care clinic and titrated against his body weight and Hb level [2]. His uremic pruritus was treated with sertraline which was then escalated to 150 mg according to clinical response [3]. His limb edema was reduced after using a combination of diuretic and reinforcement of drug and fluid compliance [4]. Gouty attack was treated with analgesics and ice pack. Diet advice and allopurinol were given to prevent further attack.

Home care nurse was referred for psychological interventions while social worker was referred for social support to the patient and his family members. In addition, he was arranged to join the activities in our palliative care day centre. The patient and his domestic helper highly appreciated our arrangement. In the day centre, Mr. K could have social gathering with other patients, for example, enjoying opera and music video, watching television, doing some hand-made work, and joining outdoor activities, for example, going to Disneyland. In fact, he has high attendance rates (about 2-3 times/week) in our centre.

After 6 months of care, the severity of pain, edema, and pruritus were significantly reduced (5 to 2, 7 to 3, and 8 to 2 out of 10, resp.) according to Edmonton Symptom Assessment Scale (ESAS) [5]. Hb level was raised to 10-11 mg/dL. His 6-month casualty attendance was markedly reduced from 13 to only 1 time after receiving renal PC care because his uremic symptoms and psychosocial needs could now be better managed via our interdisciplinary approach.

3. Discussion

This report demonstrated how renal palliative care could help relieve symptom, provide psychosocial care, and thus reduce healthcare cost through multidisciplinary approach.

Mr. K suffered from heavy symptom burden which was commonly found in renal palliative care patients [6]. By using ESA, it was shown to reduce fatigue for this group of patients by correcting anaemia [2]. Sertraline, a selective serotonin reuptake inhibitor, was found to be effective to relieve antihistamine refractory uremic pruritus and help reduce anxiety when the dosage is titrated to above 100 mg [3]. For treatment of refractory fluid retention, addition of low dose metolazone to furosemide could be successfully managed in the previous studies [4]. In order to prevent episodes of hyperkalemia and fluid overload, diet and drug compliance were both reinforced by doctor and our nurses visit during his PC clinic follow-up. By using collaborative care model between nephrology and palliative care team, symptom scores, depressed mood, and the rate of rehospitalization were found to be reduced in our local study [7].

A previous study found that many chronically ill people who were admitted to an ED had complex psychosocial problems and limited access to support systems and home-care services along with their medical problems [8]. PC services possess superiority over EDs and acute hospital setting for a holistic, multidisciplinary, and timely approach for addressing PC needs of renal failure patients. The role of

day hospice care to renal palliative care patients has never been mentioned previously. Apart from providing social support and respite care, regular monitoring of patient's diet and fluid compliance by our staff of day centre might alleviate fluid overload or gouty attack for this patient.

In fact, people with intellectual disabilities are among the most disadvantaged groups in society. Mild intellectual disabilities are particularly vulnerable as their intellectual disability is not always recognized [9]. They may be socially clumsy and misread during social situations, which could lead healthcare staff to adopt negative attitudes.

Pertinent issues included the fact that their somatic complaints were often thought to be related to their mental incapacitation and hence ignored. Difficulty for the family in finding medical teams which could cope with Mr. K's dual needs is as well demonstrated in this case report. A previous study had shown that medical assessment for this group of patients is difficult due to communication problems, lack of medical notes and history due to previously fragmented care, and unfamiliarity of staff in ordinary healthcare services in dealing with people with intellectual disabilities [1].

Carers who have worked closely with the person with intellectual disabilities may also have strong feelings and emotions of their own when their client becomes terminally ill, complicating the situation further [1]. Botsford suggested that the complexity of staff roles, where there is a responsibility not only to individuals and families but also to colleagues, administrations, regulating bodies, and other providers, creates conflicts and dilemmas about end-of-life care [10]. If there is a disagreement between different parties, she suggested the involvement of social workers, clergy, hospice workers, or bereavement professionals to work as mediators. Palliative care professionals can be in a good position to provide guidance and support in such situations.

It is foreseeable that as patients become frailer, multidisciplinary input will play a central role in addressing their needs, including symptom control, advance care planning, and end-of-life care. It is crucial that palliative care be well coordinated to address the needs of these patients. A similar success by using this collaborative model can be seen with hematology teams of local hospitals [11]. Our joint care model in Hong Kong provided a good learning opportunity for both specialists in palliative care and nephrology, and, hopefully, patients will benefit from our joint effort in care.

Conflict of Interests

The authors have no conflict of interests regarding the publication of this paper.

References

[1] I. Tuffrey-Wijne, "The palliative care needs of people with intellectual disabilities: a literature review," *Palliative Medicine*, vol. 17, no. 1, pp. 55–62, 2003.

[2] K.-Y. Chan, C.-W. Li, H. Wong et al., "Effect of erythropoiesis-stimulating agents on hemoglobin level, fatigue and hospitalization rate in renal palliative care patients," *International Urology and Nephrology*, vol. 46, no. 3, pp. 653–657, 2014.

[3] K. Y. Chan, C. W. Li, H. Wong et al., "Use of sertraline for anti-histamine-refractory uremic pruritus in renal palliative care patients," *Journal of Palliative Medicine*, vol. 16, no. 8, pp. 966–970, 2013.

[4] J. Rosenberg, F. Gustafsson, S. Galatius, and P. R. Hildebrandt, "Combination therapy with metolazone and loop diuretics in outpatients with refractory heart failure: an observational study and review of the literature," *Cardiovascular Drugs and Therapy*, vol. 19, no. 4, pp. 301–306, 2005.

[5] S. N. Davison, G. S. Jhangri, and J. A. Johnson, "Cross-sectional validity of a modified Edmonton symptom assessment system in dialysis patients: a simple assessment of symptom burden," *Kidney International*, vol. 69, no. 9, pp. 1621–1625, 2006.

[6] D. S. P. Yong, A. O. L. Kwok, D. M. L. Wong, M. H. P. Suen, W. T. Chen, and D. M. W. Tse, "Symptom burden and quality of life in end-stage renal disease: a study of 179 patients on dialysis and palliative care," *Palliative Medicine*, vol. 23, no. 2, pp. 111–119, 2009.

[7] K. Y. Chan, H. W. B. Cheng, D. Y. H. Yap et al., "Reduction of acute hospital admissions and improvement in outpatient attendance by intensified renal palliative care clinic follow-up: the Hong Kong experience," *Journal of Pain and Symptom Management*, vol. 49, no. 1, pp. 144–149, 2015.

[8] T. Beynon, B. Gomes, F. E. M. Murtagh et al., "How common are palliative care needs among older people who die in the emergency department?" *Emergency Medicine Journal*, vol. 28, no. 6, pp. 491–495, 2011.

[9] MENCAP, *The NHS: Health for All? People with Learning Disabilities and Healthcare*, Mencap National Centre, London, UK, 1998.

[10] A. L. Botsford, "Integrating end of life care into services for people with an intellectual disability," *Social Work in Health Care*, vol. 31, no. 1, pp. 35–48, 2000.

[11] H. W. Cheng, "Optimizing end-of-life care for patients with hematological malignancy: rethinking the role of palliative care collaboration," *Journal of Pain and Symptom Management*, 2015.

19

The Hidden Cost of Untreated Paragangliomas of the Head and Neck: Systemic Reactive (AA) Amyloidosis

Erkan Dervisoglu,[1] Murat Ozturk,[2] Mehmet Tuncay,[1] Gulhatun Kilic Dervisoglu,[3] Yesim Gurbuz,[4] and Serhan Derin[5]

[1]*Department of Nephrology, School of Medicine, Kocaeli University, 41000 Kocaeli, Turkey*
[2]*Department of Otorhinolaryngology, School of Medicine, Kocaeli University, 41000 Kocaeli, Turkey*
[3]*Department of Neurology, Kandira Government Hospital, 41600 Kocaeli, Turkey*
[4]*Department of Pathology, School of Medicine, Kocaeli University, 41000 Kocaeli, Turkey*
[5]*Department of Otorhinolaryngology School of Medicine, Muğla Sıtkı Koçman University, 48000 Muğla, Turkey*

Correspondence should be addressed to Serhan Derin; serhanderin@yahoo.com.tr

Academic Editor: Jaume Almirall

We report a case of a 51-year-old man who was diagnosed with systemic reactive (AA) amyloidosis in association with untreated glomus jugulare and glomus caroticum tumors. He refused radiotherapy and renal replacement therapy. Paragangliomas, although rare, should be considered one of the tumors that can result in AA amyloidosis.

1. Introduction

Paragangliomas are uncommon true neoplasms that arise from paraganglionic chemoreceptor cells. Other terms used to describe these lesions include glomus tumors, nonchromaffin paragangliomas, chemodectomas, and carotid body-like tumors [1]. Systemic reactive (AA) amyloidosis is usually observed during chronic infectious or inflammatory processes or rarely with benign or malignant tumors. The association of isolated paragangliomas with systemic reactive amyloidosis has been rarely reported. In this report, we present a case of systemic reactive amyloidosis associated with glomus jugulare and caroticum tumors.

2. Case Report

A 51-year-old man with a glomus jugulare tumor was referred to our nephrology clinic with suspected renal failure and proteinuria. Twenty-nine years prior, the patient had an operation for glomus jugulare tumor that resulted in extensive hemorrhaging and required a two-month hospitalization. Since the operation, the patient had not sought any follow-up care for his glomus tumor. His brother was diagnosed as having a glomus caroticum tumor. The patient complained of pulsatile tinnitus and a mass in his right external ear canal.

On admission, the patient's blood pressure was 100/70 mm Hg, pulse rate 78/min, and temperature 36.6°C. He had 1+ pitting edema in the lower extremities. On otolaryngologic exam, the patient had a red-whitish mass protruding from the middle ear to external ear, filling the external ear canal (Figure 1). Audiometry testing found an 85 dB mixed-type hearing loss on the left and a 29 dB sensorineural hearing loss on the right. The patient had a daily and urinary protein excretion of 2 g and albumin excretion of 1 g with no abnormality in urinary sedimentation. Erythrocyte sedimentation rate was 69 mm/h and C-reactive protein level was 6.4 mg/dL (normal: <0.8 mg/dL). His hemoglobin was low (9.33 g/dL), but his platelet and leukocyte counts were normal. Serum creatinine was 4.09 mg/dL, blood urea nitrogen 46 mg/dL, total protein 5.9 g/dL, and albumin 2.86 g/dL. Serum electrolytes, liver enzymes, and C3 and C4 levels were within normal range. Tests for hepatitides B and C, HIV, anti-nuclear antibody, and anti-double-stranded DNA were also negative. Chest X-ray and EKG were normal. Abdominal ultrasonography showed normal sized kidneys with bilateral grade 2 echogenicity.

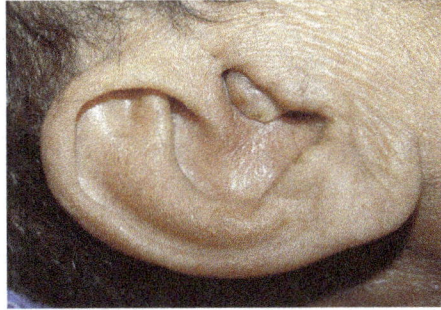

FIGURE 1: A red-whitish mass protruding from the middle ear to external ear, filling the external ear canal.

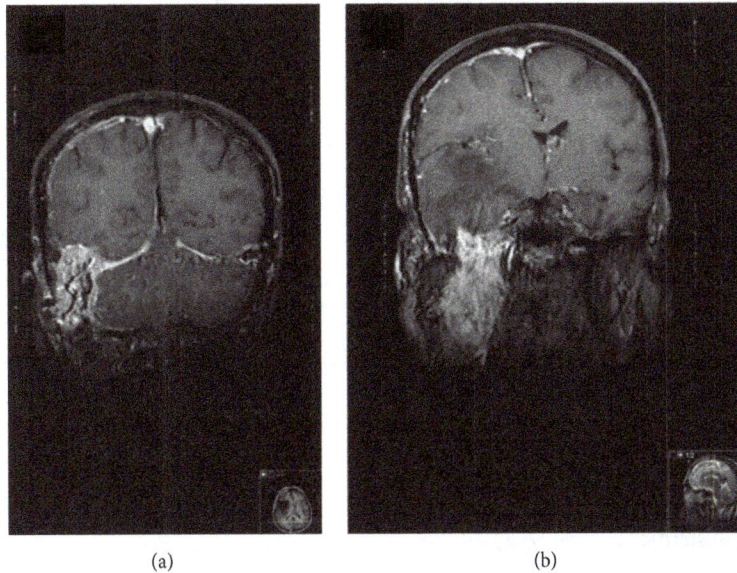

(a)   (b)

FIGURE 2: Cranial magnetic resonance images demonstrate (a) a mass lesion that arises from the right jugular foramen, extending to the medial cranial fossa, consistent with glomus jugulare, and (b) a mass lesion at the carotid bifurcation, consistent with glomus caroticum.

After placement of a dual-lumen hemodialysis (HD) catheter into the right internal jugular vein, HD treatment three times weekly was started. Cranial magnetic resonance imaging (MRI) showed a mass lesion arising from the right jugular foramen, extending to medial cranial fossa (consistent with a glomus jugulare), and a mass lesion at the carotid bifurcation, consistent with a glomus caroticum (Figure 2). The tumors were deemed unresectable and radiotherapy was suggested.

We suspected amyloidosis as the underlying cause of his renal failure and proteinuria. Due to his severe renal failure, we performed a rectal biopsy without complication. A homogenous, amorphous, and eosinophilic material was seen in the walls of submucosal vessels on light microscopy. The material was positive on Congo red staining and was digested by $KMnO_4$ (Figure 3). Immunohistochemical analysis showed positive staining for AA amyloid. Based on these results, we made a diagnosis of AA amyloidosis. Neither he nor his family had a history of Mediterranean fever (MEFN), and he had no clinical signs of MEFN. Treatment was started with colchicine 1 mg/day and the patient continued with regular HD three times weekly. He refused to receive radiotherapy for his tumors and died 3 months after the commencement of HD.

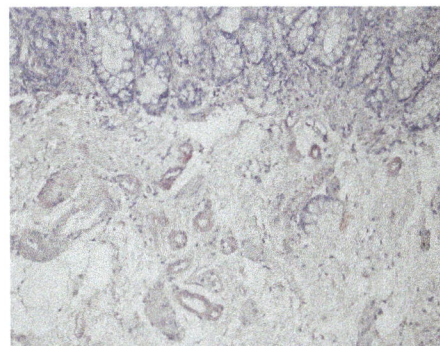

FIGURE 3: Amyloid is noted in the submucosal vessels (Congo red stain ×100).

3. Discussion

Paraganglionic tissue is derived from the neural crest and is found in several locations in the body: in the carotid body, along the course of Jacobson's nerve, within the adventitia of the jugular bulb at the jugular foramen, and within the adrenal medulla [2]. Jugular foramen paragangliomas are deep-seated, extremely vascular lesions that involve vital neurovascular skull base structures. First line treatment is total surgical excision of the tumor. If excision is not possible because of the particular anatomy or because of factors associated with a high risk of surgical complications, radiation therapy may be used. Irradiation induces a vasculitis, which halts tumor progression [3]. In the present case, because clinical and radiographic findings revealed tumor spread to several different locations, we offered radiotherapy as treatment, but the patient refused.

The association of isolated paragangliomas with systemic reactive amyloidosis has been rarely reported. Amongst paragangliomas associated amyloidosis there were two reports of glomus caroticum tumors [4, 5]. In one of them tumor was isolated unilaterally [4], and, in the other, tumor was a part of familial multiple endocrine neoplasia [5]. To our knowledge, we present the first documented case of systemic reactive amyloidosis associated with glomus jugulare and caroticum tumors.

Serum amyloid A (SAA) is formed in the liver as an acute-phase reactant secondary to provocation of inflammation by cytokines [6]. The tumor-initiated inflammatory response prompts the hepatic production of SAA protein, resulting in AA deposition in both systemic vasculature and highly vascular organs such as the spleen, kidney, and liver [7]. Inflammatory cytokines inhibit monocyte-mediated SAA degradation in vitro, which underscores the importance of adequate SAA degradation and the influence of cytokines in secondary amyloid deposition [8]. In this case, since no other inflammatory, infectious, or neoplastic cause could be detected, we speculated that systemic reactive (AA) amyloidosis was induced by the tumor-related inflammation itself.

In patients with AA amyloidosis, if the underlying pathologic condition is controlled or eliminated, deposition of AA fibrils may be halted and perhaps even reversed [7]. This is also valid for tumor-associated AA amyloidosis based on reports [9, 10] in which resection of the AA amyloidosis-inciting tumor was followed by a marked decline in proteinuria and improvement in renal function. In the present case, since neither surgery nor radiotherapy was performed, we were not able to evaluate the response to therapy.

In conclusion, this patient had long-standing paragangliomas that resulted in eventual complications due to tumor-associated systemic amyloidosis. Paragangliomas, although rare, should be considered one of the tumors that can result in AA amyloidosis.

4. Summary

The patient presented here had long-standing paragangliomas that resulted in eventual complications due to tumor-associated systemic amyloidosis. Paragangliomas, although rare, should be considered one of the tumors that can result in AA amyloidosis.

Conflict of Interests

The authors report no conflict of interests. The authors alone are responsible for the content and writing of the paper.

References

[1] S. C. Prasad, N. Thada, Pallavi, and K. C. Prasad, "Paragangliomas of the Head & Neck: the KMC experience," *Indian Journal of Otolaryngology and Head & Neck Surgery*, vol. 63, no. 1, pp. 62–73, 2011.

[2] O. Makiese, S. Chibbaro, M. Marsella, P. T. B. Huy, and B. George, "Jugular foramen paragangliomas: management, outcome and avoidance of complications in a series of 75 cases," *Neurosurgical Review*, vol. 35, no. 2, pp. 185–194, 2012.

[3] J. Reiser, K. S. Danielson, J. M. Levy, R. D. Zonis, and F. K. Christensen, "A 36-year-old woman with pulsatile mass of the left tympanic membrane," *Western Journal of Medicine*, vol. 152, no. 4, pp. 439–440, 1990.

[4] A. Gupta, A. Khaira, D. Bhowmik, S. K. Agarwal, and S. C. Tiwari, "Carotid body tumor and amyloidosis: an uncommon association," *Saudi Journal of Kidney Diseases and Transplantation*, vol. 21, no. 2, pp. 337–338, 2010.

[5] O. Larraza-Hernandez, J. Albores-Saavedra, G. Benavides, L. G. Krause, J. C. Perez-Merizaldi, and A. Ginzo, "Multiple endocrine neoplasia. Pituitary adenoma, multicentric papillary thyroid carcinoma, bilateral carotid body paraganglioma, parathyroid hyperplasia, gastric leiomyoma, and systemic amyloidosis," *The American Journal of Clinical Pathology*, vol. 78, no. 4, pp. 527–532, 1982.

[6] E. Dervisoglu, K. Yildiz, A. Hacihanefioglu, and A. Yilmaz, "Systemic reactive (AA) amyloidosis in a patient with Glanzmann thrombasthenia," *Amyloid*, vol. 14, no. 4, pp. 309–311, 2007.

[7] A. Ersoy, G. Filiz, C. Ersoy et al., "Synchronous carcinomas of stomach and bladder together with AA amyloidosis," *Nephrology*, vol. 11, no. 2, pp. 120–123, 2006.

[8] K. Migita, S. Yamasaki, K. Shibatomi et al., "Impaired degradation of serum amyloid A (SAA) protein by cytokine-stimulated monocytes," *Clinical and Experimental Immunology*, vol. 123, no. 3, pp. 408–411, 2001.

[9] A. L. Tang, D. R. Davies, and A. J. Wing, "Remission of nephrotic syndrome in amyloidosis associated with a hypernephroma," *Clinical Nephrology*, vol. 32, no. 5, pp. 225–229, 1989.

[10] I. Agha, R. Mahoney, M. Beardslee, H. Liapis, R. G. Cowart, and I. Juknevicius, "Systemic amyloidosis associated with pleomorphic sarcoma of the spleen and remission of nephrotic syndrome after removal of the tumor," *The American Journal of Kidney Diseases*, vol. 40, no. 2, pp. 411–415, 2002.

20

Biopsy Induced Arteriovenous Fistula and Venous Stenosis in a Renal Transplant

Sridhar R. Allam,[1,2] **Balamurugan Sankarapandian,**[1,2] **Imran A. Memon,**[1,2] **Patrick C. Nef,**[1,2] **Tom S. Livingston,**[3] **and George Rofaiel**[4]

[1] *Tarrant Nephrology Associates, 1001 Pennsylvania Avenue, Fort Worth, TX 76104, USA*
[2] *Division of Transplant Nephrology, Fort Worth Transplant Institute, Plaza Medical Center, 900 Eighth Avenue, Fort Worth, TX 76104, USA*
[3] *Department of Interventional Radiology, Plaza Medical Center, 900 Eighth Avenue, Fort Worth, TX 76104, USA*
[4] *Division of Transplant Surgery, Fort Worth Transplant Institute, Plaza Medical Center, 900 Eighth Avenue, Fort Worth, TX 76104, USA*

Correspondence should be addressed to Sridhar R. Allam; sallam@tarrantnephrology.com

Academic Editor: Rumeyza Kazancioglu

Renal transplant vein stenosis is a rare cause of allograft dysfunction. Percutaneous stenting appears to be safe and effective treatment for this condition. A 56-year-old Caucasian female with end stage renal disease received a deceased donor renal transplant. After transplant, her serum creatinine improved to a nadir of 1.2 mg/dL. During the third posttransplant month, her serum creatinine increased to 2.2 mg/dL. Renal transplant biopsy showed BK nephropathy. Mycophenolate was discontinued. Over the next 2 months, her serum creatinine crept up to 6.2 mg/dL. BK viremia improved from 36464 copies/mL to 15398 copies/mL. A renal transplant ultrasound showed lower pole arteriovenous fistula and abnormal waveforms in the renal vein. Carbon dioxide (CO_2) angiography demonstrated severe stenosis of the transplant renal vein. Successful coil occlusion of fistula was performed along with angioplasty and deployment of stent in the renal transplant vein. Serum creatinine improved to 1.5 mg/dL after.

1. Introduction

Renal transplant vein stenosis is a rare cause of allograft dysfunction. It can result from damage to the vein during organ procurement or from surgical complications like hematoma, lymphocele, or torsion of renal vein. Other reported etiologies include allograft rejection [1], renal vein thrombophlebitis from adjacent infected fluid collection [2], high-pressure turbulent flow in the presence of arteriovenous fistula in the renal allograft [3], external compression from the crossing iliac artery [4], preexisting renal vein stenosis in the donor kidney [5], or idiopathic [6]. Renal transplant vein stenosis should be considered in the differential diagnosis of unexplained allograft dysfunction. The use of balloon venoplasty and/or stent placement seems to be a safe and effective approach. Herein, we report a case of biopsy induced arteriovenous fistula that led to renal transplant vein stenosis and allograft dysfunction.

2. Case Presentation

A 56-year-old Caucasian female with end stage renal disease due to hypertension, who was on hemodialysis for about 5 years, received 1A 2B 1DR antigen mismatch deceased donor renal transplant. The donor was a 50-year-old lady that died of streptococcal meningitis with terminal creatinine of 0.8 and kidney donor profile index score of 47%. The cold ischemia time was 3 hours and 22 minutes and warm ischemia time was 29 minutes. Surgery was uncomplicated with implantation of kidney in the right lower quadrant of abdomen with end-to-side anastomosis to external iliac vessels. Patient received thymoglobulin (6 mg/kg total) induction therapy followed by triple immunosuppressive regimen of tacrolimus, mycophenolate, and prednisone. Patient had immediate graft function with improvement in serum creatinine to a nadir of 1.2 mg/dL. During 3-month posttransplant office visit, her serum creatinine increased to 1.6 mg/dL. She was

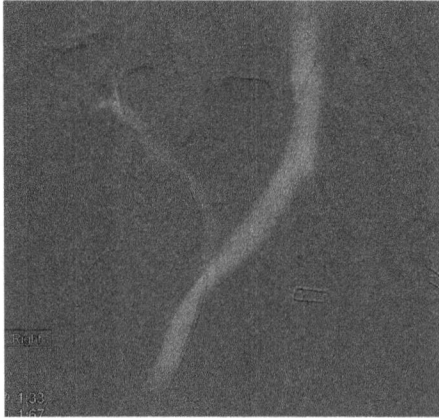

FIGURE 1: CO_2 angiogram showed high-grade stenosis of renal transplant vein.

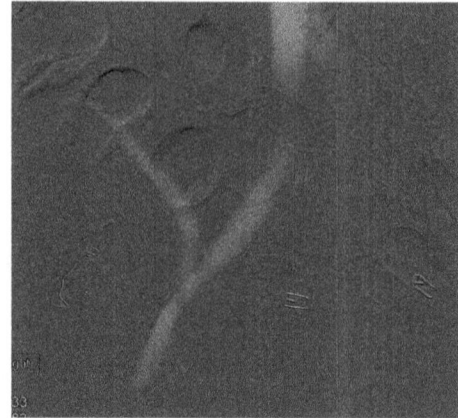

FIGURE 2: CO_2 angiogram obtained after placement of stent in renal transplant vein showed no residual stenosis.

noted to have BK viremia of 13920 copies/mL. Mycophenolate was reduced from 720 mg twice daily to 360 mg twice daily. About 2 weeks later, serum creatinine further increased to 2.2 mg/dL. Blood BK PCR increased to 36464 copies/mL. Renal transplant ultrasound showed elevated resistive indices. Renal transplant biopsy was performed that showed focal severe acute tubular injury with isolated small foci of inflammation surrounding the affected tubules. There was no evidence of tubulitis, arteritis, or significant interstitial inflammation. There was mild tubular atrophy and interstitial fibrosis. SV40 stain showed clusters of weak to very strong staining of tubular epithelial nuclei. Mycophenolate was discontinued and tacrolimus dose was adjusted to maintain trough level of 3 to 5.

Over the next month, her serum creatinine increased to 3.1 to 3.5 mg/dL range. During her fifth posttransplant month office visit, she reported progressive oliguria and lower extremity edema. She was noted to be fluid overloaded on exam. Serum creatinine further increased to 6.2 mg/dL. Random urine protein by creatinine ratio showed nephrotic range proteinuria with a ratio of 4.5, which was a significant increase from 1.1 a month prior. She was hospitalized at that point and was dialyzed on two consecutive days for fluid overload. Blood BK PCR actually improved to 15398 copies/mL. A renal transplant ultrasound showed lower pole arteriovenous fistula, increased velocities, and abnormal waveforms in the renal vein. Given dialysis dependent allograft dysfunction despite improvement in BK viremia and abnormal findings of the ultrasound, we proceeded with interventional radiological procedures. Common iliac angiography with CO_2 demonstrated patent common and external iliac arteries. There was a widely patent end-to-side renal artery anastomosis. Arteriovenous fistula was demonstrated in the lower pole of the transplant kidney with early filling of the renal vein. There was severe stenosis of the main renal vein. Successful coil occlusion of fistula was performed using a 3 mm × 50 mm microcoil. Then, renal venography using CO_2 was performed that confirmed a high-grade stenosis of the renal vein for a length of approximately 30 mm (Figure 1). Angioplasty was initially performed with 8 mm × 4 cm balloon followed by

10 mm × 4 cm balloon. Repeat venography again demonstrated moderately severe stenosis of the renal vein. Then, 8 mm × 30 mm self-expanding stent was deployed across the renal vein stenosis. Repeat venography demonstrated no significant residual stenosis (Figure 2). Percutaneous renal transplant biopsy performed at the same time showed moderate to severe acute tubular injury with mild interstitial infiltrate consisting of lymphocytes and plasma cells. There was mild arteriosclerosis, interstitial fibrosis, and tubular atrophy (about 10%). There was positive tubular epithelial nuclear staining for SV40. In addition, there was extensive interstitial edema, likely a consequence of significant venous outflow obstruction. Her urine output significantly improved after renal vein stenting and dialysis was discontinued after a total of three dialysis sessions. Serum creatinine eventually stabilized around 1.5 mg/dL range. Patient was given oral anticoagulation combined with antiplatelet therapy Aspirin 81 mg daily for 6 months after the procedure followed by long-term administration of Aspirin 325 mg daily.

3. Discussion

This patient's course is consistent with biopsy induced arteriovenous fistula that likely led to renal vein stenosis in the allograft. Although not reported in the literature before, another potential reason for development of venous stenosis in our patient could be BK virus induced inflammation. Progressive rise in serum creatinine despite improvement in BK viremia/nephropathy, extensive interstitial edema on biopsy that is indicative of venous outflow obstruction, and prompt improvement in allograft function following renal vein stenting support venous stenosis as the predominant etiology of her allograft dysfunction. A series of 8 cases of renal transplant vein stenosis causing allograft dysfunction was first reported in 1991 [3]. Of these 8 cases, 5 were causally related to development of arteriovenous fistula following renal transplant biopsies. Arteriovenous fistula causes high-pressure turbulent blood flow in the vein that may lead to spasm and stenosis of vein over time. Progression of venous stenosis can lead to complete occlusion and allograft loss [3]. There are no specific clinical symptoms or signs to suspect allograft dysfunction from renal vein stenosis. It can present weeks to years after renal transplantation. Diagnosis can be made by duplex ultrasound in some cases by visualization of reduced caliber and increased velocities in the vein. CT and MR angiography are other imaging modalities that can be used for diagnosis [2, 5]. Conventional or CO_2 based venography may be required to diagnose or confirm renal vein stenosis suggested by other imaging modalities. Once the diagnosis is confirmed by venography, the balloon venoplasty and stent placement can be performed at the same time. This percutaneous technique holds promise by successful treatment of this condition and avoidance of open surgical procedure.

In summary, renal transplant vein stenosis should be considered in the differential diagnosis of unexplained allograft dysfunction. Percutaneous venoplasty and/or stenting appear to be safe and effective treatment for this rare condition.

Conflict of Interests

The authors declare that there is no conflict of interests regarding the publication of this paper.

Acknowledgments

The authors thank Denise S. Young, RN, and Jennifer A. Johnson, APRN, for their contribution to this work.

References

[1] J. P. Cercueil, D. Chevet, C. Mousson, E. Tatou, D. Krause, and G. Rifle, "Acquired vein stenosis of renal allograft—percutaneous treatment with self-expanding metallic stent," *Nephrology Dialysis Transplantation*, vol. 12, no. 4, pp. 825–826, 1997.

[2] K. K. Jeong, J. H. Duck, and K.-S. Cho, "Post-infectious diffuse venous stenosis after renal transplantation: duplex ultrasonography and CT angiography," *European Radiology*, vol. 12, no. 3, pp. S118–S120, 2002.

[3] S. Olliff, R. Negus, C. Deane, and H. Walters, "Renal transplant vein stenosis: demonstration and percutaneous venoplasty of a new vascular complication in the transplant kidney," *Clinical Radiology*, vol. 43, no. 1, pp. 42–46, 1991.

[4] A. Obed, D. C. Uihlein, N. Zorger et al., "Severe renal vein stenosis of a kidney transplant with beneficial clinical course after successful percutaneous stenting," *American Journal of Transplantation*, vol. 8, no. 10, pp. 2173–2176, 2008.

[5] J. Pine, R. Rajaganeshan, R. Baker et al., "Early postoperative renal vein stenosis after renal transplantation: a report of two cases," *Journal of Vascular and Interventional Radiology*, vol. 21, no. 2, pp. 303–304, 2010.

[6] Q. Mei, X. He, W. Lu, and Y. Li, "Renal vein stenosis after renal transplantation: treatment with stent placement," *Journal of Vascular and Interventional Radiology*, vol. 21, no. 5, pp. 756–758, 2010.

21

Plotting of Ethylene Glycol Blood Concentrations Using Linear Regression before and during Hemodialysis in a Case of Intoxication and Pharmacokinetic Review

Youngho Kim

Division of Nephrology, Department of Internal Medicine, University of New Mexico, 901 University Boulevard SE, Suite 150, MSC 04-2785, Albuquerque, NM 87106, USA

Correspondence should be addressed to Youngho Kim; ablapia@gmail.com

Academic Editor: Aikaterini Papagianni

Introduction. As blood concentration measurement of commonly abused alcohol is readily available, the equation was proposed in previous publication to predict the change of their concentration. The change of ethylene glycol (EG) concentrations was studied in a case of intoxication to estimate required time for hemodialysis (HD) using linear regression. *Case Report.* A 55-year-old female with past medical history of seizure disorder, bipolar disorder, and chronic pain was admitted due to severe agitation. The patient was noted to have metabolic acidosis with elevated anion gap and acute kidney injury, which prompted blood concentration measurement of commonly abused alcohol. Her initial EG concentration was 26.45 mmol/L. Fomepizole therapy was initiated, soon followed by HD to enhance clearance. *Discussion.* Plotting of natural logarithm of EG concentrations over time showed that EG elimination follows first-order kinetics and predicts the change of its concentration well. Pharmacokinetic review revealed minimal elimination of EG by alcohol dehydrogenase (ADH) which could be related to genetic predisposition for ADH activity and home medications as well as presence of propylene glycol. Pharmacokinetics of EG is relatively well studied with published parameters. Consideration and application of pharmacokinetics could assist in management of EG intoxication including HD planning.

1. Introduction

Ethylene glycol is sweet-tasting chemical compound without odour or color found in many commercially available products such as automobile antifreeze, deicing fluids, paint, and cosmetics. American Association of Poison Control Centers reports 2070 cases of ethylene glycol exposure from automotive products alone that were treated in health care facility in 2012. Alcohols are rather benign in their original form and they become toxic by being metabolized into organic acids that consume buffering capacity with development of metabolic acidosis and cause tissue injury. Hepatic metabolism accounts for approximately 80% of ethylene glycol elimination, with the remaining 20% being eliminated unchanged in urine [1, 2]. Ethylene glycol is metabolized via alcohol dehydrogenase (ADH) to glycoaldehyde which is rapidly metabolized to glycolate, the metabolite mainly responsible for the metabolic acidosis in ethylene glycol intoxication. Glycolate is metabolized by various pathways,

including one to oxalate which rapidly precipitates with calcium in various tissues and in the urine [3]. Tissue toxicity of ethylene glycol and its metabolites has been reported to show following gradient: glyoxalate > glycoaldehyde > glycolate > ethylene glycol [4]. For nephrotoxicity, glycoaldehyde and glyoxylate are the principal metabolites responsible for causing ATP depletion and phospholipid and enzyme destruction in renal tubular cell [5]. Treatment recommendation for ethylene glycol intoxication includes alcohol dehydrogenase inhibition by fomepizole (4-methylpyrazole, Antizol) to prevent biotransformation of ethylene glycol to its toxic metabolites and enhanced clearance by hemodialysis. Hemodialysis is recommended when severe metabolic acidosis (pH < 7.3) is unresponsive to therapy or renal failure exists, or if the ethylene glycol concentration is greater than 50 mg/dL unless fomepizole is being administered and the patient is asymptomatic with a normal arterial pH [1, 6]. However, ethylene glycol elimination was directly proportional to the remaining renal function as estimated by creatinine clearance, with median fractional excretion of 25.5%, and patients with normal serum creatinine concentration at the initiation of fomepizole therapy had rapid rates of renal elimination that rationalize selective hemodialysis therapy in patients treated with fomepizole when renal elimination pathway is intact [7]. As measurement of blood concentration of commonly abused alcohols is readily available in many clinical circumstances at the time of care, the equation was proposed and validated in previous publications to plan the duration of hemodialysis therapy [8, 9]. A case of intoxication was encountered during inpatient consultation service rotation that was treated with fomepizole therapy and hemodialysis. Pharmacokinetic aspect of ethylene glycol concentration during clinical course was studied and applied to predict the change of its concentration using linear regression and to estimate the required duration of hemodialysis and its efficacy.

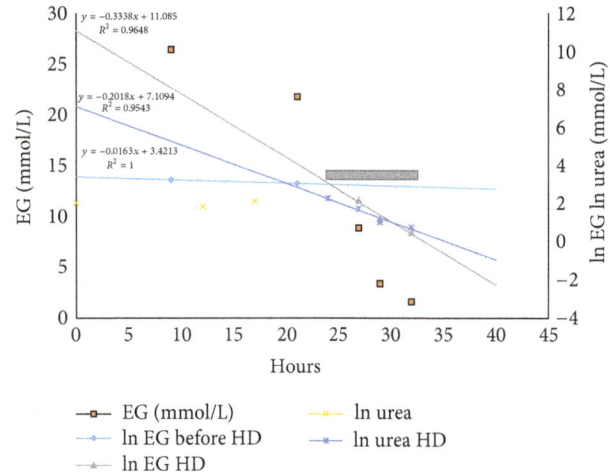

FIGURE 1: Gray bar represents hemodialysis.

2. Case Report

A 55-year-old female with past medical history of seizure disorder, bipolar disorder, and chronic pain was admitted to ICU due to severe agitation. The patient complained of dizziness along with nausea shortly before hospitalization which was first reported to home physical therapist. There was no neurological deficit besides becoming agitated progressively over time for which she was given several doses of benzodiazepines. Her initial vital signs were blood pressure 119/75 mmHg, pulse rate 58/min, tympanic temperature 98.5, and body weight 99 kg. The second set of laboratory data after ICU admission revealed following: sodium 148 mEq/L, potassium 5.6 mEq/L, chloride 108 mEq/L, carbon dioxide 6 mEq/L, urea nitrogen 24 mg/dL, creatinine 1.85 mg/dL, calcium 8.7 mg/dL, and albumin 4.0 mg/dL. The serum anion gap was elevated at 34. Serum osmolality was not obtained. The patient was intubated for airway protection using lorazepam and rocuronium. Arterial blood gas revealed pH 7.22 and PCO_2 17 mmHg. Her baseline creatinine before admission was noted as 1.1 mg/dL. Blood concentrations of commonly abused alcohols were sought given anion gap metabolic acidosis and additional history of psychosocial issues from family. Urinalysis was negative for crystals. Ethylene glycol level became available 169 mg/dL (26.45 mmol/L) 19 hours after admission and other alcohols were negative. Glycolic acid or glyoxylic acid blood concentration was not obtained. Quantification of consumed ethylene glycol was not possible due to the lack of reliable consumption history. Plotting of blood concentrations of ethylene glycol and urea and their corresponding natural logarithm with trend lines using linear regression function is shown in Figure 1. Fomepizole therapy was initiated and, within 2 hours, hemodialysis followed. The patient was treated using Polyflux Revaclear MAX dialyzer (Gambro, 1.8 m² membrane surface area) via right internal jugular vascular catheter. Blood flow and dialysate flow were set 300–400 mL/min and 1.5 times blood flow, respectively. Total volume treated was 138.6 L for 8 hours with average blood flow 290 mL/min. The patient was maintained on continuous IV drip of lorazepam for sedation along with several doses

of IV phenytoin for subtherapeutic drug level noted upon admission.

3. Discussion

During hemodialysis, solute elimination occurs via the first-order kinetic process, and the distribution of a drug in a dialyzed, renal failure patient can be expressed by the one-compartment model [7, 10]. Change of concentration over time in first-order kinetics could be expressed as below and integrated to encompass the times of sampling and measurement to evaluate kinetic process and natural logarithm of concentration change would show linear relation over time:

$$\text{rate} = -\frac{d[C]}{dt} = k[C]$$

$$\longrightarrow \frac{d[C]}{[C]} = -k \cdot dt$$

$$\longrightarrow \int \frac{d[C]}{[C]} = \int -k \cdot dt \tag{1}$$

$$\longrightarrow \int_0^t \frac{1}{[C]} \cdot d[C] = -k \int_0^t dt$$

$$\longrightarrow \ln[C]\,t - \ln[C]\,o = -kt$$

$$\longrightarrow \ln[C]\,t = -kt + \ln[C]\,o,$$

where C is concentration, t is time, and k is elimination rate constant.

Ethylene glycol concentrations during hemodialysis show exponential decrease over time and their corresponding natural logarithm exhibits linear relation suggesting first-order kinetic elimination of ethylene glycol. Fomepizole therapy was started only 2 hours prior to hemodialysis which makes its impact on ethylene glycol concentration in our case minimal. Total elimination rate constant before hemodialysis, sum of renal and hepatic elimination by ADH ($k^{\text{total before HD}} = k^{\text{renal}} + k^{\text{ADH}}$), is calculated to be 0.0163 h⁻¹, expressed as a slope of function of natural logarithm of ethylene glycol concentrations over time. Ethylene glycol elimination is known to follow first-order kinetics in the absence of treatment, with an estimated serum half-life of between 3 and 9 hours [7, 11] and it was 42.5 hours in our case. k^{renal} was estimated as $0.0128\,\text{h}^{-1}$ based on creatinine clearance by Cockcroft-Gault formula, suggested fractional excretion, and volume of distribution. It would leave much smaller k^{ADH} than previously observed which could be due to her genetic predisposition for ADH activity and home medications including morphine and methylphenidate that were known to inhibit ADH activity in vitro [12, 13]. Interestingly, propylene glycol level became positive later in the course and its concentration peaked to 88 mg/dL. Continuous IV drips of lorazepam and phenytoin were thought to be sources. Propylene glycol, though considered generally safe, can cause intoxication when large quantities are ingested. Several cases of lactic acidosis after inadvertent propylene glycol intoxication were reported in patients with renal dysfunction [14]. Propylene glycol shares the same metabolic pathway with ethylene glycol and may compete for ADH interfering with hepatic elimination of ethylene glycol in our case. Total elimination rate constant during hemodialysis was significantly increased to $0.3338\,\text{h}^{-1}$. Manufacturer's box inlet indicates in vitro urea clearance of 293 mL/min with blood flow at 300 mL/min which we achieved close in our case. Actual urea elimination rate constant and clearance in our case were $0.2018\,\text{h}^{-1}$ and 133.5 mL/min, respectively, based on Watson estimate of total body water and the difference of urea clearance could be partly from in vivo urea generation in catabolic state of critically ill patient. Using the assumption that toxic alcohols would have a dialysis clearance similar to urea and the volume of distribution of toxin is the total body water as determined by the Watson formula, the following equation was proposed to estimate the required dialysis time in hours to reach a 5 mmol/L toxin concentration target [8]:

From the above equations, $\ln[C]t = -kt + \ln[C]o$ and since $K(\text{clearance}) = k \cdot Vd$,

$$-\frac{V \ln (5/Co)}{0.06K}, \tag{2}$$

where V is Watson estimate of total body water, Co is the initial concentration (mmol/L), K is clearance of toxin that is assumed to be 80% of the manufacturer-specified dialyzer urea clearance (mL/min) at the initial observed blood flow rate to allow estimates to be made at the start of dialysis [8], and 0.06 is conversion factor to have product in hour. There was significant difference in the manufacturer's in vitro urea clearance, actual urea, and ethylene clearance during hemodialysis, the equation produced 4.3 hours of required dialysis time which was overestimated approximately by 1 in our case when compared to linear regression plot of actual concentration change of ethylene glycol. Half of the hemodialysis after initial 4 hours out of total 8-hour treatment did not contribute much in regard to ethylene glycol concentration reduction clinically.

In conclusion, plotting of ethylene glycol blood concentrations and their natural logarithm showed that ethylene glycol elimination during hemodialysis followed first-order kinetics and predicted the change of its concentration well. In our case, hepatic elimination of ethylene glycol by ADH was minimal which could be related to genetic predisposition for ADH activity and home medications as well as presence of propylene glycol. Pharmacokinetics of ethylene glycol is relatively well studied as one of the commonly abused alcohols with published parameters. Consideration and application of pharmacokinetics could assist with hemodialysis planning in clinical practice.

Conflict of Interests

The author declares that there is no conflict of interests regarding the publication of this paper.

References

[1] N. Vasavada, C. Williams, and R. N. Hellman, "Ethylene glycol intoxication: case report and pharmacokinetic perspectives," *Pharmacotherapy*, vol. 23, no. 12 I, pp. 1652–1658, 2003.

[2] D. G. Barceloux, G. R. Bond, E. P. Krenzelok, H. Cooper, and J. A. Vale, "American Academy of Clinical Toxicology practice guidelines on the treatment of methanol poisoning," *Journal of Toxicology. Clinical Toxicology*, vol. 40, no. 4, pp. 415–446, 2002.

[3] D. Jacobsen and K. E. McMartin, "Methanol and ethylene glycol poisonings. Mechanism of toxicity, clinical course, diagnosis and treatment," *Medical Toxicology and Adverse Drug Experience*, vol. 1, no. 5, pp. 309–334, 1986.

[4] P. A. Gabow, K. Clay, J. B. Sullivan, and R. Lepoff, "Organic acids in ethylene glycol intoxication," *Annals of Internal Medicine*, vol. 105, no. 1, pp. 16–20, 1986.

[5] V. Poldelski, A. Johnson, S. Wright, V. D. Rosa, and R. A. Zager, "Ethylene glycol-mediated tubular injury: idenitification of critical metabolites and injury pathways," *American Journal of Kidney Diseases*, vol. 38, no. 2, pp. 339–348, 2001.

[6] D. G. Barceloux, E. P. Krenzelok, K. Olson, W. Watson, and H. Miller, "American academy of clinical toxicology practice guidelines on the treatment of ethylene glycol poisoning. Ad Hoc committee," *Journal of Toxicology—Clinical Toxicology*, vol. 37, no. 5, pp. 537–560, 1999.

[7] M. L. A. Sivilotti, M. J. Burns, K. E. McMartin, and J. Brent, "Toxicokinetics of ethylene glycol during fomepizole therapy: implications for management," *Annals of Emergency Medicine*, vol. 36, no. 2, pp. 114–125, 2000.

[8] D. J. Hirsch, K. K. Jindal, P. Wong, and A. D. Fraser, "A simple method to estimate the required dialysis time for cases of alcohol poisoning," *Kidney International*, vol. 60, no. 5, pp. 2021–2024, 2001.

[9] G. M. Youssef and D. J. Hirsch, "Validation of a method to predict required dialysis time for cases of methanol and ethylene glycol poisoning," *American Journal of Kidney Diseases*, vol. 46, no. 3, pp. 509–511, 2005.

[10] M. Brvar, M. Vrtovec, D. Kovač, G. Kozelj, T. Pezdir, and M. Bunc, "Haemodialysis clearance of baclofen," *European Journal of Clinical Pharmacology*, vol. 63, no. 12, pp. 1143–1146, 2007.

[11] A. F. Eder, C. M. McGrath, Y. G. Dowdy et al., "Ethylene glycol poisoning: toxicokinetic and analytical factors affecting laboratory diagnosis," *Clinical Chemistry*, vol. 44, no. 1, pp. 168–177, 1998.

[12] M. G. Roig, F. Bello, F. J. Burguillo, J. M. Cachaza, and J. F. Kennedy, "In vitro interaction between psychotropic drugs

and alcohol dehydrogenase activity," *Journal of Pharmaceutical Sciences*, vol. 80, no. 3, pp. 267–270, 1991.

[13] W. F. Bosron, L. Lumeng, and T.-K. Li, "Genetic polymorphism of enzymes of alcohol metabolism and susceptibility to alcoholic liver disease," *Molecular Aspects of Medicine*, vol. 10, no. 2, pp. 147–158, 1988.

[14] A. Zosel, E. Egelhoff, and K. Heard, "Severe lactic acidosis after an iatrogenic propylene glycol overdose," *Pharmacotherapy*, vol. 30, no. 2, article 219, 2010.

22

Blockade of Alternative Complement Pathway in Dense Deposit Disease

Aurore Berthe-Aucejo,[1] Mathieu Sacquépée,[2] Marc Fila,[3] Michel Peuchmaur,[4] Emilia Perrier-Cornet,[1] Véronique Frémeaux-Bacchi,[5] and Georges Deschênes[3]

[1] Service de Pharmacie, Hôpital Robert Debré, 48 boulevard Sérurier, 75019 Paris, France
[2] Service de Néphrologie, Centre Hospitalier Territorial de Nouvelle Calédonie, Gaston Bourret, BP J5, 98849 Nouméa, New Caledonia
[3] Service de Néphrologie Pédiatrique, Hôpital Robert Debré, 48 boulevard Sérurier, 75019 Paris, France
[4] Laboratoire d'Anatomopathologie, Hôpital Robert Debré, 48 boulevard Sérurier, 75019 Paris, France
[5] Laboratoire d'Immunologie, Hôpital Européen Georges-Pompidou, 20-40 rue Leblanc, 75015 Paris, France

Correspondence should be addressed to Aurore Berthe-Aucejo; aurore.berthe84@gmail.com

Academic Editors: R. Enríquez, H. Matsukura, and K. Nozu

A patient aged 17 with dense deposit disease associated with complement activation, circulating C3 Nef, and Factor H mutation presented with nephrotic syndrome and hypertension. Steroid therapy, plasma exchange, and rituximab failed to improve proteinuria and hypertension despite a normalization of the circulating sC5b9 complex. Eculizumab, a monoclonal antibody directed against C5, was used to block the terminal product of the complement cascade. The dose was adapted to achieve a CH50 below 10%, but proteinuria and blood pressure were not improved after 3 months of treatment.

1. Introduction

Dense deposit disease or DDD (formerly referred to as membranoproliferative glomerulonephritis type II) is a rare disease affecting less than 2 people per million, both adults and children. Nephrotic syndrome, severe hypertension, and progression to chronic renal failure are usually observed in patients with DDD. The histological pattern in light microcopy is limited to an enlargement of the mesangium with a mild mesangial cell hypercellularity [1]. Electron microscopy allows us to evidence electron-dense enlargement of the glomerular basement membrane that specially affects the lamina densa. Paradoxically, the precise composition of the dense deposits is not really known [2], while C3 fraction is only seen in the margin of the dense deposits but not within the dense deposits [1]. Complement activation with low C3 levels due to complement alternative pathway dysregulation is mostly due to the presence of a circulation C3 nephritic factor (C3 NeF) which is an autoantibody that stabilizes C3 convertase. In addition, mutations in the factor H gene have also been reported in a few patients [3]. Steroid therapy can be used but the efficacy was not proven. Specific treatment can be proposed like plasma exchanges. They is used to clear the C3 NeF and restore a normal complement balance. They have also shown encouraging results. New therapeutic approaches such as rituximab (anti-CD20) or eculizumab (anti-C5) could be proposed [1]. Eculizumab, a monoclonal antibody directed against complement C5 that blocks the final products of complement activation, might subsequently be considered as a relevant treatment in DDD. Here, we present the case of a patient presenting with DDD, in whom eculizumab was tried during 3 months.

2. Case Presentation

The patient was a young man aged 17 and born from unrelated parents. In September 2007, at the age of 15, hypertension

(a)

(b)

(c)

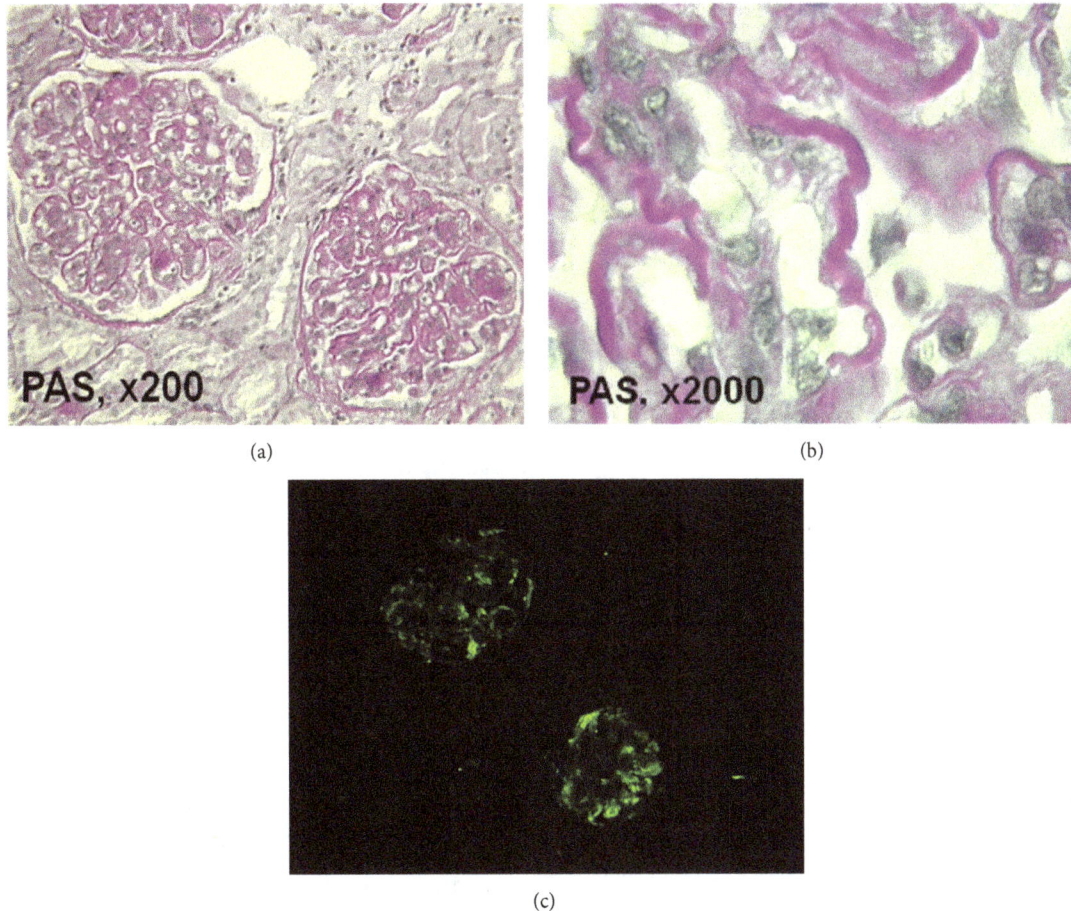

FIGURE 1: (a) Type II membranoproliferative glomerulonephritis characterized by mesangial matrix and cellular increases is responsible for a lobular accentuation associated with a diffuse and intense staining of the peripheral basement membrane (periodic acid-Schiff [PAS], magnification [G]: ×200). (b) The diffuse and intense staining of the peripheral basement membrane indicates the presence of dense deposit material (PAS, G ×2000). (c) Immunofluorescence techniques show segmental pseudo linear and granular IgM deposits along the peripheral capillary wall (fluorescein isothiocyanate anti-IgM, G ×100).

and nephrotic syndrome (proteinuria = 2.14 g/24 h, plasma albumin = 25 g/L) led to performing a renal biopsy and he was diagnosed with a DDD in October 2007. Hepatitis C virus (HCV) and human immunodeficiency virus (HIV) tests were negative and the patient was vaccinated against hepatitis B virus (HBV). Low C3 (538 mg/L; normal value 660–1250) with normal C4 (160 mg/L; normal values 93–380) levels were evidenced and related to a circulating C3 NeF. Plasma level of antigenic factor H was 54% (normal value 65–140), while those of factor B and factor I were normal. In addition, gene sequencing analysis of complement factor H gene showed an heterozygous mutation (p. R232X) located in SCR 4 (short consensus repeats) leading to a deficiency in factor H. Renal function was within normal limits at this period (serum creatinine = 59 μmol/L). The patient received 10 plasma exchanges against fresh frozen plasma from April 2008 to June 2008 and then four injections of rituximab, a monoclonal antibody directed against CD20, that led to B cell depletion during several months and was supposed to control the C3 NeF. This treatment showed no efficacy on nephrotic syndrome. The plasma level of sC5b9

complex level was high at 755 ng/mL in February 2008 and was normalized (<600 ng/mL) before plasma exchange. Oral alternative-day steroid therapy (prednisolone 40 mg/48 h) as well as ramipril and irbesartan was given from June 2008, but the patient disrupted the medical follow-up during 2 years. In March 2010, the blood pressure was 132/85, proteinuria was 2.55 g/L (0.26 g/mmol of creatinine), serum albumin was 16.7 g/L, and eGFR was 93 mL/min/1.73/m^2 according to the 2009 Schwartz formula. A second renal biopsy was realized and showed dense deposits in 100% of glomerulus and 15% of interstitial fibrosis (Figures 1(a), 1(b), and 1(c)). The patient was vaccinated with Menactra to prevent *Neisseria meningitidis* infection as a preparation prior to introduce eculizumab. Initial schedule was similar to those proposed in patients with atypical haemolytic uremic syndrome, namely, 900 mg every week for 4 weeks and then 1200 mg on week 5 and every 2 weeks. Treatment was associated with penicillin V treatment. After 5 weeks of treatment, CH50 level decreased from 146% to an undetectable plasma level. From week 8, CH50 resumed to be 25% and the dose of eculizumab was subsequently increased to 1500 mg every week and by day

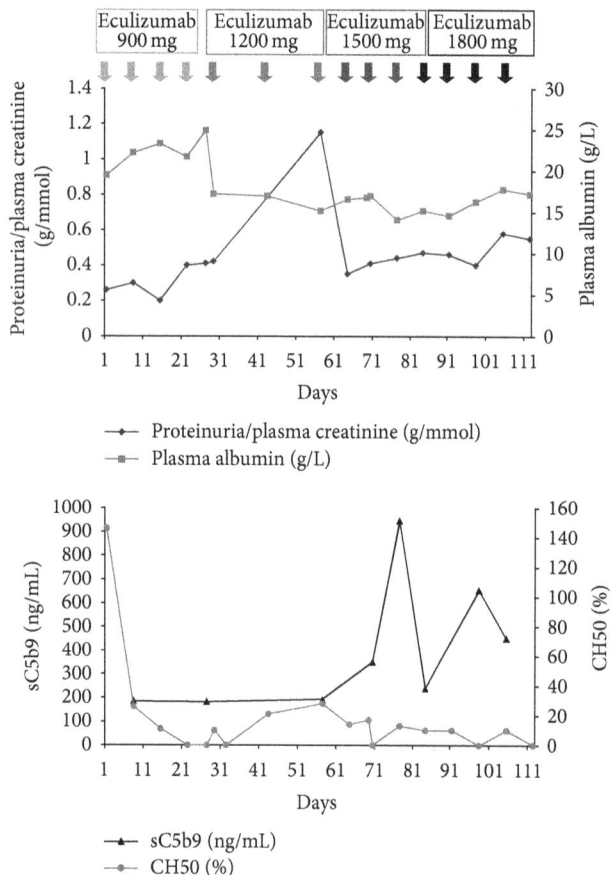

FIGURE 2: Response to eculizumab therapy in dense deposit disease.

84 to 1800 mg every week in order to achieve a complete and continuous blockade of CH50 (below 10%, Figure 2). At the time of the first injection, the plasma level of sC5b9 was normal and remained in the normal range during the first 7 injections. Paradoxically, the level rose up to 945 ng/mL, while the dose of eculizumab was increased to 1500 mg per week and more. Renal function, blood pressure, and proteinuria were unchanged after 3 months of treatment (Figure 2). Plasma albumin transiently increased to 25 g/L by day 25 and then after return to the initial level or below (Figure 1). Subsequently, eculizumab was stopped after 14 injections and 3.5 months of continuous treatment. No side effect was observed during the treatment.

The patient is lost to follow-up for one year. At last control, nephrotic syndrome was persistent and the patient was considered to have a normal renal function.

3. Discussion

The diagnosis of DDD is frequently done in children below 15 years of age, with half of them progressing to end-stage renal failure in less than 10 years. In immunofluorescence, C3 deposits feature a "railroad track" on both sides of dense deposits, while IgG deposits are lacking. In most patients, a positive C3 NeF, an autoantibody that stabilizes the C3 convertase, is associated with an alternative pathway C3

consumption. Therefore, the fluid phase-restricted complement alternative pathway dysregulation with a continuously activated and consumed C3 should be a prerequisite for the development of DDD [4]. Most treatments of DDD are based on results obtained in short case series due to the rarity of the disease [5]. Steroids are usually considered as ineffective in DDD although several pediatric case reports showed improvement of proteinuria. Plasma replacement therapy has also been reported in single case reports and might stabilize the creatinine clearance in the rapidly progressive forms of the disease. According to the permanent activation of the complement alternative pathway, the treatment of DDD with eculizumab could be a relevant alternative treatment and has been reported to reduce the level of proteinuria in the first case reports [6–9]. Nevertheless, the most recent series of 6 patients treated with eculizumab, whose 3 patients were diagnosed with DDD, showed variability of responses from no effect to a partial or a transient effect [7]. Consistently, our patient did not show any benefit of this very expensive drug, despite the close control of a complete blockade of the final complement byproducts during 3.5 months. Among the many causes of failure, the duration of the disease over 2 years prior to the treatment and a period of active therapy limited to 3 months are the main limits in the interpretation of this case report. Moreover, discordance between sC5b9 and CH50 levels was observed and not explained. Indeed, sC5b9 level paradoxically rose after 10 injections of eculizumab, while CH50 level was undetectable suggesting a complete blockade of the alternative pathway. Failure can be explained by a normal level of sC5b9 at the time of the first injection of eculizumab, while previous reports showing an efficacy of eculizumab include patients with an initial high plasma level of sC5b9 complex [7, 9].

We conclude that the short-term blockade of complement is not systematically successful in all patients with DDD. As previously suggested, additional research is needed to isolate the subgroup of patients, in whom eculizumab could be used with success and will certainly improve our understanding of the disease.

Conflict of Interests

The authors declare that there is no conflict of interests regarding the publication of this paper.

References

[1] R. J. H. Smith, J. Alexander, P. N. Barlow et al., "New approaches to the treatment of dense deposit disease," *Journal of the American Society of Nephrology*, vol. 18, no. 9, pp. 2447–2456, 2007.

[2] S. Sethi, J. D. Gamez, J. A. Vrana et al., "Glomeruli of Dense Deposit Disease contain components of the alternative and terminal complement pathway," *Kidney International*, vol. 75, no. 9, pp. 952–960, 2009.

[3] A. Servais, L.-H. Noël, L. T. Roumenina et al., "Acquired and genetic complement abnormalities play a critical role in dense deposit disease and other C3 glomerulopathies," *Kidney International*, vol. 82, no. 4, pp. 454–464, 2012.

[4] R. Martínez-Barricarte, M. Heurich, F. Valdes-Cañedo et al., "Human C3 mutation reveals a mechanism of dense deposit disease pathogenesis and provides insights into complement activation and regulation," *Journal of Clinical Investigation*, vol. 120, no. 10, pp. 3702–3712, 2010.

[5] G. B. Appel, H. T. Cook, G. Hageman et al., "Membranoproliferative glomerulonephritis type II (dense deposit disease): an update," *Journal of the American Society of Nephrology*, vol. 16, no. 5, pp. 1392–1403, 2005.

[6] M. Vivarelli, A. Pasini, and F. Emma, "Eculizumab for the treatment of dense-deposit disease," *New England Journal of Medicine*, vol. 366, no. 12, pp. 1163–1165, 2012.

[7] A. S. Bomback, R. J. Smith, G. R. Barile et al., "Eculizumab for dense deposit disease and C3 glomerulonephritis," *Clinical Journal of the American Society of Nephrology*, vol. 7, no. 5, pp. 748–756, 2012.

[8] E. Daina, M. Noris, and G. Remuzzi, "Eculizumab in a patient with dense-deposit disease," *New England Journal of Medicine*, vol. 366, no. 12, pp. 1161–1163, 2012.

[9] S. Radhakrishnan, A. Lunn, M. Kirschfink et al., "Eculizumab and refractory membranoproliferative glomerulonephritis," *New England Journal of Medicine*, vol. 366, no. 12, pp. 1165–1166, 2012.

23

Association of Acute Interstitial Nephritis with Carnivora, a Venus Flytrap Extract, in a 30-Year-Old Man with Hodgkin's Lymphoma

Susan Ziolkowski and Catherine Moore

University of Rochester Medical Center, 601 Elmwood Avenue, P.O. Box MED, Rochester, NY 14642, USA

Correspondence should be addressed to Susan Ziolkowski; susan_ziolkowski@urmc.rochester.edu

Academic Editor: Theodore I. Steinman

Acute interstitial nephritis (AIN) is a common cause of acute kidney injury and has been associated with a variety of medications. This is the case of 30-year-old man with Hodgkin's lymphoma who on routine labs before chemotherapy was found to have acute nonoliguric renal failure. A kidney biopsy was performed and confirmed the diagnosis of acute interstitial nephritis. The patient had taken several medications including a higher dose of Carnivora, a Venus flytrap extract, composed of numerous amino acids. The medication was discontinued and kidney function improved towards the patient's baseline indicating that this may be the possible cause of his AIN. Proximal tubular cell uptake of amino acids increasing transcription of nuclear factor-kappaB is a proposed mechanism of AIN from this compound.

1. Introduction

Acute interstitial nephritis (AIN) is a common cause of acute kidney injury (AKI) causing immune-mediated tubulointerstitial injury with an overall incidence of 15–27% of all renal biopsies performed for AKI [1]. Medications, most notably NSAIDs and antibiotics, are the most common cause of AIN representing >75% of cases. Systemic diseases such as sarcoidosis and systemic lupus erythematosus are other causes, while about 5–10% of cases are idiopathic [1]. Cases of AIN commonly present with nonspecific signs such as nausea, vomiting, and malaise. Other findings such as fever, rash, eosinophilia, oliguria, and arthralgia present at varying frequencies [2]. Renal manifestations of AIN generally occur within three weeks of the inciting drug with an average delay of ten days [3].

Patients who discontinue the inciting medication within two weeks of the onset of AIN are more likely to recover renal function than those who continue the medication for a longer period of time [4]. Therefore, new medications that are thought to cause AIN should be reported and promptly discontinued by a clinician to improve a patient's chance of recovery.

Carnivora is a supplement that is extracted from *Dionaea muscipula*, a species of the Venus flytrap plant. The product is manufactured in Germany, sold via the internet, and marketed as an "immune modulator" and antioxidant that selectively kills "primitive cells" that intrude the human body without harming the body's own cells. The physiologic effect is much like the Venus flytrap where foreign animal and vegetable products are digested without harming the plant's own cells. Numerous compounds including droserone, hydroplumbagin, quercetin, formic acid, myricetin, gallic acid, and several amino acids are naturally present in this compound. There have been no reported cases of AIN associated with Carnivora, exposure to Venus flytraps, or any of the above compounds [5]. The patient presented had other types of drug exposure such as metoclopramide, promethazine, and baclofen; however, a likely association with Carnivora is discussed below.

2. A Case Report

The patient is a 30 year old man with recurrent Hodgkin's lymphoma originally diagnosed in January 2010 who

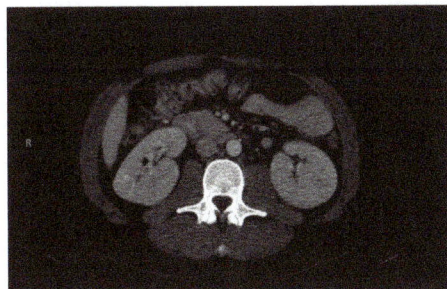

FIGURE 1: CT scan with oral contrast showing enlarged 15 cm right kidney and 14.5 cm left kidney with no hydronephrosis.

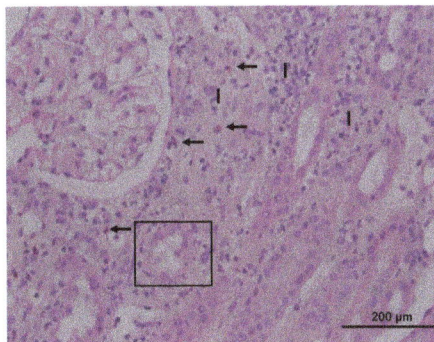

FIGURE 2: Photomicrograph showing active interstitial nephritis with acute tubulitis and mixed interstitial inflammation including numerous eosinophils. I: interstitial inflammation, arrows: eosinophils, and box: active tubulitis (H&E 30x magnification).

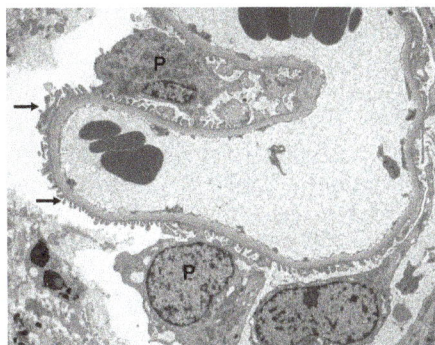

FIGURE 3: Electron microscopy showing lack of podocyte effacement or glomerular basement membrane changes. Arrows: intact foot processes, P: podocytes (original mag. = 3500x).

underwent an autologous stem cell transplant at that time. Routine restaging scans revealed a recurrence in abdominal lymph nodes and the patient underwent an exploratory laparotomy and mesenteric lymph node biopsy, which confirmed a recurrence of Hodgkin lymphoma. During this hospitalization, he had two doses of ampicillin-sulbactam and limited doses of promethazine, metoclopramide, and baclofen. He admitted to taking a supplement, Carnivora, at home for about one year, which he discontinued during his hospital stay. He was discharged from the hospital with a creatinine of 0.94 mg/dL. After leaving the hospital, he resumed Carnivora at a higher dose (4 capsules, three times a day). Four weeks later, the creatinine was noted to be acutely elevated to 2.78 mg/dL prior to starting treatment with brentuximab vedotin, a CD30 antibody-drug conjugate. CT scan of the abdomen also revealed bilateral enlargement of the kidneys (from 11 to 14 cm) not associated with hydronephrosis compared to a CT scan two months ago (Figure 1). The patient received his dose of brentuximab despite these findings and was referred to the Nephrology department several days later for progressive renal insufficiency.

When seen by the Nephrology department, he was reporting a several-day history of fevers, nausea, and vomiting. He denied NSAID use, gross hematuria, dysuria, or decreased urinary frequency. Physical exam was remarkable only for dry mucous membranes with stable vital signs. Labs were notable for creatinine of 3.42 mg/dL, BUN of 32 mg/dL, and white blood cell count of 10,900 with normal eosinophils. Urate, lactate dehydrogenase, and phosphorus were all normal at 4.3 mg/dL, 195 U/L, and 3.8 mg/dL, respectively. Urinalysis revealed <1 eosinophil, 4+ WBC, and 30+ protein. Urine : protein creatinine ratio was 0.76. The patient was admitted to the hospital for intravenous fluids and for kidney biopsy. Carnivora was again discontinued during this hospitalization.

His kidney biopsy revealed acute tubulointerstitial nephritis with no evidence of glomerular injury or fibrosis. Light microscopy revealed diffuse interstitial inflammation with edema, which was predominantly lymphocytic with occasional plasma cells, polymorphic leukocytes, and frequent prominent clusters of eosinophils. Moderately extensive cortical tubular necrosis and injury with some dilated tubules were noted (Figure 2). Immunofluorescence

was 1+ to 3+ positive for C3 in the arterioles and mesangium, tubular basement membranes, and Bowman's capsule. Immunofluorescence was negative for IgA, IgG, IgM, kappa, lambda, C1q, albumin, and fibrin. Electron microscopy showed the glomerular basement membranes were intact. He was treated with intravenous methylprednisolone 250 mg for 3 days, followed by a slow steroid taper. Creatinine improved to 2.99 mg/dL at discharge and continued to decline as an outpatient. The patient has not resumed Carnivora and creatinine has since remained stable at ~1.5 mg/dL (Figure 3).

3. Discussion

This case represents a previously unreported association of AIN in a patient using Carnivora extract. When considering the differential in this case, some considerations included uric acid nephropathy from tumor lysis syndrome, renal vein thrombosis, and obstruction from an enlarged lymph node or tumor. These diagnoses were effectively excluded through CT scan of the abdomen and phosphorus, urate, potassium, and calcium levels. Lymphomatous renal infiltration, seen in one-third of lymphoma patients on autopsy, was also a strong possibility due to bilateral enlargement on CT scan.

However, few of these patients develop renal failure with only 12 reported cases in the literature [6, 7]. The absence of atypical lymphoid cells and prominent eosinophils on his renal biopsy argues against this process. Finally, ampicillin-sulbactam, promethazine, metoclopramide, and baclofen in the previous month are possible culprits; however they did not fit the typical temporal relationship as well as Carnivora and were given in limited doses. The reintroduction of Carnivora at a higher dose also makes it the more likely triggering factor. Finally, the discontinuation of Carnivora, along with initiation of steroids, did lead to improvement of his renal function making this the more likely cause. Penicillins such as ampicillin-sulbactam have been associated with AIN; however, there have been no reports of AIN with promethazine, metoclopramide, and baclofen.

The mechanism of AIN is not completely understood. One proposed mechanism is that absorption of various plasma proteins and molecules by tubular cells causes secretion of chemotactic and inflammatory mediators in the interstitium. Nuclear factor-kappaB (NF-kappaB) is a protein complex that regulates DNA transcription and upregulates inflammatory mediators and is overexpressed in the kidneys of proteinuric animals [8–14]. Increased trafficking of protein has been seen to upregulate RANTES production which is a chemoattractant molecule stimulated by NF-kappaB [15]. The inhibition of NF-kappaB has been shown to reduce cortical tubulointerstitial injury in rat models [16]. Carnivora is marketed as an immune suppressant primarily due to a compound plumbagin in the product that inhibits factor-kappaB (NF-kappaB) in lymphocytes [17]. Based on these findings, Carnivora would presumably decrease the incidence of interstitial nephritis. However, Carnivora is also largely composed of a variety of amino acids which when absorbed by the tubular cells can upregulate transcription of NF-kappaB and RANTES and stimulate an inflammatory reaction [18, 19]. Therefore, the components of Carnivora can both suppress and incite inflammation within the renal interstitium. This is similar to another case report of creatine, a high amino acid supplement, as the cause of interstitial nephritis in one patient; however this correlation is currently under debate [20].

Therefore, this case illustrates the potential for acute interstitial nephritis in a patient taking Carnivora and how early discontinuation of this medication can improve kidney recovery. The mechanism by which acute interstitial nephritis develops may similarly occur for other high protein supplements.

Conflict of Interests

The authors declare that there is no conflict of interests regarding the publication of this paper.

Acknowledgments

The authors would like to thank Dr. Bernard Panner and Dr. Bruce Goldman for their assistance providing pathologic images.

References

[1] M. Praga and E. González, "Acute interstitial nephritis," *Kidney International*, vol. 77, no. 11, pp. 956–961, 2010.

[2] M. R. Clarkson, L. Giblin, F. P. O'Connell et al., "Acute interstitial nephritis: clinical features and response to corticosteroid therapy," *Nephrology Dialysis Transplantation*, vol. 19, no. 11, pp. 2778–2783, 2004.

[3] J. Rossert, "Drug-induced acute interstitial nephritis," *Kidney International*, vol. 60, no. 2, pp. 804–817, 2001.

[4] C. M. Kodner and A. Kudrimoti, "Diagnosis and management of acute interstitial nephritis," *The American Family Physician*, vol. 67, no. 12, pp. 2527–2534, 2003.

[5] "What Is Carnivora?" Carnivora Research Inc, 2013, http://www.carnivora.com/about-carnivora.html.

[6] G. T. Obrador, B. Price, Y. O'Meara, and D. J. Salant, "Acute renal failure due to lymphomatous infiltration of the kidneys," *Journal of the American Society of Nephrology*, vol. 8, no. 8, pp. 1348–1354, 1997.

[7] L. Sellin, C. Friedl, G. Klein, R. Waldherr, L. C. Rump, and S. M. Weiner, "Acute renal failure due to a malignant lymphoma infiltration uncovered by renal biopsy," *Nephrology Dialysis Transplantation*, vol. 19, no. 10, pp. 2657–2660, 2004.

[8] M. Gomez-Chiarri, A. Ortiz, J. L. Lerma et al., "Involvement of tumor necrosis factor and platelet-activating factor in the pathogenesis of experimental nephrosis in rats," *Laboratory Investigation*, vol. 70, no. 4, pp. 449–459, 1994.

[9] M. Gómez-Chiarri, A. Ortiz, S. González-Cuadrado et al., "Interferon-inducible protein-10 is highly expressed in rats with experimental nephrosis," *The American Journal of Pathology*, vol. 148, no. 1, pp. 301–311, 1996.

[10] J.-C. Wu, G.-M. Fan, K. Kitazawa, and T. Sugisaki, "The relationship of adhesion molecules and leukocyte infiltration in chronic tubulointerstitial nephritis induced by puromycin aminonucleoside in Wistar rats," *Clinical Immunology and Immunopathology*, vol. 79, no. 3, pp. 229–235, 1996.

[11] W. W. Tang, M. Qi, J. S. Warren, and G. Y. Van, "Chemokine expression in experimental tubulointerstitial nephritis," *Journal of Immunology*, vol. 159, no. 2, pp. 870–876, 1997.

[12] A. Nomura, Y. Morita, S. Maruyama et al., "Role of complement in acute tubulointerstitial injury of rats with aminonucleoside nephrosis," *The American Journal of Pathology*, vol. 151, no. 2, pp. 539–547, 1997.

[13] P. A. Baeuerle and T. Henkel, "Function and activation of NF-κB in the immune system," *Annual Review of Immunology*, vol. 12, pp. 141–179, 1994.

[14] P. J. Barnes and M. Karin, "Nuclear factor-κB - A pivotal transcription factor in chronic inflammatory diseases," *The New England Journal of Medicine*, vol. 336, no. 15, pp. 1066–1071, 1997.

[15] C. Zoja, R. Donadelli, S. Colleoni et al., "Protein overload stimulates RANTES production by proximal tubular cells depending on NF-κB activation," *Kidney International*, vol. 53, no. 6, pp. 1608–1615, 1998.

[16] G. K. Rangan, Y. Wang, Y.-C. Tay, and D. C. H. Harris, "Inhibition of nuclear factor-κB activation reduces cortical tubulointerstitial injury in proteinuric rats," *Kidney International*, vol. 56, no. 1, pp. 118–134, 1999.

[17] R. Checker, D. Sharma, S. K. Sandur, S. Khanam, and T. B. Poduval, "Anti-inflammatory effects of plumbagin are mediated by inhibition of NF-kappaB activation in lymphocytes," *International Immunopharmacology*, vol. 9, no. 7-8, pp. 949–958, 2009.

[18] C. Zoya and G. Remuzzi, "Interstitial nephritis," in *Principles of Molecular Medicine*, M. S. Runge and C. Patterson, Eds., pp. 636–642, Humana Press Inc., Totowa, NJ, USA, 2nd edition, 2006.

[19] J. K. Jeloka, "Pathophysiology of acute interstitial nephritis," *Clinical Queries: Nephrology*, vol. 1, no. 1, pp. 27–28, 2012.

[20] K. M. Koshy, E. Griswold, and E. E. Schneeberger, "Interstitial nephritis in a patient taking creatine," *The New England Journal of Medicine*, vol. 340, no. 10, pp. 814–815, 1999.

24

A Case of Concurrent MPO-/PR3-Negative ANCA-Associated Glomerulonephritis and Membranous Glomerulopathy

Yasuyuki Nakada,[1] **Nobuo Tsuboi,**[1] **Yasuto Takahashi,**[1] **Hiraku Yoshida,**[1] **Yoriko Hara,**[1] **Hideo Okonogi,**[1] **Tetsuya Kawamura,**[1] **Yoshihiro Arimura,**[2] **and Takashi Yokoo**[1]

[1]*Division of Nephrology and Hypertension, Department of Internal Medicine, The Jikei University School of Medicine, 3-25-8 Nishi-Shinbashi, Minato-ku, Tokyo 105-8461, Japan*
[2]*Department of Internal Medicine, Kyorin University School of Medicine, Tokyo, Japan*

Correspondence should be addressed to Yasuyuki Nakada; nakadaya_august06@hotmail.com

Academic Editor: Aikaterini Papagianni

We report a case in which antineutrophil cytoplasmic antibody- (ANCA-) associated glomerulonephritis and membranous glomerulopathy (MGN) were detected concurrently. The patient showed rapidly progressive renal deterioration. A renal biopsy showed crescentic glomerulonephritis, together with marked thickening and spike and bubbling formations in the glomerular basement membranes. Indirect immunofluorescence examination of the patient's neutrophils showed a perinuclear pattern. Enzyme-linked immunosorbent assays revealed that the ANCA in this case did not target myeloperoxidase (MPO) or proteinase 3 (PR3) but bactericidal-/permeability-increasing protein, elastase, and lysosome. The relationship between these two etiologically distinct entities, MPO-/PR3-negative ANCA-associated glomerulonephritis and MGN, remains unclear.

1. Introduction

The presence of antineutrophil cytoplasmic antibody (ANCA) in serum may be associated with small-vessel vasculitis, which occurs often in the renal glomeruli. Immunoglobulin deposits are usually absent in the glomeruli of patients with ANCA-associated glomerulonephritis (ANCA-GN), and ANCA infusion does not lead to glomerulonephritis in animal models. Based on these findings, it is proposed that ANCA does not damage the glomerulus directly, but neutrophils activated by ANCA integrate into capillary walls and release several protein-degrading enzymes, and, finally, these pathological changes may cause necrosis to glomerular capillary walls [1].

The two major antigens for ANCA, proteinase 3 (PR3) and myeloperoxidase (MPO), are usually referred to as the serological markers of ANCA-associated vasculitis and glomerulonephritis on ELISA tests, with perinuclear and cytoplasmic lesions in neutrophils, respectively. In these diseases, it is well-known that pauci-immune necrotizing

and/or crescentic glomerulonephritis are often found in renal biopsies, with nonnephrotic range proteinuria and relatively high degrees of hematuria, as well as rapid decreases in kidney function, leading to end-stage renal disease (ESRD) within several months.

In the absence of these two major antigens for ANCA, possibilities remain for minor antigens, including elastase, bactericidal-/permeability-increasing protein (BPI), and cathepsin C. Such minor antigens often indicate drug-induced ANCA. The most common ANCA-inducing drugs are antithyroid drugs (especially propylthiouracil), though it often occurs after many years of exposure [2].

Membranous glomerulopathy (MGN) is the most common cause of nephrotic syndrome in adults. It is characterized histopathologically by subepithelial deposits of immunoglobulins and complement, with microscopic changes in the glomerular basement membrane (GBM), including spike and bubbling formations. Many cases of MGN are thought to represent primary disease, while the rest represent secondary illnesses, related to systemic lupus erythematosus, drugs, malignancies, or infections. The prognosis of MGN is variable, with one-third of untreated patients slowly progressing to end-stage renal disease within 10 years [3].

To our knowledge, no case of MPO- and PR3-negative ANCA-GN concurrent with MGN has been reported previously [4].

2. Case Report

The patient was a 70-year-old male with a 20-year history of sick sinus syndrome, for which he had a permanent cardiac pacemaker. He also had a 2-year history of interstitial pneumonia. While under treatment for angina pectoris 2 years before admission, he was found to have kidney dysfunction (serum creatinine, 1.4 mg/dL; blood urea nitrogen, 30 mg/dL; and 4+ protein and 2+ occult blood on urinalysis). In early December 2008, he had orthopnea, which worsened gradually. On December 24, he had a checkup in our hospital and was admitted. The medications he was taking on admission included aspirin, ticlopidine, allopurinol, carvedilol, atorvastatin, and carbocisteine. He was 171 cm tall and weighed 61 kg. His temperature was 37.0°C. His blood pressure was 145/70 mmHg. Lung auscultation revealed bilateral coarse crackles. An abdominal examination was normal. Pretibial pitting edema was evident. Laboratory findings on admission are shown in Table 1. The kidney function test had worsened, compared with 2 years earlier. There were significant hypoalbuminemia and elevation of C-reactive protein. Results of a urinalysis were 3+ positive for protein and 3+ positive for blood, with many red blood cells, 2+ for granular casts, and 1+ for red blood cell casts in the urinary sediment. The amount of proteinuria was 5.12 g/day. Urine culture results were negative on admission. An electrocardiogram showed a ventricular pacing rhythm. A chest X-ray revealed bilateral pleural effusion and pulmonary congestion. MPO and PR3-ANCA were both negative by enzyme-linked immunosorbent assay (ELISA), but P-ANCA was detected by indirect immunofluorescence (IIF; Figure 1). Bactericidal-/permeability-increasing protein (BPI), elastase, and lysozyme antibodies were also positive on ELISA (Wieslab ANCA panel kit) despite negative results for azurocidin, cathepsin G, and lactoferrin.

After admission, we stopped the allopurinol and atorvastatin because several studies have shown a relationship between these drugs and the immediate development of ANCA-associated vasculitis. His pulmonary congestion was improved using diuretics. However, his kidney function worsened gradually. We performed a kidney biopsy on February 4, 2009. The renal biopsy specimen contained 15 glomeruli for light microscopic evaluation, of which 3 were globally sclerotic. There were 5 cellular, 3 fibrocellular, and 3 fibrotic crescents in the remaining 12 nonsclerotic glomeruli (Figure 2(a)). No necrotic lesion was found. Marked thickening and spike and bubbling formations were observed in the GBM by periodic acid-Schiff methenamine silver (PAM) staining (Figure 2(b)). There was tubular atrophy, especially around the globally sclerotic glomeruli, with interstitial fibrosis and inflammation involving numerous lymphocytes. An immunofluorescence

TABLE 1: Laboratory findings on admission.

Peripheral blood	
WBC	9800/μL
Neutro	78.1%
RBC	$311 \times 10^4/\mu$L
Hb	10.2 g/dL
Ht	31.0%
PLT	$26.3 \times 10^4/\mu$L
Blood chemistry	
AST	17 IU/L
ALT	12 IU/L
LDH	286 IU/L
ALP	209 IU/L
TP	6.6 g/dL
Alb	2.7 g/dL
BUN	43 mg/dL
Cr	3.22 mg/dL
Na	144 mEq/L
K	4.3 mEq/L
Cl	111 mEq/L
Ca	8.0 mg/dL
Pi	4.0 mg/dL
TC	183 mg/dL
LDL-C	116 mg/dL
TG	121 mg/dL
FPG	83 mg/dL
HbA1c	5.5%
Serology	
CRP	5.9 mg/dL
IgG	962 mg/dL
IgA	149 mg/dL
IgM	40 mg/dL
C3	88 mg/dL
C4	19 mg/dL
CH50	30.5 U/mL
TSH	2.42 μIU/mL
BNP	1135.7 pg/mL
KL-6	689 U/mL
ANA	×80 (speckled)
dsDNAIgG	<5.0 IU/mL
RA test	(−)
MPO-ANCA	<10 E.U.
PR3-ANCA	<10 E.U.
Azurocidin-ANCA	(−)
BPI-ANCA	(+)
Cathepsin G-ANCA	(−)
Elastase-ANCA	(+)
Lactoferrin-ANCA	(−)
Lysozyme-ANCA	(+)
SS-A/RO	(−)
SS-B/LA	(−)

TABLE 1: Continued.

Anti-GBM	<10 E.U.
Cryoglobulin	(−)
HBs-Ag	(−)
HCV-Ab	(−)
TPHA	(−)
Urine	
U-protein	5.13 g/day
24-hour-CCr	21 mL/min
Sediment	
RBC	Many/HPF
WBC	50–99/HPF
C-granule	2+
C-RBC	1+

microscopic evaluation revealed granular staining along glomerular capillary walls for immunoglobulin IgG (2+) and C3 (2+) (Figure 2(c)). There was no staining for IgA, IgM, or C1q. Electron-dense deposits in the subepithelial lesions and fused podocyte foot processes were revealed by electron microscopy (Figure 2(d)). Based on these findings, the present case was diagnosed histopathologically as crescentic glomerulonephritis, concurrent with MGN (Ehrenreich-Churg classification: Stage III).

Due to extraocular myositis, an inflammatory disease that selectively affects the muscles around the eyes, which occurred on January 26, 2009, he received oral prednisolone (30 mg/day) and the symptoms improved rapidly. Despite steroid therapy, his kidney dysfunction progressed severely (serum creatinine 6.23 mg/dL, urea nitrogen 54 mg/dL on February 3). After he started hemodialysis on February 12, his laboratory findings did not show significant signs of improvement in terms of kidney function. The dose of corticosteroid was tapered without recurrence of extraocular myositis.

3. Discussion

The pathological and physiological roles of ANCA to minor antigens, other than PR3 and MPO, have not been determined, but some cases have been reported in relation to systemic vasculitis. Our patient was positive for multiple ANCAs, including elastase, BPI, and lysozyme. Wiesner et al. reported that human neutrophil elastase antibodies (HNE-ANCA) are often found in cocaine-induced midline destructive lesions [5]. Seidowsky et al. reported three cases that developed HNE-ANCA-associated vasculitis with rapidly progressive glomerulonephritis [6]. Interestingly, both of these reports also had ANCAs for bactericidal-/permeability-increasing protein (BPI), as observed in our case. Schultz et al. reported about BPI-ANCA; the prevalence of BPI-ANCA was 5–45% in all ANCA-associated vasculitides. Other conditions with BPI-ANCA sometimes involve prolonged lower airway infection with Gram-negative bacteria [7]. Although the features of HNE-/BPI-ANCA described above were similar to our case, the typical staining pattern by IIF in HNE-/BPI-ANCA is a cytoplasmic pattern, unlike our case (perinuclear pattern).

ANCAs to multiple antigens can be seen in drug-induced ANCA-associated vasculitis, including those caused by propylthiouracil, hydralazine, penicillamine, sulfasalazine, allopurinol, and atorvastatin [2, 8, 9]. In our case, allopurinol and atorvastatin, as causal drugs of ANCA-associated vasculitis, had been prescribed many years earlier. Haroon and Devlin reported a case of ANCA-associated systemic vasculitis induced by atorvastatin but without vasculitic glomerulonephritis [8]. In addition, in the cases of atorvastatin or allopurinol, only MPO-ANCA-associated vasculitis has been reported previously. Although the possibility remains, it thus seems unlikely that the ANCA-GN observed in our case was induced by atorvastatin or allopurinol. In addition, a previous study found an association between ANCA-associated vasculitis and minor-target antigens, and the authors showed that almost 80% of cases of ANCA-associated vasculitis that were positive by immunofluorescence but negative for MPO-/PR3-ANCA by ELISA had minor targeted antigen-ANCA (BPI, elastase, cathepsin B, and lysozyme) [10]. A study on the origin and development of ANCA-associated glomerulonephritis with LAMP-2 and LAMP-2 ANCA suggested that infection and molecular mimicry may trigger autoimmunity by inducing antibodies to bacterial adhesion protein FimH and the development of AAV [11]. Indeed, the authors showed that the frequency of LAMP-2 ANCA in patients with untreated AAV was 80–91% [12]. Unfortunately, we were unable to analyze the presence of LAMP-2 ANCA in this patient because of a lack of samples.

ANCA-associated vasculitis with glomerular immune complex deposits may be associated with heavier proteinuria [13]. However, ANCA-associated glomerulonephritis rarely induces nephrotic-range proteinuria, even when immune complex deposits are demonstrated by electron microscopy (EM) in glomeruli; if present, most immune complex deposits are found in the mesangial area [13]. These observations contrast with our case, in which most of the dense deposits were found in the subepithelial area. This further supports that our case was complicated by membranous glomerulopathy.

Concurrent MGN and ANCA-associated glomerulonephritis have rarely been reported. Tse et al. reported 10 cases of MGN superimposed with vasculitic glomerulonephritis, and four of them were ANCA-positive [14]. Their kidney function recovered with immunosuppressive therapy and/or plasma exchange, except one patient in whom the renal pathological findings were especially severe. Recently, Nasr et al. reported 14 patients with MGN and ANCA-GN and identified the rate of crescent formation as a risk factor for developing ESRD [4]. However, they found that the stage of MGN was not associated with ESRD. In our case, most of the remaining glomeruli (92%) were affected by crescent formations, indicating that the kidney damage was irreversible, even with aggressive therapy.

At present, any association between MGN and ANCA-GN is unclear. Matsumoto et al. reported an interesting hypothesis that MPO demonstrated in epimembranous deposits (this lesion is anionic) is highly cationic. Because BPI, elastase, and lysozyme are all cationic, ANCAs for these minor antigens might be related to the formation of immune complexes [15]. Because of the lack of renal biopsy

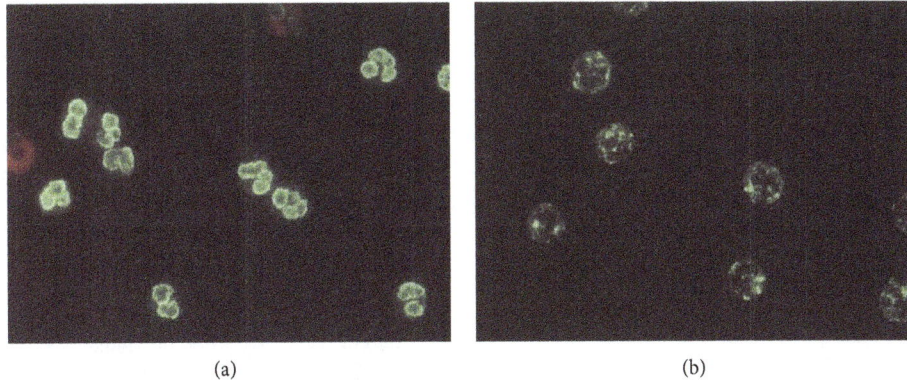

(a)

(b)

FIGURE 1: Indirect immunofluorescence reaction pattern of the patient's serum. (a) Fixed with ethanol, neutrophils showed a perinuclear pattern. (b) Fixed with formalin, neutrophils showed a cytoplasmic pattern.

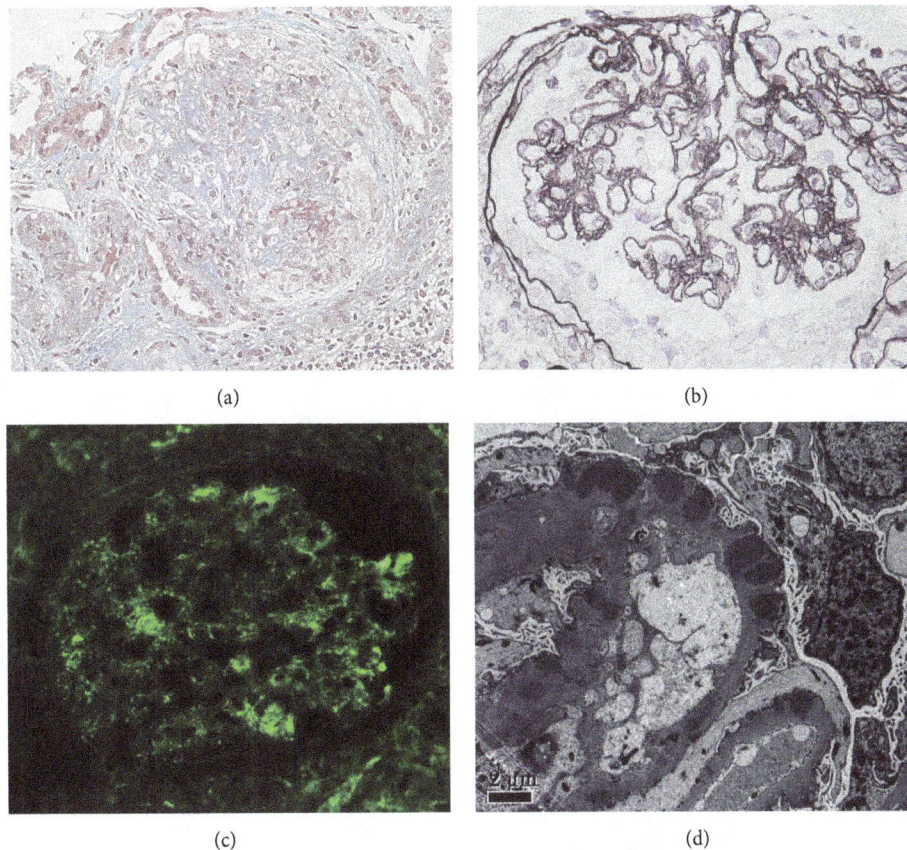

(a)

(b)

(c)

(d)

FIGURE 2: (a) Fibrocellular crescent in Bowman's space with significant collapse of glomerular tufts and the presence of glomerular-fibrinoid necrosis (Masson-trichrome stain). (b) GBM thickening including spike and bubbling formations in the subepithelial lesions (PAM stain). (c) Granular staining for IgG along glomerular capillary walls (IgG immunofluorescence stain). (d) Electron-dense deposits in the subepithelial lesions (electron microscopy).

material, we were unable to demonstrate the presence of epimembranous deposits composed of ANCAs including BPI, elastase, and/or lysozyme, which might have revealed a correlation between ANCA-associated vasculitis and MGN in this case.

On the other hand, Nasr et al. suggested that the concurrence of MGN and ANCA-GN may just be by chance, because they occur together too infrequently to be related pathologically [4].

In our case, the presence of proteinuria, microscopic hematuria, and mild renal dysfunction two years earlier are signs of either vasculitis or more possible membranous nephropathy, which existed before the present disease. The amount of cellular crescents and the presence of interstitial inflammation suggest that vasculitis is the second disease occurring in a preexisting membranous nephropathy.

Although AAV might be associated with the development of extraocular myositis, no case of AAV with extraocular myositis has been previously reported. Thus, we also could not clarify the relationship in this case.

In conclusion, we report a rare case of MGN concurrent with ANCAGN, in which the targeted ANCA antigens were neither MPO nor PR3. Whether there is any relationship between these two etiologically distinct entities remains unclear.

Conflict of Interests

The authors have declared that no conflict of interests exists.

References

[1] X. Bosch, A. Guilabert, and J. Font, "Antineutrophil cytoplasmic antibodies," *The Lancet*, vol. 368, no. 9533, pp. 404–418, 2006.

[2] H. K. Choi, P. A. Merkel, A. M. Walker, and J. L. Niles, "Drug-associated antineutrophil cytoplasmic antibody-positive vasculitis," *Arthritis & Rheumatology*, vol. 43, no. 2, pp. 405–413, 2000.

[3] S. L. Hogan, K. E. Muller, J. C. Jennette, and R. J. Falk, "A review of therapeutic studies of idiopathic membranous glomerulopathy," *The American Journal of Kidney Diseases*, vol. 25, no. 6, pp. 862–875, 1995.

[4] S. H. Nasr, S. M. Said, A. M. Valeri et al., "Membranous glomerulonephritis with ANCA-associated necrotizing and crescentic glomerulonephritis," *Clinical Journal of the American Society of Nephrology*, vol. 4, no. 2, pp. 299–308, 2009.

[5] O. Wiesner, K. A. Russell, A. S. Lee et al., "Antineutrophil cytoplasmic antibodies reacting with human neutrophil elastase as a diagnostic marker for cocaine-induced midline destructive lesions but not autoimmune vasculitis," *Arthritis & Rheumatism*, vol. 50, no. 9, pp. 2954–2965, 2004.

[6] A. Seidowsky, M. Hoffmann, S. Ruben-Duval et al., "Elastase-ANCA-associated idiopathic necrotizing crescentic glomerulonephritis—a report of three cases," *Nephrology Dialysis Transplantation*, vol. 22, no. 7, pp. 2068–2071, 2007.

[7] H. Schultz, J. Weiss, S. F. Carroll, and W. L. Gross, "The endotoxin-binding bactericidal/permeability-increasing protein (BPI): a target antigen of autoantibodies," *Journal of Leukocyte Biology*, vol. 69, no. 4, pp. 505–512, 2001.

[8] M. Haroon and J. Devlin, "A case of ANCA-associated systemic vasculitis induced by atorvastatin," *Clinical Rheumatology*, vol. 27, no. 2, supplement, pp. 75–77, 2008.

[9] F. Yu, M. Chen, Y. Gao et al., "Clinical and pathological features of renal involvement in propylthiouracil-associated ANCA-positive vasculitis," *The American Journal of Kidney Diseases*, vol. 49, no. 5, pp. 607–614, 2007.

[10] M. V. Talor, J. H. Stone, J. Stebbing, J. Barin, N. R. Rose, and C. L. Burek, "Antibodies to selected minor target antigens in patients with anti-neutrophil cytoplasmic antibodies (ANCA)," *Clinical and Experimental Immunology*, vol. 150, no. 1, pp. 42–48, 2007.

[11] R. Kain, M. Exner, R. Brandes et al., "Molecular mimicry in pauci-immune focal necrotizing glomerulonephritis," *Nature Medicine*, vol. 14, no. 10, pp. 1088–1096, 2008.

[12] R. Kain, H. Tadema, E. F. McKinney et al., "High prevalence of autoantibodies to hLAMP-2 in anti-neutrophil cytoplasmic antibody-associated vasculitis," *Journal of the American Society of Nephrology*, vol. 23, no. 3, pp. 556–566, 2012.

[13] M. Haas and J. A. Eustace, "Immune complex deposits in ANCA-associated crescentic glomerulonephritis: a study of 126 cases," *Kidney International*, vol. 65, no. 6, pp. 2145–2152, 2004.

[14] W. Y. Tse, A. J. Howie, D. Adu et al., "Association of vasculitic glomerulonephritis with membranous nephropathy: a report of 10 cases," *Nephrology Dialysis Transplantation*, vol. 12, no. 5, pp. 1017–1027, 1997.

[15] K. Matsumoto, H. Honda, T. Shibata et al., "MPO-ANCA crescentic glomerulonephritis complicated by membranous nephropathy: MPO demonstrated in epimembranous deposits," *NDT Plus*, vol. 2, no. 6, pp. 461–465, 2009.

25

Subphrenic Abscess as a Complication of Hemodialysis Catheter-Related Infection

Fernando Caravaca, Victor Burguera, Milagros Fernández-Lucas, José Luis Teruel, and Carlos Quereda

Department of Nephrology, Hospital Ramón y Cajal, 28034 Madrid, Spain

Correspondence should be addressed to Fernando Caravaca; fcaravacaf@gmail.com

Academic Editor: Yoshihide Fujigaki

We describe an unusual case of subphrenic abscess complicating a central venous catheter infection caused by *Pseudomonas aeruginosa* in a 59-year-old woman undergoing hemodialysis. The diagnosis was made through computed tomography, and *Pseudomonas aeruginosa* was isolated from the purulent drainage of the subphrenic abscess, the catheter tip and exit site, and the blood culture samples. A transesophageal echocardiography showed a large tubular thrombus in superior vena cava, extending to the right atrium, but no evidence of endocarditis or other metastatic infectious foci. Catheter removal, percutaneous abscess drainage, anticoagulation, and antibiotics resulted in a favourable outcome.

1. Introduction

Infection is a common complication of central venous catheters (CVC) used for vascular access in hemodialysis patients. Gram-positive bacteremia is the typical clinical presentation of CVC related infectious complications. *Pseudomonas aeruginosa* is a less frequent pathogen associated with catheter infection, accounting for 4–16% of isolates [1]. Nevertheless, this pathogen should always be considered as one potential causative agent of CVC related infections, especially in immunocompromised hosts. Metastatic infectious foci are important determinants of the morbidity and mortality of CVC related infections. Endocarditis, septic embolism, and visceral abscesses are rare but serious complications whose mere suspicion demands careful clinical and radiological search.

We report a case of a subphrenic abscess and CVC related bloodstream infection with *Pseudomonas aeruginosa* in a 59-year-old woman on haemodialysis.

2. Case Report

A 59-year-old woman with a history of mild intellectual disability and chronic renal allograft dysfunction was admitted to our hospital with a febrile syndrome and a progressive ten-day history of nonproductive cough. She was receiving haemodialysis at a satellite dialysis unit, through a jugular permanent catheter, which had been placed 93 days before. She was not taking corticosteroids or any other immunosuppressive agents, and she had no history of any intra-abdominal disease or recent surgical procedure. The patient complained of intermittent chills and fever up to 39°C for the last few days, with no close temporal relationship with the dialysis session. The rest of anamnesis was anodyne. Physical examination showed a blood pressure of 100/50 mmHg, respiratory rate of 19 breaths/min, and temperature of 38.4°C. Chest auscultation revealed regular heart sounds with a pansystolic murmur, which had already been described in her clinical history, and the breath sounds were absent in the lower third of the right lung. The abdominal exam did not reveal tenderness, hepatomegaly, or masses. Jugular catheter inspection showed inflammatory signs and mild purulent discharge around the exit site.

Her initial WBC was 16×10^9 cells/L (normal range: $4.5–10.5 \times 10^9$ cells/L), and she had an absolute neutrophil count of 13×10^9 cells/L. C-reactive protein was 230 mg/L (normal range: 1–5 mg/dL) and procalcitonin was 1.2 ng/mL (<0.05 ng/mL). No abnormalities were found on the liver

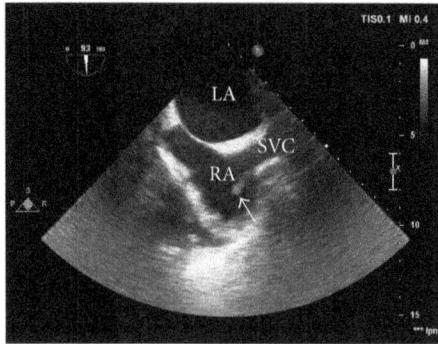

FIGURE 1: Transesophageal echocardiography showing a tubular 4 × 0.5 cm thrombus (arrow) in superior vena cava (SVC) to the right atrium (RA); left atrium (LA).

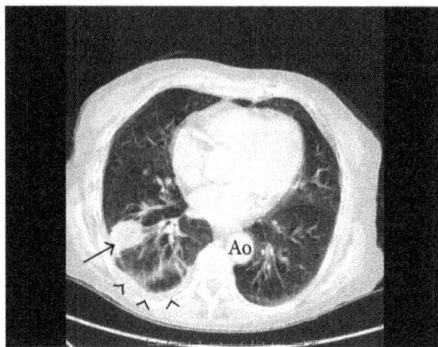

FIGURE 2: Computed tomography of the chest (lung window) showing a small focal consolidation within the posterior segment of the right lower lobe (arrow) and mild pleural effusion (arrowheads).

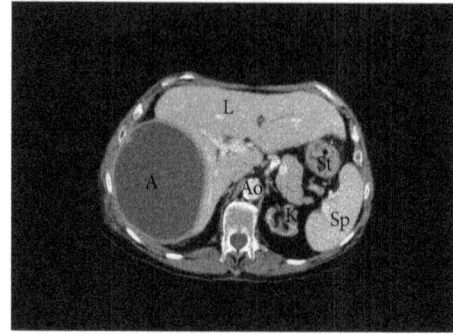

FIGURE 3: Computed tomography showing a 13 × 10 × 16 cm abscess (A), compressing the liver (L); abdominal aorta (Ao); kidney (K); spleen (Sp); stomach (St).

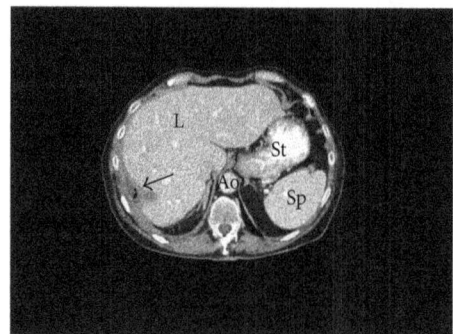

FIGURE 4: Computed tomography showing a complete healing of the subphrenic abscess (arrow); aorta (Ao); liver (L); spleen (Sp); stomach (St).

function panel. A chest X-ray showed an elevation of the right diaphragm. Cultures from catheter exit site and blood samples were taken, and empiric vancomycin plus gentamicin was prescribed. Forty-eight hours later, the microbiologist reported the isolation of *Pseudomonas aeruginosa* both in exit site and in blood samples. We decided to remove the catheter and to use an arteriovenous fistula, which had been created 64 days before, and it seemed fairly mature. Maki's semiquantitative culture technique of the catheter tip also isolated *Pseudomonas aeruginosa*.

A transthoracic and transesophageal echocardiography revealed a tubular 4 × 0.5 cm thrombus in superior vena cava extending to the right atrium, but no signs of endocarditis (Figure 1).

A computed tomography was done for a better definition of the thrombus, with unexpected findings: a small focal consolidation within the posterior segment of the right lower lobe and mild pleural effusion were described in the lung window (Figure 2), as well as a collection of 13 × 10 × 16 cm in the right hypochondrium and subphrenic space, compressing both the right lung and the liver (Figure 3). The abscess was drained by percutaneous catheter placement, and approximately 800 mL of purulent effluent was obtained in the next few days. *Pseudomonas aeruginosa* was also isolated in the cultures of this purulent drainage.

According to sensitivity pattern, the patient was treated with oral ciprofloxacin, intravenous tobramycin, and anticoagulation with low molecular weight heparin. The clinical course was favourable, the fever disappeared, and her condition improved rapidly. A transesophageal echocardiogram performed four weeks after admission revealed no thrombus, and another computed tomography confirmed the complete healing of the subphrenic abscess (Figure 4).

3. Discussion

To the best of our knowledge, this case described for the first time the association of a subphrenic abscess complicating a central venous catheter infection in a patient on haemodialysis.

Central venous catheters (CVC) have been increasingly used for vascular access in haemodialysis, these devices being the only option in a large percentage of patients [1]. CVC related infectious complications are common and they are associated with high morbidity, mortality, and healthcare costs [2]. The incidence of catheter-related bacteraemia ranges between 0.6 and 6.5 episodes per 1000 catheter-days, being higher in nontunneled catheters compared with tunneled catheters [1]. Gram-positive bacteria are responsible for the majority of CVC related infections in haemodialysis patients. *Staphylococcus aureus* and coagulase negative *Staphylococcus* are isolated in 50 to 80 percent of these cases. In addition, gram-negative species account for 20 to 40 percent of catheter-related bacteremia [3–6], and *Pseudomonas/Stenotrophomonas* species are isolated in 4 to 16 percent of these episodes [1, 7, 8].

Pseudomonas aeruginosa is a nonfermentative gram-negative aerobic rod, commonly isolated in the environment, which is responsible for a myriad of infections, especially those of nosocomial origin. This microorganism has a predilection for devitalized tissues and nonbiological materials, such as catheters, prosthesis, and other medical devices [9].

In the case described here, the isolation of *Pseudomonas aeruginosa* in the exit site and tip of the catheter, blood samples, and purulent drainage from the subphrenic abscess suggests a pathogenetic cascade in which the contamination of catheter may have acted as primary source of the infection followed by a haematogenous dissemination, probably with septic emboli formation and, finally, abscess formation in a very unusual location.

Subphrenic abscess formation is a more common complication of intra-abdominal processes (i.e., appendicitis, diverticulitis, etc.) or surgical procedures, although cases of unknown origin have also been described [10]. Isolation of more than one microorganism, especially mixed gram-negative and anaerobic microorganisms, would suggest the intra-abdominal origin of the abscess formation. On the contrary, the isolation of only one microorganism, as in the present case, may rather suggest that the infection was of haematogenous origin.

In our case, the finding of a large thrombus in superior vena cava and right atrium may suggest that the dissemination of the infection could have occurred through pulmonary septic embolisms with abscess formation in the right lower lobe and extension to the subphrenic space by contiguity (subphrenic or hypophrenic empyema).

In this patient, despite bacteraemia and systemic dissemination of *Pseudomonas*, the clinical course was relatively benign without developing septic shock and with a rapid favourable response to antibiotics and abscess drainage. A remarkably good outcome has already been described in *Pseudomonas* bacteraemia associated with CVC in haemodialysis patients [11]. It is likely that prompt catheter removal contributes to the favourable outcome observed in these patients, and, in this regard, the mere fact of *Pseudomonas* isolation and its well-known virulence prevent attempts at catheter salvage, an important risk factor for adverse outcomes after an initial episode of CVC bacteraemia.

The description of this case highlights also the critical importance of a careful clinical and radiological search for metastatic septic foci, especially in those CVC related infections in which a source of septic emboli has been detected (venous thrombus or endocarditis).

Conflict of Interests

The authors declare that there is no conflict of interests regarding the publication of this paper.

References

[1] M. G. H. Betjes, "Prevention of catheter-related bloodstream infection in patients on hemodialysis," *Nature Reviews Nephrology*, vol. 7, no. 5, pp. 257–265, 2011.

[2] C. E. Lok and M. H. Mokrzycki, "Prevention and management of catheter-related infection in hemodialysis patients," *Kidney International*, vol. 79, no. 6, pp. 587–598, 2011.

[3] D. Mitchell, Z. Krishnasami, and M. Allon, "Catheter-related bacteraemia in haemodialysis patients with HIV infection," *Nephrology Dialysis Transplantation*, vol. 21, no. 11, pp. 3185–3188, 2006.

[4] M. R. Saleem, S. Mustafa, P. J. T. Drew et al., "Endophthalmitis, a rare metastatic bacterial complication of haemodialysis catheter-related sepsis," *Nephrology Dialysis Transplantation*, vol. 22, no. 3, pp. 939–941, 2007.

[5] L. K. Kairaitis and T. Gottlieb, "Outcome and complications of temporary haemodialysis catheters," *Nephrology Dialysis Transplantation*, vol. 14, no. 7, pp. 1710–1714, 1999.

[6] D. M. Silverstein and K. Moylan, "Cause and outcome of central venous catheter infections in paediatric haemodialysis patients," *Nephrology Dialysis Transplantation*, vol. 25, no. 10, pp. 3332–3337, 2010.

[7] G. A. Beathard, "Management of bacteremia associated with tunneled-cuffed hemodialysis catheters," *Journal of the American Society of Nephrology*, vol. 10, no. 5, pp. 1045–1049, 1999.

[8] T. F. Saad, "Bacteremia associated with tunneled, cuffed hemodialysis catheters," *American Journal of Kidney Diseases*, vol. 34, no. 6, pp. 1114–1124, 1999.

[9] L. D. Christensen, M. V. Gennip, M. T. Rybtke et al., "Clearance of *Pseudomonas aeruginosa* foreign-body biofilm infections through reduction of the cyclic Di-GMP level in the bacteria," *Infection and Immunity*, vol. 81, no. 8, pp. 2705–2713, 2013.

[10] G. H. Wooler, "Subphrenic abscess," *Thorax*, vol. 11, no. 3, pp. 211–222, 1956.

[11] L. Golestaneh, J. Laut, S. Rosenberg, M. Zhang, and M. H. Mokrzycki, "Favourable outcomes in episodes of *Pseudomonas* bacteraemia when associated with tunnelled cuffed catheters (TCCs) in chronic haemodialysis patients," *Nephrology Dialysis Transplantation*, vol. 21, no. 5, pp. 1328–1333, 2006.

26

Long-Term Therapeutic Plasma Exchange to Prevent End-Stage Kidney Disease in Adult Severe Resistant Henoch-Schonlein Purpura Nephritis

Patrick Hamilton,[1] **Olumide Ogundare,**[1] **Ammar Raza,**[1] **Arvind Ponnusamy,**[1] **Julie Gorton,**[1] **Hana Alachkar,**[1] **Jamil Choudhury,**[2] **Jonathan Barratt,**[3] **and Philip A. Kalra**[1]

[1]*Renal Department, Salford Royal NHS Foundation Trust, Salford, Greater Manchester M6 8HD, UK*
[2]*Histopathology Department, Salford NHS Foundation Trust, Salford, Greater Manchester M6 8HD, UK*
[3]*John Walls Renal Unit, Leicester General Hospital, Gwendolen Road, Leicester LE5 4PW, UK*

Correspondence should be addressed to Patrick Hamilton; patrick.hamilton@cmft.nhs.uk

Academic Editor: Kouichi Hirayama

A 27-year-old man presented with a palpable purpuric skin rash and joint and abdominal pain in April 2010. He had acute kidney injury and his creatinine quickly deteriorated to 687 μmol/L, with associated nephrotic range proteinuria. Kidney biopsy showed crescentic Henoch-Schonlein nephritis. He was treated with intravenous cyclophosphamide and prednisolone despite which his renal function deteriorated; he required haemodialysis for a short duration and seven sessions of therapeutic plasma exchange (TPE). Renal function improved, but after discharge from hospital he suffered 2 further relapses, each with AKI, in 4 months. Cyclophosphamide was not effective and therefore Rituximab was introduced. He initially had a partial response but his renal function deteriorated despite continued therapy. TPE was the only treatment that prevented rapid renal functional deterioration. A novel long-term treatment strategy involving regular TPE every one to two weeks was initiated. This helped to slow his progression to end-stage kidney disease over a 3-year period and to prolong the need for renal replacement therapy over this time.

1. Background

Henoch-Schonlein Purpura (HSP) is a nonthrombocytopenic, purpuric, and systemic vasculitis characterised by the deposition of immune complexes containing IgA in small venules, capillaries, and arterioles. It classically presents with the tetrad of skin, joint, and gastrointestinal and renal manifestations with approximately 90% of patients under the age of 10 years [1, 2]. In adults, although rare, it represents a more severe clinical syndrome, with a higher frequency of renal involvement [3–5]. Various treatment modalities have been used, including steroids and immunosuppression, but there is currently no consensus on the most effective treatment [6]. Therapeutic plasma exchange (TPE) has also been used in adults and children for a number of years but has been limited to short-term therapy only [7–22]. Here we present a young adult with HSP and rapidly progressive

kidney disease in whom we established long-term regular TPE for over three years to successfully hold off progression to end-stage renal disease (ESRD).

2. Case Report

In April 2010 a 27-year-old male with well controlled asthma presented to his local hospital with abdominal pain, palpable purpuric skin rash, bloating, sore throat, and joint swelling. He was diagnosed with HSP and commenced on oral steroids. Creatinine on admission was 104 μmol/L but three weeks later he transferred to our tertiary renal centre with a creatinine of 181 μmol/L, serum albumin 19 g/L, and haematoproteinuria, with a urinary protein: creatinine ratio (uPCR) of 6.19 g/g (700 g/mol). A renal immunological screen and ultrasound of the renal tract (including renal vein Doppler sonography) were normal. IgA levels were

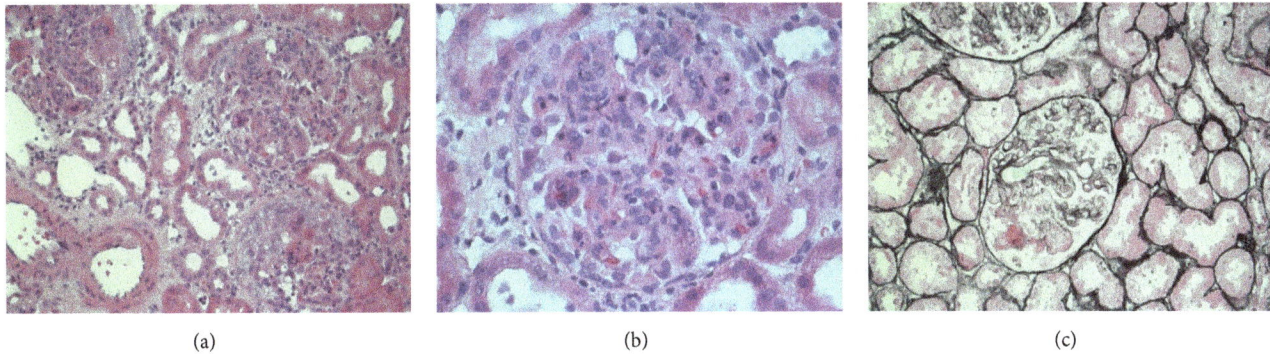

(a) (b) (c)

FIGURE 1: First native renal biopsy. (a and b) H&E slides from showing diffuse proliferative changes in all glomeruli, with neutrophils and foci of fibrinoid necrosis associated with epithelial crescents. (c) Silver stain showing obliteration of capillary loops, fibrinoid necrosis, and double contouring. Immunofluorescence showed a prominent granular positivity within the mesangium and to some extent within the membranes for IgA and C3. Oxford classification $M = 1$, $E = 1$, $S = 0$, and $T = 0$.

normal (2.21 g/L) with no evidence of IgA paraprotein. He had three pulses of methylprednisolone, and an urgent renal biopsy revealed appearances suggestive of HSP/IgAN with a prominent membranoproliferative pattern (Figure 1). Three of 15 (20%) glomeruli showed foci of fibrinoid necrosis associated with epithelial crescents and no evidence of fibrosis. Immunofluorescence demonstrated prominent granular positivity within the mesangium and within the membranes for IgA and C3. Electron microscopy showed prominent mesangial, paramesangial, and subendothelial deposits with associated patchy effacement of epithelial foot processes. The basement membranes appeared unremarkable. Oxford classification was $M = 1$, $E = 1$, $S = 0$, and $T = 0$. A mesangial hypercellularity score of 1 was originally shown to be an independent risk factor of renal decline [23]. In the Oxford classification validation study, the endocapillary hypercellularity score was shown to be associated with worsening renal function [24]. In the original Oxford classification study and the validation study both segmental glomerulosclerosis (S) and tubular atrophy/interstitial fibrosis (T) score were also shown to be associated with a poor renal outcome although these were not present on our patient's initial biopsy.

With the severity of the biopsy features and deteriorating renal function he was escalated to intravenous (IV) cyclophosphamide which stabilised his creatinine at around 280 μmol/L for one week before deteriorating rapidly to 687 μmol/L, after which he started haemodialysis and TPE. His creatinine improved to 300 μmol/L after 7 sessions of TPE; he stopped haemodialysis and was discharged on oral steroids, Ramipril, and IV cyclophosphamide. The IV cyclophosphamide was given monthly for 6 months, starting at a dose of 1200 mg (0.75 g/m^2), with a reduction to 1000 mg following the initial infusion due to renal function decline.

In July and August 2010 he was admitted twice with relapses characterised by acute kidney injury (AKI, creatinine 519 μmol/L); each of these relapses was heralded by a worsening of his rash but with no reduction in serum albumin or deterioration in uPCR (serum albumin 37 g/L and uPCR 2.40 g/g (271 g/mol) in August). During each episode of AKI, other causes such as infection, nephrotoxic therapy,

or change in therapy were ruled out and hence the episodes were attributed to active HSP disease; further evidence for this was provided by the fact that the renal function improved following TPE.

A repeat biopsy during the first relapse showed less severe acute glomerular lesions compared to his first biopsy: 3/30 sclerosed glomeruli but predominantly global mesangial hypercellularity, 13% (4/30) crescent formation, and mild diffuse interstitial fibrosis with some tubular loss. Immunofluorescence showed predominantly mesangial IgA deposits with weak IgG and C3 staining.

He received IV methylprednisolone followed by oral prednisolone, continuation of IV cyclophosphamide (6 pulses by 14 weeks), and 7 sessions of TPE, again with an improvement in his creatinine. He relapsed two weeks later with worsening leg rash, requiring IV methylprednisolone, two sessions of haemodialysis, and 4 sessions of TPE. Following this he had Rituximab which led to an improvement both clinically and biochemically with creatinine dropping to 181 μmol/L and uPCR to 0.88 g/g (100 g/mol) (Figure 2). His immunoglobulin levels were normal but dropped after commencing Rituximab with IgA levels falling to 0.54 g/L. From July 2010 to January 2011 he had a total of six doses but four weeks after his last dose his renal function was clearly deteriorating again. He initially received 1 g Rituximab in July 2010 followed by three doses of 700 mg at weekly intervals with the last dose on 29 September 2010. He received a further 700 mg Rituximab in October 2010 and another 1 g in January 2011.

Given the previous beneficial responses to TPE it was felt that regular long-term TPE was the most likely way to safely avoid further episodes of AKI. No evidence base was available to guide frequency and so he was empirically treated with a session every 1 or 2 weeks depending on symptoms and response of creatinine. The regular TPE regime was commenced 11 months after initial presentation and he was maintained on 5 mg prednisolone and Ramipril daily which kept his blood pressure well controlled.

In view of the long-term treatment plan he had an arteriovenous fistula fashioned to facilitate the TPE. Joint care

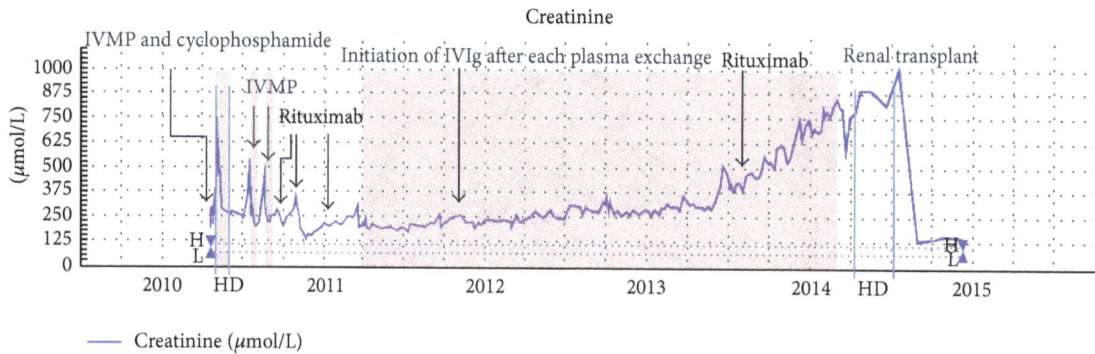

FIGURE 2: Therapy timeline with serum creatinine level from presentation to December 2014. Shaded area represents TPE therapy. IVMP, intravenous methylprednisolone; HD, haemodialysis; IVIg, intravenous immunoglobulin; PLEX, TPE.

with the immunology team helped to reduce the infection risk and he received daily prophylactic azithromycin, as well as intravenous immunoglobulin (initially 15 g but increased to 20 g due to low serum IgG levels in January 2012) with every session.

For 3 years, between March 2011 and March 2014, he had a total of 108 sessions of TPE with no further AKI episodes. There was however a steady decline in renal function (approximately 9 mL/min/1.73 m^2/year) and persistent haematoproteinuria with proteinuria in the range of 1.77–2.65 g/g (200–300 g/mol) with no significant improvement if the frequency of TPE was increased. Over this period his main extrarenal manifestation of leg rash settled.

From the middle of 2013 there was acceleration in his renal decline and associated rise in uPCR to 6.44 g/g (729 g/mol) but there were no extrarenal manifestations (Figure 2). This could not be halted despite increasing his TPE frequency to alternate days and reintroduction of Rituximab in July and October 2013 (1 g for each infusion). He started regular haemodialysis in March 2014 and had a live related renal transplant from his brother in August 2014. The graft functioned well from the outset with creatinine stabilizing at 150 μmol/L.

3. Discussion

Less than 10% of cases of HSP occur in adults, but this condition can have catastrophic implications with up to 11% reaching ESRD and 13% exhibiting severe renal impairment (creatinine clearance < 30 mL/min) [1–3]. Most studies investigating HSP in adults have been limited by small numbers but the consistency of disease severity and the nature of renal involvement is striking [3–5].

Unfortunately treatment options are limited, with little convincing evidence for immunosuppressive therapy; other than steroids, the Kidney Disease: Improving Global Outcomes (KDIGO) guidelines do not suggest the addition of immunosuppressive agents [6] and a meta-analysis concluded that data for any interventions that might improve kidney outcomes were sparse except for short-term prednisolone [25]. Rituximab has shown some promise although at present

there have only been three case reports in adult onset HSP, albeit all successful in controlling AKI and extrarenal manifestations and preventing ESRD [26–28].

The use of TPE alone or in combination with immunomodulation therapies in the acute phase of HSP is well reported in the literature [7–22]. However to the best of our knowledge there has been no previous report of the long-term use of TPE to prevent the onset of ESRD. Our patient received over 100 sessions of TPE in the more chronic progressive phase of his condition.

Since Berger and Hinglais described the mesangial deposition of IgA, the importance of this immunoglobulin in the disease pathogenesis has become ever clearer [29]. The body produces IgA at a daily rate which is more than all other immunoglobulins combined, but due to its short half-life and loss in secretions it is the second most prevalent class of antibody after IgG [30]. In patients with HSP and IgAN there appears to be abnormal glycosylation of polymeric IgA1 [31–33] with these molecules having a predilection for self-aggregation and for combining with IgG molecules to form antigenic circulating IgA-containing complexes [34, 35]. These circulating complexes, and in particular the high molecular weight complexes and those with high levels of aberrantly glycosylated IgA1, become deposited in the glomerular mesangium with high affinity and with subsequent stimulation of cellular proliferation, cytokine release, immune cell infiltration, and glomerular injury [36–40].

Following the discovery of the presence of circulating immune complexes in HSP over 30 years ago [36], reports began to emerge of the use of TPE in treatment of HSP. The benefit of this therapy lies in its ability to remove circulating immune complexes as found in HSP and IgAN [8]. Since that time, TPE has been used successfully in both adults and children and also for conditions associated with HSP such as cerebral vasculitis, intracerebral haemorrhage, haemorrhagic pancolitis, and skin manifestations but generally as a temporary measure [12, 13, 16, 17, 19, 21, 41]. The successful outcomes described in the literature may be due to the high proportion of patients, children especially, whose disease is self-limiting and also because of a degree of positive reporting bias. Given the 6-day half-life of IgA molecules, it could be hypothesised that in patients with a more severe phenotype of the disease more regular and long-term therapy with TPE should be necessary to remove the circulating immune complexes. Here we have shown that, in a patient with rapidly progressive renal disease resistant to traditional therapy, the long-term use of TPE can hold off the need for dialysis for a number of years.

Conflict of Interests

The authors declare no conflict of interests regarding the publication of this paper.

References

[1] J. M. M. Gardner-Medwin, P. Dolezalova, C. Cummins, and T. R. Southwood, "Incidence of Henoch-Schönlein purpura, Kawasaki disease, and rare vasculitides in children of different ethnic origins," *The Lancet*, vol. 360, no. 9341, pp. 1197–1202, 2002.

[2] F. T. Saulsbury, "Henoch-Schönlein purpura in children. Report of 100 patients and review of the literature," *Medicine*, vol. 78, no. 6, pp. 395–409, 1999.

[3] E. Pillebout, E. Thervet, G. Hill, C. Alberti, P. Vanhille, and D. Nochy, "Henoch-Schönlein Purpura in adults: outcome and prognostic factors," *Journal of the American Society of Nephrology*, vol. 13, no. 5, pp. 1271–1278, 2002.

[4] R. Coppo, S. Andrulli, A. Amore et al., "Predictors of outcome in Henoch-Schönlein nephritis in children and adults," *American Journal of Kidney Diseases*, vol. 47, no. 6, pp. 993–1003, 2006.

[5] S. Shrestha, N. Sumingan, J. Tan, H. Althous, L. McWilliam, and F. Ballardie, "Henoch Schönlein purpura with nephritis in adults: adverse prognostic indicators in a UK population," *QJM*, vol. 99, no. 4, pp. 253–265, 2006.

[6] G. Eknoyan, K. U. Eckardt, and B. L. Kasiske, "KDIGO clinical practice guideline for glomerulonephritis," *Kidney International Supplements*, vol. 2, no. 2, pp. 139–274, 2012.

[7] R. Coppo, B. Basolo, D. Roccatello et al., "Immunological monitoring of plasma exchange in primary IgA nephropathy," *Artificial Organs*, vol. 9, no. 4, pp. 351–360, 1985.

[8] R. Coppo, B. Basolo, O. Giachino et al., "Plasmapheresis in a patient with rapidly progressive idiopathic IgA nephropathy: removal of IgA-containing circulating immune complexes and clinical recovery," *Nephron*, vol. 40, no. 4, pp. 488–490, 1985.

[9] J.-F. Augusto, J. Sayegh, L. Delapierre et al., "Addition of plasma exchange to glucocorticosteroids for the treatment of severe Henoch-Schönlein purpura in adults: a case series," *American Journal of Kidney Diseases*, vol. 59, no. 5, pp. 663–669, 2012.

[10] D. Donghi, U. Schanz, U. Sahrbacher et al., "Life-threatening or organ-impairing Henoch-Schönlein purpura: plasmapheresis may save lives and limit organ damage," *Dermatology*, vol. 219, no. 2, pp. 167–170, 2009.

[11] K. Chaudhary, J.-Y. Shin, G. Saab, and A. M. Luger, "Successful treatment of Henoch-Schonlein purpura nephritis with plasma exchange in an adult male," *NDT Plus*, vol. 1, no. 5, pp. 303–306, 2008.

[12] B. Acar, F. I. Arikan, B. Alioglu, N. Oner, and Y. Dallar, "Successful treatment of gastrointestinal involvement in Henoch-Schönlein purpura with plasmapheresis," *Pediatric Nephrology*, vol. 23, no. 11, p. 2103, 2008.

[13] L. Karamadoukis, L. Ludeman, and A. J. Williams, "Henoch-Schönlein purpura with intracerebral haemorrhage in an adult patient: a case report," *Journal of Medical Case Reports*, vol. 2, no. 1, article 200, 2008.

[14] M. Shenoy, M. V. Ognjanovic, and M. G. Coulthard, "Treating severe Henoch-Schönlein and IgA nephritis with plasmapheresis alone," *Pediatric Nephrology*, vol. 22, no. 8, pp. 1167–1171, 2007.

[15] J. Rech, F. Fuchs, S. Kallert et al., "Plasmapheresis therapy in an elderly patient with rapidly progressive Henoch-Schönlein purpura with disseminated organ involvement," *Clinical Rheumatology*, vol. 26, no. 1, pp. 112–114, 2007.

[16] S. B. Wortmann, T. J. W. Fiselier, N. C. A. J. Van De Kar, R. A. H. M. Aarts, A. Warris, and J. M. T. Draaisma, "Refractory severe intestinal vasculitis due to Henoch-Schönlein Purpura: successful treatment with plasmapheresis," *Acta Paediatrica*, vol. 95, no. 5, pp. 622–623, 2006.

[17] Y.-K. Wen, Y. Yang, and C.-C. Chang, "Cerebral vasculitis and intracerebral hemorrhage in Henoch-Schönlein purpura treated with plasmapheresis," *Pediatric Nephrology*, vol. 20, no. 2, pp. 223–225, 2005.

[18] Y. Kawasaki, J. Suzuki, M. Murai et al., "Plasmapheresis therapy for rapidly progressive Henoch-Schönlein nephritis," *Pediatric Nephrology*, vol. 19, no. 8, pp. 920–923, 2004.

[19] C.-L. Chen, Y.-H. Chiou, C.-Y. Wu, P.-H. Lai, and H.-M. Chung, "Cerebral vasculitis in Henoch-Schönlein purpura: a case report with sequential magnetic resonance imaging changes and treated with plasmapheresis alone," *Pediatric Nephrology*, vol. 15, no. 3-4, pp. 276–278, 2000.

[20] T.-C. Chen, F.-R. Chung, C.-H. Lee, S.-C. Huang, J.-B. Chen, and K.-T. Hsu, "Successful treatment of crescentic glomerulonephritis associated with adult-onset Henoch-Schoenlein purpura by double-filtration plasmapheresis," *Clinical Nephrology*, vol. 61, no. 3, pp. 213–216, 2004.

[21] S. H. Eun, S. J. Kim, D. S. Cho, G. H. Chung, D. Y. Lee, and P. H. Hwang, "Cerebral vasculitis in Henoch-Schönlein purpura: MRI and MRA findings, treated with plasmapheresis alone," *Pediatrics International*, vol. 45, no. 4, pp. 484–487, 2003.

[22] A. Gianviti, R. S. Trompeter, T. M. Barratt, M. F. Lythgoe, and M. J. Dillon, "Retrospective study of plasma exchange in patients with idiopathic rapidly progressive glomerulonephritis and vasculitis," *Archives of Disease in Childhood*, vol. 75, no. 3, pp. 186–190, 1996.

[23] D. C. Cattran, R. Coppo, H. T. Cook et al., "The Oxford classification of IgA nephropathy: rationale, clinicopathological correlations, and classification," *Kidney International*, vol. 76, no. 5, pp. 534–545, 2009.

[24] R. Coppo, S. Troyanov, S. Bellur et al., "Validation of the Oxford classification of IgA nephropathy in cohorts with different presentations and treatments," *Kidney International*, vol. 86, no. 4, pp. 828–836, 2014.

[25] W. Chartapisak, S. L. Opastiraku, N. S. Willis, J. C. Craig, and E. M. Hodson, "Prevention and treatment of renal disease in Henoch-Schönlein purpura: a systematic review," *Archives of Disease in Childhood*, vol. 94, no. 2, pp. 132–137, 2009.

[26] E. Pillebout, F. Rocha, L. Fardet, M. Rybojad, J. Verine, and D. Glotz, "Successful outcome using rituximab as the only immunomodulation in Henoch-Schonlein Purpura: case report," *Nephrology Dialysis Transplantation*, vol. 26, no. 6, pp. 2044–2046, 2011.

[27] A. El-Husseini, A. Ahmed, A. Sabucedo, and E. Fabulo, "Refractory Henoch-Schönlein purpura: atypical aetiology and management," *Journal of Renal Care*, vol. 39, no. 2, pp. 77–81, 2013.

[28] T. P. Sala, J.-M. Michot, R. Snanoudj et al., "Successful outcome of a corticodependent Henoch-Schönlein purpura adult with rituximab," *Case Reports in Medicine*, vol. 2014, Article ID 619218, 4 pages, 2014.

[29] J. Berger and N. Hinglais, "Les dépôts intercapillaires d'IgA-IgG," *Journal d'Urologie et de Néphrologie*, vol. 74, pp. 694–695, 1968.

[30] J. M. Woof and M. A. Ken, "The function of immunoglobulin A in immunity," *Journal of Pathology*, vol. 208, no. 2, pp. 270–282, 2006.

[31] A. C. Allen, F. R. Willis, T. J. Beattie, and J. Feehally, "Abnormal IgA glycosylation in Henoch-Schonlein purpura restricted to patients with clinical nephritis," *Nephrology Dialysis Transplantation*, vol. 13, no. 4, pp. 930–934, 1998.

[32] K. K. Lau, R. J. Wyatt, Z. Moldoveanu et al., "Serum levels of galactose-deficient IgA in children with IgA nephropathy and Henoch-Schönlein purpura," *Pediatric Nephrology*, vol. 22, no. 12, pp. 2067–2072, 2007.

[33] K. K. Lau, H. Suzuki, J. Novak, and R. J. Wyatt, "Pathogenesis of Henoch-Schönlein purpura nephritis," *Pediatric Nephrology*, vol. 25, no. 1, pp. 19–26, 2010.

[34] M. Tomana, J. Novak, B. A. Julian, K. Matousovic, K. Konecny, and J. Mestecky, "Circulating immune complexes in IgA nephropathy consist of IgA1 with galactose-deficient hinge region and antiglycan antibodies," *The Journal of Clinical Investigation*, vol. 104, no. 1, pp. 73–81, 1999.

[35] J. Novak, Z. Moldoveanu, M. B. Renfrow et al., "IgA nephropathy and henoch-schoenlein purpura nephritis: aberrant glycosylation of IgA1, formation of IgA1-containing immune complexes, and activation of mesangial cells," *Contributions to Nephrology*, vol. 157, pp. 134–138, 2007.

[36] R. Levinsky and T. M. Barratt, "IgA immune complexes in Henoch-Schonlein Purpura," *The Lancet*, vol. 314, no. 8152, pp. 1100–1103, 1979.

[37] J. Novak, M. Tomana, K. Matousovic et al., "IgA1-containing immune complexes in IgA nephropathy differentially affect proliferation of mesangial cells," *Kidney International*, vol. 67, no. 2, pp. 504–513, 2005.

[38] J. Novak, L. Raskova Kafkova, H. Suzuki et al., "IgA1 immune complexes from pediatric patients with IgA nephropathy activate cultured human mesangial cells," *Nephrology Dialysis Transplantation*, vol. 26, no. 11, pp. 3451–3457, 2011.

[39] J. Novak, H. L. Vu, L. Novak, B. A. Julian, J. Mestecky, and M. Tomana, "Interactions of human mesangial cells with IgA and IgA-containing immune complexes," *Kidney International*, vol. 62, no. 2, pp. 465–475, 2002.

[40] T. Ootaka, T. Saito, J. Soma, A. Yusa, and K. Abe, "Mechanism of infiltration and activation of glomerular monocytes/macrophages in IgA nephropathy," *American Journal of Nephrology*, vol. 17, no. 2, pp. 137–145, 1997.

[41] O. Basaran, B. C. Acar, N. Uncu et al., "Plasma exchange therapy for severe gastrointestinal involvement of Henoch Schonlein purpura in children," *Pediatric Rheumatology*, vol. 12, supplement 1, article P357, 2014.

27

Concomitant Persistent Left Superior Vena Cava and Horseshoe Kidney

Faraz Jaffer and Vijay Chandiramani

University of Arizona, South Campus, Tucson, AZ 85715, USA

Correspondence should be addressed to Faraz Jaffer; farazjaffer@uahealth.com

Academic Editor: Yoshihide Fujigaki

Persistent left superior vena cava (PLSVC) and horseshoe kidney (HSK) are common congenital abnormalities; however presence of both in the same person is extremely rare. A patient with hepatitis C cirrhosis awaiting transplant presented with worsening liver dysfunction, diagnosed with acute renal failure secondary to hepatorenal syndrome, and required X-ray fluoroscopy guided tunneled venous catheter placement for hemodialysis. Review of imaging studies demonstrated coexistence of PLSVC and HSK. PLSVC in adulthood is usually incidental with the most common drainage pattern being without physiologic dysfunction. Isolated horseshoe kidney is still the most common of renal fusion anomalies; however etiology of coexistent PLSVC remains unknown.

1. Introduction

Persistent left superior vena cava (PLSVC) and horseshoe kidney (HSK) are common congenital abnormalities. The prevalence of PLSVC and HSK in the general population is 0.3–0.5% and 0.1–0.3%, respectively. Both PLSVC and HSK are known to be physiologically insignificant in most patients. The presence of both PLSVC and horseshoe kidney arising in the same person is extremely rare with concurrent prevalence estimates unknown.

2. Case Description

A 58-year-old female with medical history significant for liver cirrhosis secondary to hepatitis C infection, chronic obstructive pulmonary disease, diabetes mellitus, and hypertension presented to the hospital for increasing abdominal distension, weakness, and confusion. She was first diagnosed with chronic nonhepatitis B hepatitis in 1983, later revised to hepatitis C cirrhosis in 1992, and underwent pegylated interferon plus ribavirin treatment for three months in 2002; however, she ceased treatment due to adverse effects leading to noncompliance. Since 2011, the patient has been undergoing evaluation for liver transplantation on outpatient basis and no prior hospitalizations were reported due to complications from liver disease.

At presentation, patient's encephalopathic and physical examination was remarkable for abdominal distension with tenderness. Laboratory findings demonstrated serum sodium of 118 mMol/L, potassium of 6.4 mMol/L, chloride of 114 mMol/L, blood urea nitrogen of 57 mg/dL, and creatinine of 4.8 mg/dL (baseline: 0.8 mg/dL). The patient was found to be oliguric, urine microscopy demonstrated "muddy brown casts" consistent with acute tubular necrosis, and after extensive workup this was determined as secondary to hepatorenal physiology. Patient's renal status continued to deteriorate to eventual anuria, hyperkalemia refractory to medical management, and encephalopathy, for which a vascular catheter was fitted into the right internal jugular vein under ultrasound guidance without difficulty and care, and the patient was transferred to the intensive care unit for continuous venous-venous hemofiltration (CVVH) therapy. The patient received a 5-day total of CVVH and, on hospital day 7, with creatinine clearance of 15.32 mL/min, the patient shuttled to catheterization lab, where 15 mL of Isovue-300 contrast was used for safe placement of a right-sided tunneled venous catheter for scheduled triweekly hemodialysis sessions. Contrast enhanced X-ray fluoroscopy demonstrated persistent left superior vena cava (Figure 1). Upon careful review of current and past imaging studies, a contrast enhanced computed tomography (CT) of the thorax, abdomen, and pelvis and a magnetic resonance

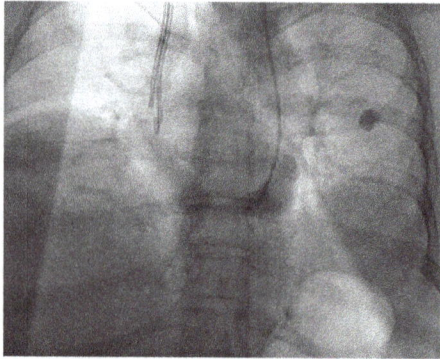

FIGURE 1: Persistence of left superior vena cava during X-ray fluoroscopic placement of tunnel dialysis catheter.

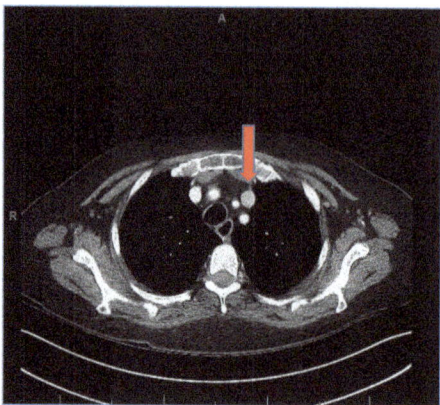

FIGURE 2: CT thorax visualizing persistent left superior vena cava.

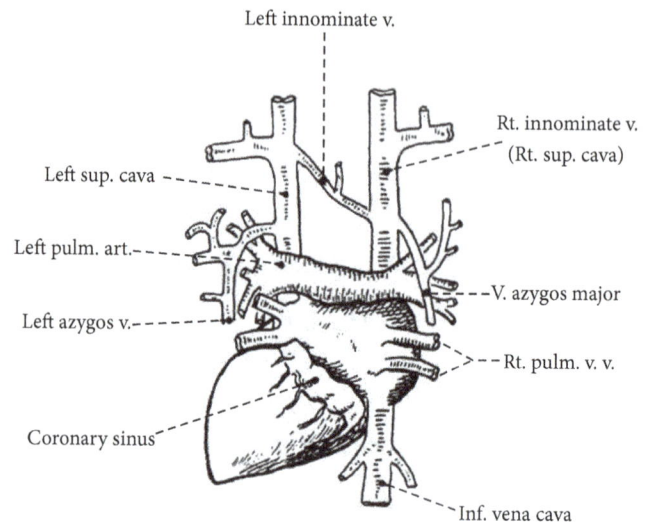

FIGURE 3: Diagram of the heart and great veins from behind, showing the arrangement in a case of persistence of the left superior cava. Credit: Sharpey-Schafer et al. [2].

imaging (MRI) of abdomen which were conducted as part of outpatient workup for liver transplantation corroborated the existence of both PLSVC and HSK (Figure 2).

3. Discussion

Genesis of PLSVC is due to failed regression of left anterior cardinal with or without persistent left innominate vein. Our patient presentation is consistent with the most common type of PLSVC which demonstrates both left and right SVCs draining into the right atrium via coronary sinus without physiological consequence (Figure 3). The less common presenting drain pattern, seen in 10–20% of patients with PLSVC, results in communication with left atrium leading to right-to-left shunt that can create paradoxical emboli leading to neurologic, mesenteric, and/or peripheral sequelae. Most are incidental findings on chest imaging with widened mediastinum on plain chest film, and computed tomography of chest provides a more defined image. In our case, prior CT imaging documented left superior vena cava and however was not readily available for review when patient underwent catheter placement. Intraoperative venography can be utilized to map venous abnormality. Cognizant of the patient's impaired creatinine clearance, we scheduled the procedure to precede patient's scheduled dialysis session and elected to conservatively use contrast in our fluoroscopy to ensure safe and appropriate placement of catheter and thus minimizing complications such as fatal perforation of superior vena cava reported in the setting of unrecognized stenosis due to prior trauma from intravenous catheter [1]. Although the most common types of PLSVC have not been known to be symptomatic, intravenous placement and their implications in these rare anomalies are yet to be demonstrated.

Concomitant presence of horseshoe kidney highlights the rarity of finding two common congenital abnormalities in the same person. Isolated horseshoe kidney is the most common of renal fusion anomalies and patients clinically present with acute renal failure due to anatomic complications of ureteropelvic junction obstructions, nephrolithiasis, and less commonly malignancies, which can all be treated successfully through endourological intervention. A retrospective analysis of patients with known history of HSK compared with general population demonstrated significantly increased prevalence of PLSVC; however, patients were asymptomatic and no reasons for their coexistence were identified. Even though there are no complications reported due to concurrent HSK with PLSVC, the etiology of their coexistence is unknown and thus warrants further investigation. In addition, it would be of use to investigate whether prevalence of horseshoe kidney retards recovery from acute kidney injury compared to general population.

Interventionists frequently utilize the left internal jugular as site of access for tunnel catheter placement; thus, identification and knowledge of anomalous vascular anatomy are vital to safe placement of tunneled central venous dialysis catheter.

Conflict of Interests

The authors declare that there is no conflict of interests regarding the publication of this paper.

References

[1] W. Schummer, C. Schummer, and H. Fritz, "Perforation der V. cava superior bei unerkannter Stenose Fallbericht einer letalen Komplikation einer zentralvenösen Katheterisierung," *Der Anaesthesist*, vol. 50, no. 10, pp. 772–777, 2001, English Abstract.

[2] E. Sharpey-Schafer, J. Symington, and T. H. Bryce, Eds., *Quain's Anatomy, Part III, The Heart*, vol. 4, Longmans, Green, and Co., London, UK, 11th edition, 1919.

28

Neonatal Urinary Ascites: A Report of Three Cases

Adaobi Solarin,[1] **Priya Gajjar,**[2] **and Peter Nourse**[2]

[1]Department of Paediatrics, Babcock University Teaching Hospital, PMB 21244, Ilishan-Remo, Ogun State, Nigeria
[2]Renal Unit, Red Cross Children's Hospital, Cape Town, South Africa

Correspondence should be addressed to Adaobi Solarin; asolar234@gmail.com

Academic Editor: Aikaterini Papagianni

Urinary ascites in neonates is not a common condition. Three cases of urinary ascites are presented and each of them has a different aetiology. Neonates with urinary ascites usually present as clinical emergency, requiring resuscitation, ventilator support, and subsequent drainage of urine. The ultimate management depends on the site of extravasation and the underlying cause.

1. Introduction

Reports of urinary ascites in the neonates date back to 1681 when Mauriceau [1, 2] gave the earliest description of foetal ascites. It was in 1952 that the first successfully treated case was reported [3]. Although it is a very rare condition, various causes have been attributed. Posterior urethral valve is most common accounting for approximately 70% of the aetiology. It occurs most commonly from the rupture of calyceal fornixes secondary to raised intrarenal pressure. Rarely, urinary bladder perforation is responsible for urinary ascites in posterior urethral valve.

Perforation of the neonatal bladder is rare, with only 17 cases reported between 1956 and 1985 [4]. Predisposing factors apart from posterior urethral valves include neurogenic bladder, congenital bladder diverticulum, and detrusor areflexia [4]. The majority are the results of umbilical arterial catheterization [5] causing rupture of the dome of the bladder or of patent urachus. Spontaneous rupture of the bladder has also been reported in the literature as a result of profound hypoxia or morphine administration [6], though rupture may also occur without clear predisposing factors and is presumably associated with obstructive uropathy, abdominal trauma, neurogenic bladder, difficult obstetric delivery, and iatrogenic injuries during urethral catheterization and umbilical catheterization [7].

Diagnosis is suspected on the basis of ascites with deranged renal function and is confirmed by imaging. Ultrasound helps to establish the presence of ascites and dilatation of the upper tracts with or without associated urinomas and cystic dysplasia of the kidneys. Voiding cystourethrography (VCUG) helps to establish the leak at the level of the urinary bladder by contrast extravasation into the peritoneal cavity and provides information about the underlying disease with associated changes in the urinary tracts. Neonatal urinary ascites is a life-threatening condition as the peritoneal membrane "autodialyzes" the urine, leading to progressive increase in the blood urea nitrogen (BUN) and derangement of the serum electrolytes. Management consists of catheter drainage or surgery depending on the condition of the neonate, with the primary aim of diversion of urine from the peritoneal cavity. Prognosis depends on early diagnosis and adequate urinary drainage.

2. Case 1

Baby S, male preterm, with birth weight of 1800 gm, was delivered at 33-week gestation by SVD on 5/05/2013. He had an Apgar score of 4 in 1 minute, 7 in 5 minutes. He required ventilator support and inotropes. At birth he was oedematous with marked abdominal distension. Mother is blood group O positive and coombs negative; she had apparently normal ultrasound at 16 weeks and 28 weeks. A TORCH screen to identify intrauterine infections was negative. Placental histology showed normal cord vessels and normal membrane while sections showed focal villous oedema. The renal function was deranged with serum creatinine of 148 micromol/L. Ascetic tap performed reveals high creatinine of 249 micromol/L

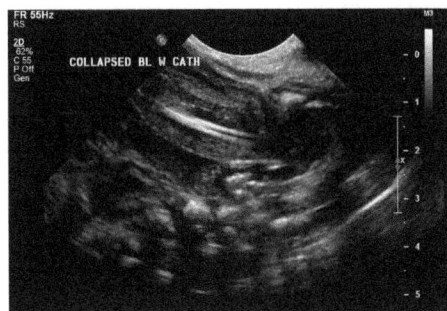

FIGURE 1: Catheter visualized with tip protruding through the dome of bladder.

compared to serum creatinine of 148. The baby was anuric; however, urinary catheter was passed and initial output improved to 4 mL/kg/hr. Ultrasonography showed catheter visualized in a collapsed bladder which appears to have a markedly thickened wall. The tip of catheter protrudes through the dome of the bladder (see Figure 1).

Blood creatinine dropped after catheterization from 148 to 42 micromol/L. Baby became polyuric and urinary losses were replaced with appropriate fluid. Cystoscopy and primary repair of posterior bladder wall were done and urinary catheter was removed on day 6 after operation. No posterior urethral valve was identified during the cystoscopy. Urine output normalized to 1 mL/kg/hr. This was a case of an isolated bladder perforation. He has been seen twice on follow-up; his creatinine remains normal, with good stream of urine. He has had one urinary tract infection; isolated organism was *Enterobacter cloacae* which was treated according to sensitivity profile. He has been discharged from urology clinic.

3. Case 2

Baby P, male, with birth weight of 3240 gms, was delivered at 36-week gestation by emergency caesarean section for macrosomia and abdominal ascites on 12/11/2013. Apgar score was 1 in 1 minute, 6 in 5 minutes, and 7 in 10 minutes. He was in marked respiratory distress attributed to the splitting of the diaphragm. There was also severe metabolic acidosis with pH of 6.78, pCO_2 17.7, pO_2 3.78, base excess of minus 19, and bicarbonate of 9.9. An ultrasound showed multicystic kidneys, marked bilateral hydronephrosis with a thickened bladder wall. Ascites was drained via a Tenckhoff catheterization. He was oliguric; urinary catheterization was done with urine output improving to 1.2 mL/kg/hr. Ascites fluid was analyzed with creatinine level of 118 micrommol/L while serum creatinine was 102 micromol/L. Micturating cystourethrogram showed a posterior urethral valve and a grade 5 vesicoureteric reflux into the right pelvicalyceal collecting system and ureter (see Figure 2). He had the valve ablated on 21/11/13, renal function normalized, and is being followed up by the nephrology and urology teams. He has four proven UTIs (*E. coli*, *Klebsiella*, *Enterococcus*, and *Pseudomonas aeruginosa,* resp.) and is treated with appropriate antibiotics according to sensitivity pattern. Renal

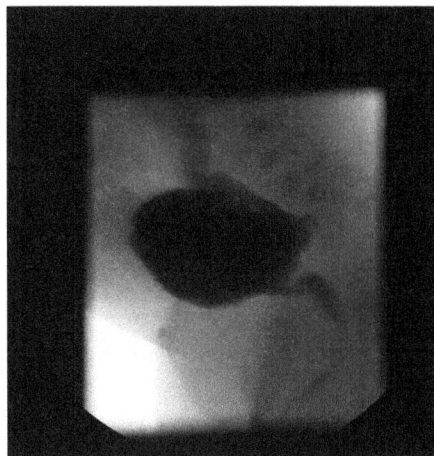

FIGURE 2: Voiding cystourethrogram confirming the posterior urethral valve.

function remains normal. He had serial ultrasounds done which showed persistent bilateral hydronephrosis and dilated ureters as well as debris in calyces of the left kidney and calcification demonstrated in the lower pole. MAG 3 diuretic renogram showed marked asymmetry of uptake, with left kidney within normal limit. Right kidney was smaller than left one and there was good Lasix response. Later image showed regular, well-defined renal margins after Lasix. Renal output efficiency was similar in both kidneys (left 90%, Rt 88%) and renal relative uptake (Lt 79%, Rt 21%).

He has been booked for reablation on 22/4/2015 by the urology team, and at last follow-up visit 27/02/15 he had no UTI and was between the 25th and 50th centile for weight and at the 50th centile for height.

4. Case 3

Baby H was delivered by caesarean section at 33 weeks and 6 days of gestation on 23/04/2013. Mother is known with type 2 diabetes mellitus, well controlled on metformin and insulin. Caesarean section was done on account of prolonged rupture of membrane and chorioamnionitis. Baby had respiratory distress at birth, requiring inotropes and ventilator support. He also had *E. coli* sepsis and was noted to develop progressively abdominal distension from the third day of life. He had oliguria with impaired renal function and hyponatremia. He was admitted at our center between 20/05/2013 and 26/05/2013. Micturating cystourethrogram showed immediate extravasation of contrast into peritoneal cavity. He had surgical repair of the bladder wall (see Figure 3). Urine output as well as renal function normalized. He was seen by the urology team on 23/08/2013 for follow-up and the renal function remained normal; weight and height are appropriate for age, and he was subsequently discharged from the unit.

5. Discussion

All the three cases presented had in common prematurity and hypoxia (see Table 1); however, there was no history of trauma

TABLE 1: Summary of the various cases and the management.

Cases (patients)	1	2	3
Gestational ages (weeks)	33	36	33
Birth weight (grams)	1800	3240	2500
Apgar score at 1, 5, and 10 mins or asphyxiated with abnormal blood gas	4, 7	1, 6, and 7	Asphyxiated
Ventilator support	Yes	Yes	Yes
Inotropes	Yes	No	Yes
Deranged renal function	Yes	Yes	Yes
Time of presentation of bladder rupture following birth	At birth	At birth	72 hrs
U/S, VCUG	Urethral catheter seen piercing dome of bladder	Bilateral hydronephrosis, hydroureters, and thickened trabeculae bladder. PUV is confirmed on VCUG	MCUG revealed extravasation of contrast into peritoneal cavity
Identifiable causes	Hypoxia, hypotension, and prematurity	PUV, hypoxia, and prematurity	Hypoxia, hypotension, and prematurity
Management of the bladder rupture	Abdominal paracentesis. Surgical repair of bladder wall tear	Conservative management. Abdominal paracentesis. Urethral catheter in situ for 10–14 days. Ablation of valve	Surgical repair of bladder wall tear
Clinical outcome	Successful	Successful, on long term follow-up	Successful

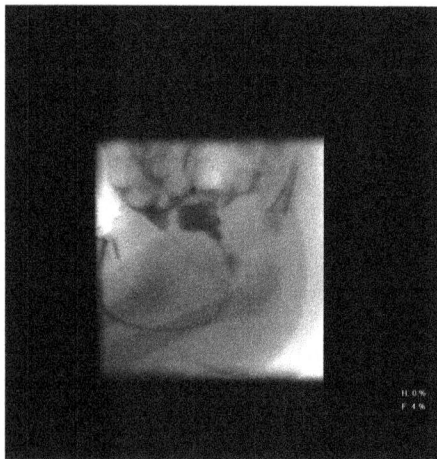

FIGURE 3: Water-soluble contrast administered via indwelling transurethral catheter. Spontaneous micturition on early filling (approximately 5 mL injected), with immediate extravasation of contrast into the peritoneal cavity. The study was therefore terminated, before the posterior urethra could be adequately evaluated. Bladder rupture is confirmed.

in any of them. One of the cases was a posterior urethral valve. Urinary ascites in posterior urethral valve can occur as a result of rupture of calyceal fornixes or transudation across the intact upper tract. It can also occur following the rupture of bladder wall. In obstructive uropathy, the upper tracts are subjected to high pressures in the intrauterine life. This affects the development of the kidneys and cystic renal dysplasia ensues. However, protective mechanisms do exist

to prevent this irreversible damage to the kidneys. These protective mechanisms include vesicoureteral reflux, bladder diverticula, and urine extravasation [8]. Extravasation at the level of the fornixes may result in urinoma formation around the kidneys, which may remain contained or communicate freely with the peritoneal cavity, leading to urinary ascites.

Urinary ascites can also occur following spontaneous or iatrogenic bladder rupture. The prolonged exposure to hypoxia that leads to ischemic visceral damage may also cause ischemic lesions to the bladder, which may lead to the rupture. Vasdev et al. [9] reported urinary ascites following bladder rupture of six cases. They attributed the rupture to hypoxia in all but one case. None of the cases Vasdev et al. [9] described was secondary to trauma and their time of presentation ranged from within 24 hours of life to 24 days. Umbilical arterial catheterization causing trauma to the dome of the bladder or to a patent urachus accounts for 75% of bladder ruptures [10]. The Foley catheter has also been reported to induce rupture [11, 12]. Morphine administration can cause urinary retention, which may lead to the rupture of the bladder [6].

Morrell et al. reported urinary ascites in a female preterm baby who had a spontaneous bladder rupture due to hypoxia [13]. Hypotension, abdominal distention, and electrolyte imbalance were observed in their patient. In this case report, Morrell et al. suggested that nontraumatic rupture of the bladder occurred as a result of hypoxia and hypotension, signifying that the bladder fundus vascular circulation is sensitive to ischemia [13]. The other case report in the literature described two preterm babies with nonobstructive urinary bladder rupture. This time, hypotension, severe respiratory distress, and umbilical artery catheterization were presented as risk factors [14]. Hypotonia and a full-stretched bladder may facilitate necrosis and spontaneous rupture of the bladder due to pressure [10].

Two of our presented cases had urinary ascites following bladder rupture. These babies had hypoxia and hypotension (requiring inotropes) and were also preterm. These are part of the identified risk factors for urinary ascites. Vasdev et al. [9] in their report highlighted the histologic appearance of the bladder following rupture. They postulated possible fetal hypoxia as reason for the ischaemic insult to the bladder. However, in our first patient who was born hydropic, histology of the placenta was morphologically abnormal while that histology of the debrided bladder was normal. This may be explained by the possibility that hypoxia could have occurred during delivery and not in utero.

The current diagnostic workup of patients with neonatal ascites consists of ultrasonography and paracentesis. The biochemical analysis of the ascites fluid should confirm the diagnosis of its origin; creatinine, urea nitrogen, and potassium concentrations are higher than the plasma levels [15]. In our cases, simultaneous plasma and ascites chemistry showed that creatinine concentrations of the ascites fluid were higher than the plasma creatinine concentrations, indicating urinary ascites in all cases. Findings on USG include hydroureteronephrosis, urinomas, ascites, changes in bladder in the form of thickening of the bladder wall, diverticula, and dilated posterior urethra.

VCUG is the modality of choice for demonstration of anatomy of the lower urinary tract, allowing confirmation of diagnosis of PUV, changes in the bladder, vesicoureteral reflux (VUR), and actual extravasation of the contrast from a rent in the bladder wall. Bladder changes for long-standing urethral obstruction include a large capacity or a contracted bladder with trabeculation, sacculation, or diverticula. There may be associated bladder neck hypertrophy seen as narrowing at the bladder neck.

Management has to be prompt with the basic aim of achieving decompression of the urinary tract. This may be accomplished by abdominal paracentesis, catheter drainage, or surgical exploration and repair of the bladder wall. One of the indications of abdominal paracentesis includes respiratory distress [16]. In cases of PUV, catheter drainage by urethral route with or without vesicostomy achieves healing in most patients in 10–14 days. Catheter drainage fails in ruptures with large rents and requires surgical repair. Our patients with identified rupture of the bladder were surgically repaired. Prognosis depends on the age at diagnosis and the extent of changes in the urinary tract.

A high degree of suspicion for urine leak as a cause of ascites when there is no clear cause of ascites should always be entertained. Once a baby without urethral obstruction has urinary ascites, this usually indicates a large bladder defect that will not close spontaneously with catheter drainage.

Conflict of Interests

The authors declared that there is no conflict of interests.

References

[1] F. Mauriceau, *Traite les maladies des femmes grosses*, Chez l'uteur, Paris, France, 3rd edition, 1681.

[2] S. J. Cywes, J. M. Wynne, and J. H. Louw, "Urinary ascites in the new-born with a report of two cases," *Journal of Pediatric Surgery*, vol. 3, no. 3, pp. 350–356, 1968.

[3] U. James and J. A. Davies, "Congenital urethral obstruction presenting in the newborn period," *Proceedings of the Royal Society of Medicine*, vol. 45, article 401, 1952.

[4] T. S. Trulock, D. P. Finnerty, and J. R. Woodard, "Neonatal bladder rupture: case report and review of literature," *Journal of Urology*, vol. 133, no. 2, pp. 271–273, 1985.

[5] P. Arora, A. Seth, D. Bagga, S. Aneja, and V. Taluja, "Spontaneous bladder rupture secondary to posterior urethral valves in a neonate," *Indian Journal of Pediatrics*, vol. 68, no. 9, pp. 881–882, 2001.

[6] A. Sayan, M. Demircan, V. S. Erikçi, A. Çelik, and A. Arikan, "Neonatal bladder rupture: an unusual complication of umbilical catheterization," *European Journal of Pediatric Surgery*, vol. 6, no. 6, pp. 378–379, 1996.

[7] J. F. Redman, J. J. Seibert, and W. Arnold, "Urinary ascites in children owing to extravasation of urine from the bladder," *The Journal of Urology*, vol. 122, no. 3, pp. 409–411, 1979.

[8] M. H. Rittenberg, W. C. Hulbert, H. M. Snyder III, and J. W. Duckett, "Protective factors in posterior urethral valves," *Journal of Urology*, vol. 140, no. 5, pp. 993–996, 1988.

[9] N. I. Vasdev, M. G. Coulthard, M. N. Delahunt, B. Stranyzk, M. Ognjanovic, and I. E. Willet, "Neonatal urinary ascites secondary to urinary bladder rupture," *Journal of Pediatric Urology*, vol. 5, no. 2, pp. 100–104, 2009.

[10] M. Basha, M. Subhani, A. Mersal, S. A. Saedi, and J. W. Balfe, "Urinary bladder perforation in a premature infant with Down syndrome," *Pediatric Nephrology*, vol. 18, no. 11, pp. 1189–1190, 2003.

[11] D. Bettelheim, W. Pumberger, J. Deutinger, and G. Bernaschek, "Prenatal diagnosis of fetal urinary ascites," *Ultrasound in Obstetrics and Gynecology*, vol. 16, no. 5, pp. 473–475, 2000.

[12] L. Löwenstein, I. Solt, R. Talmon, M. Pery, P. Suhov, and A. Drugan, "In utero diagnosis of bladder perforation with urinary ascites. A case report," *Fetal Diagnosis and Therapy*, vol. 18, no. 3, pp. 177–182, 2003.

[13] P. Morrell, M. G. Coulthard, and E. N. Hey, "Neonatal urinary ascites," *Archives of Disease in Childhood*, vol. 60, no. 7, pp. 676–678, 1985.

[14] D. A. Diamond and C. Ford, "Neonatal bladder rupture: a complication of umbilical artery catheterization," *Journal of Urology*, vol. 142, no. 6, pp. 1543–1544, 1989.

[15] W. C. Arnold, J. F. Redman, and J. J. Seibert, "Analysis of peritoneal fluid in urinary ascites," *Southern Medical Journal*, vol. 79, no. 5, pp. 591–594, 1986.

[16] C. Limas, C. Soultanidis, S. Deftereos, M. Skordala, and J. Sigalas, "A case of spontaneous rupture of the bladder," *Turkish Journal of Pediatrics*, vol. 49, no. 2, pp. 196–198, 2007.

IgG4-Related Tubulointerstitial Nephritis Associated with Membranous Nephropathy in Two Patients: Remission after Administering a Combination of Steroid and Mizoribine

Kana N. Miyata,[1,2] Hiromi Kihira,[2] Manabu Haneda,[2] and Yasuhide Nishio[2]

[1] *Division of Nephrology and Hypertension, Harbor-UCLA Medical Center, 1124 W. Carson Street, Torrance, CA 90502, USA*
[2] *Division of Nephrology, Department of Medicine, Tokyo Metropolitan Tama Medical Center, 2-8-29 Musashidai, Fuchu-shi, Tokyo 183-8524, Japan*

Correspondence should be addressed to Kana N. Miyata; kananoshiro@gmail.com

Academic Editor: Kouichi Hirayama

We report two cases of Japanese men who presented with proteinuria, eosinophilia, hypocomplementemia, and high serum immunoglobulin G4 (IgG4) concentration and were diagnosed with membranous nephropathy associated with IgG4-related tubulointerstitial nephritis on renal biopsy. The typical renal lesions of IgG4-related disease are tubulointerstitial nephritis, which improves remarkably with steroid therapy, and occasional glomerular changes. In our two cases, renal biopsy revealed IgG4-positive immune complex deposits in glomeruli in a pattern of membranous nephropathy and concurrent tubulointerstitial nephritis with IgG4 plasma cells. In both cases, proteinuria persisted with initial prednisolone treatment and was resolved only after the addition of mizoribine. We report the first two cases in which the combination of prednisolone and mizoribine was effective for treating membranous nephropathy associated with IgG4-related tubulointerstitial nephritis.

1. Introduction

Recently, attention has been drawn to immunoglobulin G4- (IgG4-) related diseases (IgG4-RD), an autoimmune disease involving multiple organs, including the pancreas, kidney, salivary and lacrimal glands, lung, lymph nodes, and retroperitoneum [1]. It is characterized by elevated serum IgG4 concentration and abundant IgG4-positive plasma cell infiltration into the tissues. In addition, renal lesions are observed, indicating IgG4-related kidney disease (IgG4-RKD). The most common pattern observed on kidney biopsy is tubulointerstitial nephritis (IgG4-TIN); the typical presentation in this case includes a gradual decrease in kidney function with mild or no hematuria and minimal or absence of proteinuria [2]. Glomerular lesions have recently been described, including membranous nephropathy, membranoproliferative glomerulonephritis, and mesangial proliferative glomerulonephritis.

We herein present two cases of membranous nephropathy with concurrent IgG4-TIN, both of which were successfully treated by a combination of prednisolone and mizoribine.

2. Case Report

2.1. Case 1. The patient was a 69-year-old Japanese man who presented with anorexia and weight loss. Five months prior to admission, he had visited a local hospital complaining of lower abdominal pain; colonoscopy revealed early-stage colon cancer, and he underwent endoscopic resection. The patient's persistent abdominal pain, anorexia, and weight loss of >10% after two months prompted a concern for recurrence of malignancy; however, computed tomography (CT), magnetic resonance imaging, and positron emission tomography scans showed no abnormalities other than mildly enlarged supraclavicular and para-aortic lymph nodes. He was referred

TABLE 1: Laboratory findings.

	Case 1	Case 2
Urinalysis; protein/blood	3+/3+	2+/2+
Urinary protein (g/day)	1.4	2.73
Urinary β2MG (μg/L)	11,080	858 (ref, 0–230)
Urinary NAG (U/L)	31.9	151.2 (ref, 0–11.5)
Creatinine (mg/dL)	1.0	0.9
CCr (mL/min)	92.4	49.1
BUN (mg/dL)	15.4	16.1
WBC (Eosinophil) ($\times 10^9$/L) (%)	11.5 (47.5)	7.4 (46.5)
Hemoglobin (g/dL)	11.9	9.5
Hematocrit (%)	35.4	28.5
Total protein (g/dL)	9.3	7.6
Albumin (g/dL)	2.2	1.7
AST (U/L)	27	43
ALT (U/L)	15	33
ALP (U/L)	492	480
Bilirubin, total (mg/dL)	0.4	0.4
Amylase (U/L)	60	N/A
CRP (mg/dL)	1.7	0.4
CH50 (U/mL)	<5	<5 (ref, 25–48)
C3 (mg/dL)	39	21 (ref, 86–160)
C4 (mg/dL)	2.0	<2 (ref, 17–45)
Antinuclear antibody	1:320 (Homo/Spec)	<1:40
Anti-dsDNA antibody	Negative	Negative
Anti-Sm antibody	Negative	Negative
Anti-RNP antibody	Negative	16.0
Anti-SSA antibody	Negative	Negative
Anti-SSB antibody	Negative	N/A
ANCA	Negative	Negative
IgA (mg/dL)	183	386 (ref, 110–410)
IgM (mg/dL)	37	468 (ref, 83–190)
IgE (mg/dL)	413	1811 (ref, 0–202)
IgG (mg/dL)	6989	6350 (ref, 870–1700)
IgG1 (mg/dL)	1710	2460 (ref, 423–1080)
IgG2 (mg/dL)	2280	1740 (ref, 265–931)
IgG3 (mg/dL)	249	1100 (ref, 5–121)
IgG4 (mg/dL)	2750	1050 (ref, 4–108)
S-IL2 receptor (U/mL)	3912	3973 (ref, 190–650)

TABLE 1: Continued.

	Case 1	Case 2
SPEP	Normal	Normal
Cryoglobulin	Negative	Negative

Note: Conversion factors for units: Creatinine in mg/dL to μmol/L, ×88.4; CCr in mL/min to mL/s, ×0.01667; BUN in mg/dL to mmol/L, ×0.357; Hemoglobin, Total protein, and Albumin in g/dL to g/L, ×10; Bilirubin in mg/dL to mol/L, ×17.1; CRP in mg/dL to mg/L, ×10; IgA, IgM, IgE in mg/dL to mg/L, ×10; IgG, IgG1, IgG2, IgG3, and IgG4 in mg/dL to g/L, ×0.01. No conversion necessary for C3, C4 in mg/dL and g/L.
Abbreviations and definitions: β2MG, β2 microglobulin; NAG, N-acetyl-beta-D-glucosaminidase; CCr, creatinine clearance; WBC, white blood cell; AST, aspartate aminotransferase; ALT, alanine aminotransferase; ALP, alkaline phosphatase; CRP, C-reactive protein; ANCA, antineutrophil cytoplasmic antibody; IgA, immunoglobulin A; S-IL2 receptor, soluble interleukin-2 receptor; SPEP, serum protein electrophoresis; ref, reference range.

to our tertiary medical center for further evaluation. His past medical history included hypertension, dyslipidemia, and glaucoma for 10 years. Physical examination was normal, except for mild hypertension (143/80 mmHg). Laboratory findings are listed in Table 1. Urinalysis showed proteinuria (3+) quantitated at 1.4 g/day and blood (3+). Urine sediment showed microhematuria (>100/high-power field) with hyaline and granular casts. Blood tests showed low levels of complement, elevated absolute eosinophil count (5.462/μL), and normal serum creatinine level 1.0 mg/dL (88.4 μmol/L). Serum total IgG and IgG4 levels were elevated at 6989 mg/dL and 2750 mg/dL, respectively. An abdominal CT scan with contrast and kidney ultrasound showed no abnormalities and showed both kidneys at 9 cm.

The renal biopsy tissue contained the cortex and medulla, with 27 glomeruli (Figure 1), and showed focal interstitial fibrosis accompanied by a patchy infiltration of mononuclear cells, eosinophils, and numerous IgG4-positive plasma cells (>10 per high-power field). The margins of the interstitial lesions were well defined. There were no glomerular scleroses or crescent formations. All glomeruli showed global thickening of the glomerular basement membrane (GBM) without duplication. There was no increase in mesangial cells, matrix, or endocapillary hypercellularity. Periodic acid silver-methenamine staining showed spikes. Immunofluorescence (IF) revealed a diffuse granular capillary wall staining of IgG and C1q without any extraglomerular deposits. IF indicated the absence of IgA, IgM, C3, and C4. Kappa and lambda staining were not performed. Immunoperoxidase stain showed weakly positive IgG4 staining along the GBM as well as interstitial inflammation, as indicated by IgG4-positive plasma cells. Electron microscopy showed subepithelial electron-dense deposits. Tubular basement membrane immune complex deposits were not seen.

Following the renal biopsy, the patient was diagnosed with IgG4-TIN and concurrent membranous nephropathy and was started on oral prednisolone 55 mg/day (0.9 mg/kg/day) with an immediate decrease in serum IgG levels and increase in serum complement. Proteinuria, however, persisted for over 2 months, fluctuating between 1.5 and 4 g/day, and oral mizoribine 100 mg/day was

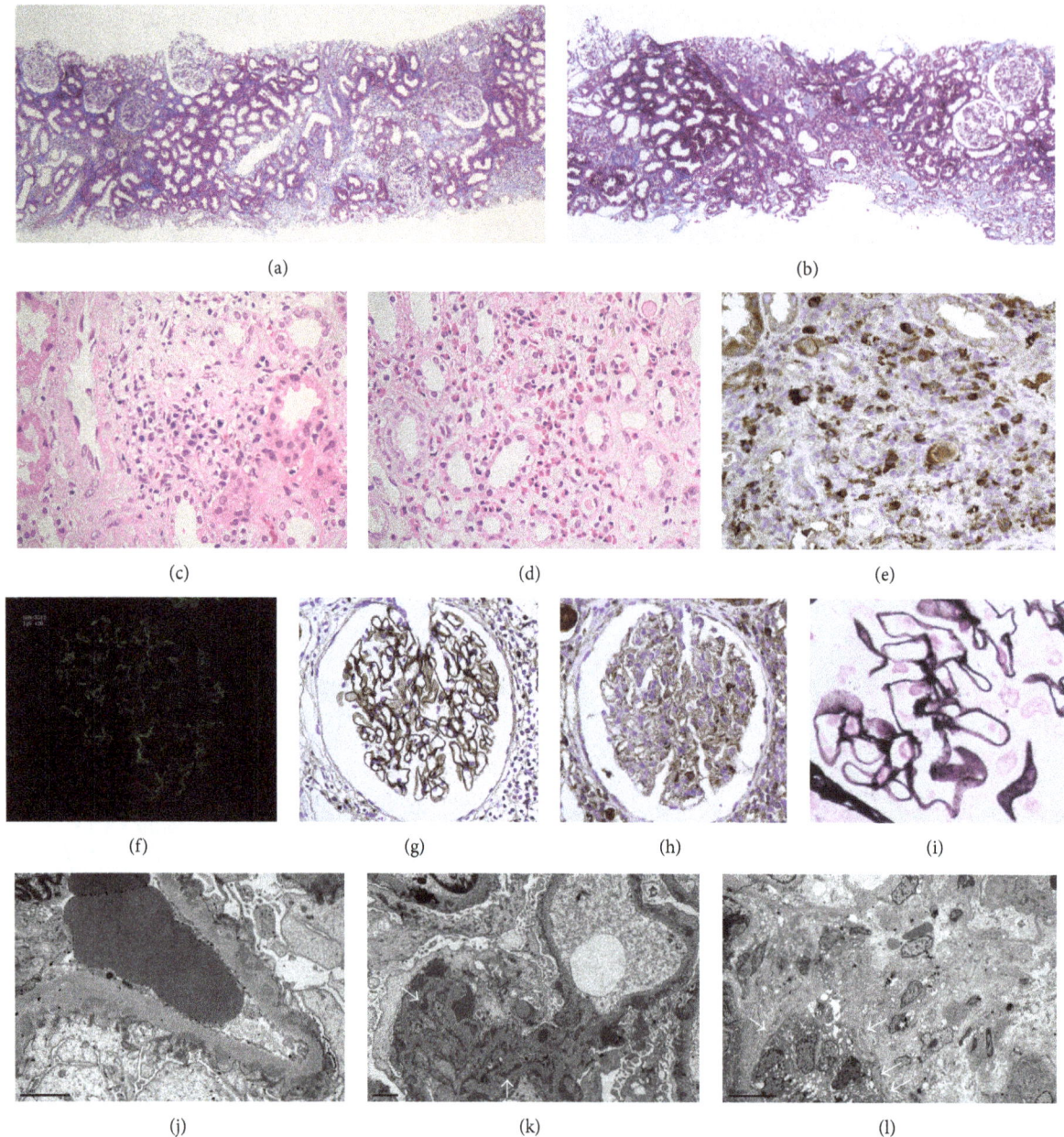

FIGURE 1: Representative microscopic histology. (a) Patchy infiltration of inflammatory cells and fibrosis in the interstitium with a clear border. Case 1. Masson trichrome stain, ×40. (b) Case 2. Masson trichrome stain, ×40. (c and d) Predominant infiltration of lymphocytes, plasma cells, and eosinophils into the interstitium. Case 1. H&E stain, ×400. (e) IgG4-positive plasma cells in the interstitium. Case 2. IgG4 immunoperoxidase stain, ×400. (f) Granular capillary wall staining for IgG. Case 1. Immunofluorescence, ×200. (g) IgG staining along the glomerular basement membrane (GBM). Case 1. IgG immunoperoxidase stain, ×400. (h) Weakly positive IgG4 staining along the GBM. Case 1. IgG4 immunoperoxidase stain, ×400. (i) Thickened GBM with spikes. Case 1. Periodic acid silver-methenamine stain, ×400. (j) Subepithelial electron-dense deposits. Case 1. ×20,000. (k) Subepithelial and mesangial electron-dense deposits. Case 2. ×10,000. (l) Scattered tubular basement membrane deposits. Case 2. ×4,000.

added. The patient's proteinuria finally trended down after initiation of mizoribine, reaching 0.4 g/day. Mizoribine was subsequently discontinued after the patient developed hepatotoxicity and was switched to azathioprine 25 mg/day. Currently, 4 years after the initial diagnosis, the patient is administered prednisolone 1 mg/day and azathioprine 25 mg/day, maintaining normal complement, normal serum creatinine level, and negative proteinuria. There were no extrarenal manifestations of IgG4-RD during this follow-up period.

2.2. Case 2. An 80-year-old Japanese man with a history of myocardial infarction, osteoarthritis, and 40-pack-year smoking was admitted to a local hospital with pancreatitis of unknown etiology 4 months prior to admission. One month after discharge, he developed leg edema on both legs and other features consistent with nephrotic syndrome, prompting referral to our medical center. Laboratory findings indicated proteinuria (2.73 g/day), eosinophilia (absolute eosinophil count 3.441/μL), hypoalbuminemia, and hypocomplementemia (Table 1). Serum creatinine was 0.9 mg/dL (79.6 μmol/L). Both IgG and IgG4 levels were elevated at 6350 mg/dL and 1350 mg/dL, respectively. Kidney ultrasound showed normal sized kidneys with small cysts. An abdominal CT scan with contrast showed a small amount of pleural effusion and ascites, without any lesions in either kidney.

Renal biopsy specimens showed interstitial infiltration of lymphocytes, plasma cells, and eosinophils, with accompanying interstitial fibrosis (Figure 1). Many of the plasma cells were positive for IgG4 staining (>10 per high-power field). All 11 glomeruli showed spikes along the glomerular capillary walls. Routine IF showed diffuse and global IgG, C3, and C1q depositions along the GBM and negative staining for IgA, IgM, and C4. Kappa and lambda staining were not performed. Granular deposition of IgG4 along the GBM was also seen on immunoperoxidase staining. Electron microscopy revealed subepithelial and mesangial electron-dense deposits and scattered tubular basement membrane deposits.

Oral prednisolone at an initial dose of 40 mg/day (0.6 mg/kg/day) reduced his serum complement and IgG levels, and proteinuria was resolved to some extent (0.3 g/day). Two months later, when the prednisolone dose was tapered, however, proteinuria recurred (2.6 g/day); mizoribine was added to his regimen, which resolved the proteinuria. He had another episode of proteinuria 10 months after the initiation of mizoribine, which was resolved with temporarily increased prednisolone dose. We followed up with this patient for 17 months after the initial diagnosis when he tested negative for proteinuria and had normal complement and serum creatinine levels, and, subsequently, we tapered the prednisolone dose to 10 mg/day with mizoribine 150 mg/day. There was no recurrence of pancreatitis or any other extrarenal manifestations of IgG4-RD during the follow-up period.

3. Discussion

While many studies have reported IgG4-RKD in the past decade, a proposal on diagnostic criteria has been only recently published [1, 13]. IgG4-TIN can be diagnosed on the basis of the histological features of plasma cell-rich TIN with >10 IgG4-positive plasma cells per high-power field in the most concentrated field and at least one other feature using imaging, serology, or other organ involvement [1]. Both our cases satisfied the criteria of histological features and serology (elevated serum total IgG and IgG4 levels). Imaging did not show any radiographic features of IgG4-TIN such as low-attenuation renal lesions or diffuse marked enlargement of the kidneys. Although other organ involvement was not apparent, mildly enlarged *supraclavicular and para-aortic* lymph nodes on CT in Case 1 and a recent history of pancreatitis of unknown etiology in Case 2 were assumed to be secondary to IgG4-RD.

It is unclear why most cases of IgG4-RKD show TIN, whereas some cases show concurrent glomerular lesions. Nishi et al. reviewed 37 cases of IgG4-RKD that presented with TIN, of which 10 cases (27%) had complicated glomerulonephritis, including mesangial proliferative glomerulonephritis, membranous nephropathy, membranoproliferative glomerulonephritis, and endocapillary proliferative glomerulonephritis [2]. Proteinuria was generally mild or absent in most solely IgG4-TIN cases; however, similar to our cases with concurrent glomerulonephritis, they had moderate proteinuria. Membranous nephropathy has been the most commonly observed glomerular lesion associated with IgG4-RD; recently, even membranous nephropathy without TIN but with other features of IgG4-RD has also been recognized as part of IgG4-RKD [9, 11, 12]. To date, 21 cases of membranous nephropathy as a manifestation of IgG4-RD (IgG4-related membranous nephropathy) have been reported (Table 2) [1, 3–16]. Interestingly, it is also recognized that primary membranous nephropathy is an IgG4-dominant disease, and it is important to distinguish IgG4-related membranous nephropathy from primary membranous nephropathy. The latest case reports showed the absence of circulating antiphospholipase A2 receptor antibodies in cases of membranous nephropathy with IgG4-RD, suggesting that the membranous nephropathy was not idiopathic but was likely secondary to IgG4-RD [10–12, 16].

Of the 15 cases in which the treatment and the outcome were reported, 13 cases were initially administered corticosteroid therapy based on the fact that typical IgG4-RD and IgG4-TIN improve remarkably with steroid therapy (Table 2). However, eventually, 3 cases required mycophenolate mofetil [11], 3 cases required rituximab [11, 12, 15], and 1 case was treated with cyclophosphamide [11]. During the follow-up period, 2 cases required maintenance hemodialysis [8, 15] and 1 case had a renal transplant [11]. Proteinuria in 7 cases remained at >1.5 g/day after treatment, though serum creatinine and proteinuria partially improved [4, 5, 11, 12]. Overall, the treatment was not completely successful in many of the IgG4-related membranous nephropathy cases.

In the two present cases, we initially failed to control proteinuria with steroids alone but observed a decrease to 0 g/day as well as maintenance of renal function after adding mizoribine. Mizoribine is an imidazole nucleoside with immunosuppressive activity, which inhibits T-cell and B-cell proliferation [17]. Its use has been associated with a low incidence of severe adverse reactions; in Japan, it is currently used widely for preventing rejection in renal transplantation and for the treatment of lupus nephritis, IgA nephropathy, and rheumatoid arthritis. Its immunosuppressive mechanism is similar to mycophenolate mofetil as an inhibitor of inosine 5'-monophosphate dehydrogenase, but it is recently proposed to have further unique properties; inhibition of renal macrophage accumulation and prevention of glomerulosclerosis and interstitial fibrosis in non-insulin-dependent diabetic kidneys [18], enhancement of glucocorticoid efficacy by binding to 14-3-3 protein and HSP60 in glomerular cells [19, 20], and better histologic outcome in IgA nephropathy in group of steroid plus mizoribine combination therapy compared to group of steroid monotherapy [21].

TABLE 2: Treatment and the effect of IgG4-related membranous nephropathy reported in previous studies.

Case	References, Year	Age (years)	Gender	IgG4/IgG (mg/dL)	TIN	S-Cr (mg/dL) Pre Tx	S-Cr (mg/dL) Post Tx	U-pro (g/day) Pre Tx	U-pro (g/day) Post Tx	f/u (months)	Treatment
1	Uchiyama-Tanaka et al. 2004 [3]	64	Male	665/5410	yes	4.5	1.5	1.5	0.1	2	mPSL
2	Watson et al. 2006 [4]	67	Male	2125/7070	yes	3.4	2.4	2.4	2.5	7	PSL
3	Saeki et al. 2009 [5], Saeki et al. 2010 [6], Saeki et al. 2013 [7]	83	Male	924/3144	yes	1.48	1.22	2.3	1.6	4	PSL
4	Saida et al. 2010 [8], Saeki et al. 2010 [6], Saeki et al. 2013 [7]	78	Male	1860/3731	yes	6.17	HD	1.38	HD	NA	PSL
5	Palmisano et al. 2010 [9]	68	Male	NA	no	1.2	NA	1.5	0.45	NA	ACEI, statins
6	Raissian et al. 2011 [1]	75	Male	NA	yes	6.6	2.5	16	NA	1.1	PSL
7	Raissian et al. 2011 [1], Fervenza et al. 2011 [10], Alexander et al. 2013 [11]	67	Female	531/1581	yes	1.2	1.3	4	0.2	7	PSL
8	Craveri et al. 2011 [12]	54	Male	730/2022	no	1.15	NA	7.3	8	11	PSL, Rituximab
9	Kawano et al. 2011 [13]	NA	NA	NA	yes	NA	NA	NA	NA	NA	NA
10	Yamaguchi et al. 2012 [14]	60	Female	142/1706	yes	1.05	NA	14	NA	NA	NA
11	Yamaguchi et al. 2012 [14]	64	Male	260/4292	yes	1.4	NA	0.67	NA	NA	NA
12	Jindal et al. 2012 [15]	72	Male	750/1511	yes	4.7	HD	15	HD	NA	PSL, Rituximab
13	Alexander et al. 2013 [11]	75	Male	NA	yes	6.6	2.5	16	3.1	6	PSL
14	Alexander et al. 2013 [11]	53	Male	NA	no	0.8	0.8	16	3.1	46	PSL, MMF
15	Alexander et al. 2013 [11]	50	Male	NA	no	1.3	1.3	3.5	1.5	20	ACEI/ARB, Rituximab, MMF
16	Alexander et al. 2013 [11]	46	Female	NA	yes	NA	Transplant	Nephrotic	0	184	none
17	Alexander et al. 2013 [11]	67	Male	NA	yes	1.8	1.4	4.5	0.7	7	PSL, Cy, ACEI
18	Alexander et al. 2013 [11]	65	Female	NA	yes	0.7	0.8	8.5	2.6	4	PSL, MMF
19	Alexander et al. 2013 [11]	64	Male	NA	yes	3.4	NA	1.7	NA	NA	NA
20	Alexander et al. 2013 [11]	34	Male	NA	no	1.6	NA	12.4	NA	NA	NA
21	Li et al. 2014 [16]	55	Male	1926/5305	yes	0.8	NA	5.5	0.2	20	PSL
22	Miyata et al. 2014 (Case 1)	69	Male	2750/6989	yes	1.0	1.17	1.4	0	48	PSL, MZR, AZA
23	Miyata et al. 2014 (Case 2)	80	Male	1050/6350	yes	0.9	0.78	2.73	0	17	PSL, MZR

Abbreviations: ACEI, angiotensin-converting enzyme inhibitor; ARB, angiotensin receptor blocker; AZA, Azathioprine; Cy, cyclophosphamide; f/u, follow up; HD, hemodialysis; mPSL, methylprednisolone; MMF, Mycophenolate mofetil; MZR, mizoribine; PSL, prednisone/prednisolone; S-Cr, serum creatinine; TIN, tubulointerstitial nephritis; U-Pro, urine protein.

While IgG4-RD is generally known to have a favorable response to steroid treatment, a poor response in cases of proteinuria with steroid therapy suggests that, although TIN subsides with steroids, the membranous nephropathy may linger. In such cases, it is justified to treat patients with immunosuppressants.

In summary, we describe two cases of IgG4-TIN with concurrent membranous nephropathy that responded favorably to the combination of prednisolone and mizoribine. When renal function or proteinuria in IgG4-RKD does not respond well to steroid therapy, particularly when these conditions are associated with membranous nephropathy, the administration of immunosuppressants should be considered.

Conflict of Interests

The authors declare that there is no conflict of interests regarding the publication of this paper.

References

[1] Y. Raissian, S. H. Nasr, C. P. Larsen et al., "Diagnosis of IgG4-related tubulointerstitial nephritis," *Journal of the American Society of Nephrology*, vol. 22, no. 7, pp. 1343–1352, 2011.

[2] S. Nishi, N. Imai, K. Yoshida, Y. Ito, and T. Saeki, "Clinicopathological findings of immunoglobulin G4-related kidney disease," *Clinical and Experimental Nephrology*, vol. 15, no. 6, pp. 810–819, 2011.

[3] Y. Uchiyama-Tanaka, Y. Mori, T. Kimura et al., "Acute tubulointerstitial nephritis associated with autoimmune-related pancreatitis," *The American Journal of Kidney Diseases*, vol. 43, no. 3, pp. e18–e25, 2004.

[4] S. J. W. Watson, D. A. S. Jenkins, and C. O. S. Bellamy, "Nephropathy in IgG4-related systemic disease," *The American Journal of Surgical Pathology*, vol. 30, no. 11, pp. 1472–1477, 2006.

[5] T. Saeki, N. Imai, T. Ito, H. Yamazaki, and S. Nishi, "Membranous nephropathy associated with IgG4-related systemic disease and without autoimmune pancreatitis," *Clinical Nephrology*, vol. 71, no. 2, pp. 173–178, 2009.

[6] T. Saeki, S. Nishi, N. Imai et al., "Clinicopathological characteristics of patients with IgG4-related tubulointerstitial nephritis," *Kidney International*, vol. 78, no. 10, pp. 1016–1023, 2010.

[7] T. Saeki, M. Kawano, I. Mizushima et al., "The clinical course of patients with IgG4-related kidney disease," *Kidney International*, vol. 84, pp. 826–833, 2013.

[8] Y. Saida, N. Homma, H. Hama et al., "A case of IgG4-related tubulointerstitial nephritis showing the progression of renal dysfunction after a cure for autoimmune pancreatitis," *Japanese Journal of Nephrology*, vol. 52, no. 1, pp. 73–79, 2010.

[9] A. Palmisano, D. Corradi, M. L. Carnevali et al., "Chronic periaortitis associated with membranous nephropathy: clues to common pathogenetic mechanisms," *Clinical Nephrology*, vol. 74, no. 6, pp. 485–490, 2010.

[10] F. C. Fervenza, G. Downer, L. H. Beck Jr., and S. Sethi, "IgG4-related tubulointerstitial nephritis with membranous nephropathy," *The American Journal of Kidney Diseases*, vol. 58, no. 2, pp. 320–324, 2011.

[11] M. P. Alexander, C. P. Larsen, I. W. Gibson et al., "Membranous glomerulonephritis is a manifestation of IgG4-related disease," *Kidney International*, vol. 83, no. 3, pp. 455–462, 2013.

[12] P. Cravedi, M. Abbate, E. Gagliardini et al., "Membranous nephropathy associated with IgG4-related disease," *The American Journal of Kidney Diseases*, vol. 58, no. 2, pp. 272–275, 2011.

[13] M. Kawano, T. Saeki, H. Nakashima et al., "Proposal for diagnostic criteria for IgG4-related kidney disease," *Clinical and Experimental Nephrology*, vol. 15, no. 5, pp. 615–626, 2011.

[14] Y. Yamaguchi, Y. Kanetsuna, K. Honda, N. Yamanaka, M. Kawano, and M. Nagata, "Characteristic tubulointerstitial nephritis in IgG4-related disease," *Human Pathology*, vol. 43, no. 4, pp. 536–549, 2012.

[15] N. Jindal, D. Yadav, C. Passero et al., "Membranous nephropathy: a rare renal manifestation of IgG4-related systemic disease," *Clinical Nephrology*, vol. 77, no. 4, pp. 321–328, 2012.

[16] X. L. Li, T. K. Yan, H. F. Li et al., "IgG4-related membranous nephropathy with high blood and low urine IgG4/IgG ratio: a case report and review of the literature," *Clinical Rheumatology*, vol. 33, pp. 145–148, 2014.

[17] H. Tanaka, K. Tsuruga, T. Aizawa-Yashiro, S. Watanabe, and T. Imaizumi, "Treatment of young patients with lupus nephritis using calcineurin inhibitors," *World Journal of Nephrology*, vol. 1, pp. 177–183, 2012.

[18] Y. Kikuchi, T. Imakiire, M. Yamada et al., "Mizoribine reduces renal injury and macrophage infiltration in non-insulin-dependent diabetic rats," *Nephrology Dialysis Transplantation*, vol. 20, no. 8, pp. 1573–1581, 2005.

[19] S. Takahashi, H. Wakui, J.-Å. Gustafsson, J. Zilliacus, and H. Itoh, "Functional interaction of the immunosuppressant mizoribine with the 14-3-3 protein," *Biochemical and Biophysical Research Communications*, vol. 274, no. 1, pp. 87–92, 2000.

[20] H. Itoh, A. Komatsuda, H. Wakui, A. B. Miura, and Y. Tashima, "Mammalian HSP60 is a major target for an immunosuppressant mizoribine," *Journal of Biological Chemistry*, vol. 274, no. 49, pp. 35147–35151, 1999.

[21] Y. Kawasaki, M. Hosoya, J. Suzuki et al., "Efficacy of multidrug therapy combined with mizoribine in children with diffuse IgA nephropathy in comparison with multidrug therapy without mizoribine and with methylprednisolone pulse therapy," *The American Journal of Nephrology*, vol. 24, no. 6, pp. 576–581, 2004.

30

A Case of Nephrotic Syndrome, Showing Evidence of Response to Saquinavir

Giles Walters,[1,2] **Faisal A. Choudhury,**[3] **and Budhima Nanayakkara**[3]

[1]*Department of Renal Medicine, Canberra Hospital, Garran, ACT 2605, Australia*
[2]*Australian National University Medical School, Canberra, Australia*
[3]*The Canberra Hospital, Australia*

Correspondence should be addressed to Faisal A. Choudhury; drfaisal56@gmail.com

Academic Editor: Patrick Honoré

The treatment of primary nephrotic syndrome such as minimal change nephropathy, membranous nephropathy, and focal segmental glomerulosclerosis nephropathy remains challenging. Whilst most cases of idiopathic nephrotic syndrome respond to steroid therapy and experience a limited number of relapses prior to complete remission, some cases suffer from frequent relapses and become steroid dependent or are primarily steroid resistant. Treatment options are limited to immunosuppressive drugs with significant side effect profiles. New modalities targeting novel pathways in the pathogenesis of nephrotic syndrome are actively sought. Here we report the case of a patient with steroid dependent focal segmental glomerulosclerosis (FSGS) nephrotic syndrome with a favourable response to a novel proteasome inhibitor saquinavir.

1. Introduction

This case study highlights the potential use of saquinavir, a proteasome inhibitor, to treat a difficult case of steroid dependent nephrotic syndrome. Saquinavir as long-term therapy is well tolerated amongst seropositive HIV patients [1, 2] and is known to reduce HIV induced proteinuria [3]. In addition to its HIV protease inhibition, it also acts to inhibit the proteasome, a key factor in the regulation of NF-κB activity [4–6]. The proteasome was implicated in pathogenesis by studies showing that NF-κB is elevated in circulating peripheral blood mononuclear cells in patients with idiopathic nephrotic syndrome [7, 8]. This was confirmed by T-cell transcriptome analysis [9]. Elevation of NF-kappa beta in T cells and its subsequent translocation into the nucleus lead to synthesis of circulating T-cell factors causing podocyte cytoskeleton disorganisation, increased glomerular permeability, and eventual proteinuria [10].

2. Case Study: Nephrotic Syndrome, Showing Evidence of Response to Saquinavir

The patient is a 23-year-old male of African Caucasian background first diagnosed with nephrotic syndrome at

the age of 4. He has been on multiple immunosuppressive regimes including cyclophosphamide, levamisole, rituximab, cyclosporine, tacrolimus, and mycophenolate mofetil. During his lifetime he has been a frequent relapser showing poor response to many steroid sparing medications. At his latest admission for relapse of nephrotic syndrome (biopsy confirmed FSGS) he was given a trial of antiretroviral proteasome inhibitor saquinavir and prednisolone followed by maintenance with saquinavir, prednisolone, and low dose cyclosporine. We report an initial response to this regime, adding support to the small number of existing cases regarding the therapeutic efficacy of saquinavir in the treatment of nephrotic syndrome.

This patient was initially seen at the Department of Renal Medicine at the Canberra Hospital in 2009 as an 18-year-old male, who otherwise had no major medical or surgical comorbidities. He had his first episode of nephrotic syndrome at the age of 4 in another centre, and since then he had been a frequent relapser but steroid responsive. Prior to being seen at our clinic, he had received two courses of cyclophosphamide in 1995 (2 mg/kg for 72 days and then 1.7 mg/kg for 90 days). Initial biopsy in 1995 revealed only minimal change. Levamisole was started as a steroid sparing agent, but after 4 years he developed a serum-sickness-like syndrome. Subsequently, levamisole was switched to cyclosporine. He was maintained on therapeutic cyclosporine for 2 years. A repeat biopsy showed prominent peritubular calcification consistent with calcineurin inhibitor toxicity. A decision to decrease cyclosporine was made and in early 2007 he had a further relapse with resistant nephrotic syndrome despite methylprednisolone and high dose diuretics. His admission was complicated by hypertension and pulmonary oedema. A biopsy at admission showed FSGS. Following his discharge from hospital his oedema and hypoalbuminaemia persisted. A decision was made to initiate rituximab therapy and he was given 3 doses in October 2007. Despite the depletion of his CD19 cells there was no remission in his clinical symptoms and he remained oedematous. He was restarted on cyclosporine and high dose prednisolone achieving remission. From this time onwards he was reviewed in clinic at the Canberra Hospital, with nearly monthly reviews following his renal function, fluid status, and blood pressure. A further relapse occurred in April 2010, after which cyclosporine was switched to tacrolimus. This resulted in remission, and the patient was able to taper his prednisolone to doses of 5 mg daily. A repeat biopsy in 2010 showed FSGS. Unfortunately from 2010 until 2012 this patient had 2 further relapses, and in-between relapses could not be weaned off prednisolone. Monthly clinical reviews revealed persistent hypoalbuminaemia, proteinuria, raised creatinine trending above baseline, and hypertension. Mycophenolate mofetil (1 g BD) was considered as a possibility given the already exhaustive list of immunosuppressive medications trialled with limited effect. Initiation of this purine synthesis inhibitor in addition to tacrolimus leads to normalisation of creatinine and serum albumin levels. During this trial period he had an episode of acute renal impairment with creatinine rising to 220 micromol/L and albumin falling to 25 mg/dL. Additionally the patient complained of intolerable gastrointestinal side effects with worsening hypertension. Mycophenolate mofetil was ceased, which unfortunately led to acute renal impairment in December 2012 with creatinine levels rising to 267, albumin of 21, and increased tissue oedema. He was admitted for in-patient management where tacrolimus was ceased and hypervolemia was treated with aggressive frusemide therapy and fluid restriction. A trial of saquinavir 1 g BD with prednisolone 75 mg daily was started. Approximately one month following discharge from hospital, this patient's oedema had fully resolved and creatinine resolved to near baseline levels. Prednisolone was gradually weaned to 15 mg daily with the introduction of low dose cyclosporine (10 mg BD), much lower than previous doses used in maintaining remission. The patient remained in remission for 2 months. Unfortunately in May 2013 he had a further relapse into nephrotic syndrome and high dose prednisolone (75 mg daily) was required for remission. He is currently maintained in a state of remission with the following medications and doses: prednisolone 5 mg daily, saquinavir 1 gm BD, and cyclosporine 10 mg BD. Apart from his steroid dependent nephrotic syndrome, his only other medical comorbidity is gout which is well controlled on

allopurinol 100 mg daily. He remains hypertensive requiring multiple antihypertensive medications including ramipril, minoxidil, and atenolol.

3. Discussion

The combination of saquinavir with high dose prednisolone as induction therapy, followed by a maintenance regime of saquinavir, low dose prednisolone, and low dose cyclosporine, allowed for a period of remission in this patient, which was unfortunately interrupted with a brief relapse. We speculate that saquinavir's unique mechanism of action on proteasome, in combination with glucocorticoid and calcineurin inhibitor, promotes the improvement and stabilisation of biochemical parameters and control of clinical symptoms by downstream inhibition of NF-κB changes.

Indeed, the proteasome is a vital component in controlling NF-κB nuclear translocation and therefore transcriptional regulation [4]. Following activation of NF-κB by cytokines such as TNF-alpha and IL-1, I-kappa-beta, the inhibitory regulator of NF-κB that keeps this protein localised to the cytoplasm, is first phosphorylated then ubiquitinated [4]. Ubiquitination targets I-kappa-b for proteosomal degradation, allowing the nuclear localisation sequence of NF-kappa beta to be unveiled [4]. Addition of saquinavir to peripheral blood mononuclear cells isolated from patients with idiopathic nephrotic syndrome has been shown to reduce the nuclear fraction of NF-kappa beta [10]. Coppo et al. (2012) [10] were the first to trial saquinavir as therapy for difficult cases of idiopathic nephrotic syndrome in children and young adults. Coppo et al. (2012) used saquinavir in addition to other immunosuppressive medications to treat 10 patients with idiopathic nephrotic syndrome. Eight patients continued the treatment for between 12 and 68 months and six of these patients responded to this agent [10]. In addition, there was a 63% reduction in prednisone use associated with a significant reduction in steroid toxicity [10]. This study also reported that saquinavir was effective when used with calcineurin inhibitors at doses much lower than required to induce remission when used without saquinavir [10]. Furthermore, given that therapeutic levels of cyclosporine inhibitors were within the therapeutic range during treatment (as was true in this case), it is unlikely that remission induced by the saquinavir/cyclosporine regime was solely attributable to pharmacokinetic modification of calcineurin inhibitors by saquinavir [11]. Remission induced in this patient following the latest relapse occurred with combination of glucocorticoid, calcineurin inhibitor, and saquinavir. Glucocorticoids act on glucocorticoid receptors promoting nuclear translocation, binding to NF-κB, and repressing its function [12, 13]. Furthermore, cyclosporine A has been shown to be a noncompetitive inhibitor of the proteasome [14], with *in vivo* suppression of lipopolysaccharide induced I-κB degradation [14]. Therefore, it is tempting to speculate that the combined suppressive effects of cyclosporine, prednisolone, and saquinavir on NF-kappa beta nuclear translocation are, at least in part, responsible for reduction in proteinuria and induction of remission in our patient [10].

4. Conclusion

The case demonstrates that the introduction of saquinavir and high dose prednisolone followed by maintenance therapy with saquinavir and low dose prednisolone and cyclosporine has the potential to induce and perhaps maintain remission in patients with difficult-to-treat steroid responsive nephrotic syndrome. Care must be taken, however, in recommending the addition of saquinavir to the treatment regime of such patients. The numbers of absolute cases treated with saquinavir that have been published remain small. Randomised control trials with greater power are required in order to clarify whether treatment with saquinavir will reach statistical significance in reducing relapse frequency and decreasing steroid use/dependence in this difficult-to-treat condition. This case study adds to the growing evidence showing that saquinavir may be useful in inducing remission by decreasing proteinuria and hypoalbuminuria in patients with steroid dependent or steroid resistant idiopathic nephrotic syndrome. We would only recommend this as rescue therapy currently or as a further step in managing difficult nephrotic patients.

Conflict of Interests

The authors declare that there is no conflict of interests regarding the publication of this paper.

References

[1] S. G. Deeks, M. Smith, M. Holodniy, and J. O. Kahn, "HIV-1 protease inhibitors: a review for clinicians," *Journal of the American Medical Association*, vol. 277, no. 2, pp. 145–153, 1997.

[2] S. G. Deeks and P. A. Volberding, "HIV-1 protease inhibitors," *AIDS Clinical Review*, pp. 145–185, 1997.

[3] R. Valle and L. Haragsim, "Nephrotoxicity as a complication of antiretroviral therapy," *Advances in Chronic Kidney Disease*, vol. 13, no. 3, pp. 314–319, 2006.

[4] S. H. Lecker and W. E. Mitch, "Proteolysis by the ubiquitin-proteasome system and kidney disease," *Journal of the American Society of Nephrology*, vol. 22, no. 5, pp. 821–824, 2011.

[5] M. Piccinini, M. T. Rinaudo, A. Anselmino et al., "The HIV protease inhibitors nelfinavir and saquinavir, but not a variety of HIV reverse transcriptase inhibitors, adversely affect human proteasome function," *Antiviral Therapy*, vol. 10, no. 2, pp. 215–223, 2005.

[6] J. van der Vlag and J. H. M. Berden, "Proteasome inhibition: a new therapeutic option in lupus nephritis?" *Nephrology Dialysis Transplantation*, vol. 23, no. 12, pp. 3771–3772, 2008.

[7] C. Cao, S. Lu, C. Dong, and R. Zhao, "Abnormal DNA-binding of transcription factors in minimal change nephrotic syndrome," *Pediatric Nephrology*, vol. 16, no. 10, pp. 790–795, 2001.

[8] D. Sahali, A. Pawlak, S. Le Gouvello et al., "Transcriptional and post-transcriptional alterations of IκBα in active minimal-change nephrotic syndrome," *Journal of the American Society of Nephrology*, vol. 12, no. 8, pp. 1648–1658, 2001.

[9] H. Mansour, L. Cheval, J.-M. Elalouf et al., "T-cell transcriptome analysis points up a thymic disorder in idiopathic nephrotic syndrome," *Kidney International*, vol. 67, no. 6, pp. 2168–2177, 2005.

[10] R. Coppo, R. Camilla, M. G. Porcellini et al., "Saquinavir in steroid-dependent and -resistant nephrotic syndrome: a pilot study," *Nephrology Dialysis Transplantation*, vol. 27, no. 5, pp. 1902–1910, 2012.

[11] H. Izzedine, V. Launay-Vacher, A. Baumelou, and G. Deray, "Antiretroviral and immunosuppressive drug-drug interactions: an update," *Kidney International*, vol. 66, no. 2, pp. 532–541, 2004.

[12] R. F. Ransom, N. G. Lam, M. A. Hallett, S. J. Atkinson, and W. E. Smoyer, "Glucocorticoids protect and enhance recovery of cultured murine podocytes via actin filament stabilization," *Kidney International*, vol. 68, no. 6, pp. 2473–2483, 2005.

[13] R. F. Ransom, V. Vega-Warner, W. E. Smoyer, and J. Klein, "Differential proteomic analysis of proteins induced by glucocorticoids in cultured murine podocytes," *Kidney International*, vol. 67, no. 4, pp. 1275–1285, 2005.

[14] S. Meyer, N. G. Kohler, and A. Joly, "Cyclosporine A is an uncompetitive inhibitor of proteasome activity and prevents NF-κB activation," *FEBS Letters*, vol. 413, no. 2, pp. 354–358, 1997.

31

Purple Urine Bag Syndrome in Two Elderly Men with Urinary Tract Infection

Jan Van Keer,[1] **Daan Detroyer,**[1] **and Bert Bammens**[1,2]

[1]*Department of Nephrology, Dialysis and Renal Transplantation, University Hospitals Leuven, Herestraat 49, 3000 Leuven, Belgium*
[2]*Department of Microbiology and Immunology, KU Leuven, Minderbroedersstraat 10, 3000 Leuven, Belgium*

Correspondence should be addressed to Bert Bammens; bert.bammens@uzleuven.be

Academic Editor: Ze'ev Korzets

Purple urine bag syndrome is a rare condition in which purple discoloration of urine inside its collection bag occurs. We describe two illustrative cases. The first patient is an 81-year-old man who was hospitalized for a newly diagnosed lymphoma with acute obstructive renal failure for which a nephrostomy procedure was performed. During the hospitalization, a sudden purple discoloration of the suprapubic catheter urine was noted, while the nephrostomy urine had a normal color. Urine culture from the suprapubic catheter was positive for *Pseudomonas aeruginosa* and *Enterococcus faecalis*; urine from the nephrostomy was sterile. The second case is an 80-year-old man who was admitted for heart failure with cardiorenal dilemma and who was started on intermittent hemodialysis. There was a sudden purple discoloration of the urine in the collection bag from his indwelling catheter. He was diagnosed with an *E. coli* urinary infection and treated with amoxicillin and removal of the indwelling catheter. These two cases illustrate the typical characteristics of purple urine bag syndrome.

1. Introduction

Purple urine bag syndrome is a rare condition characterized by a purple discoloration of urine inside the urine collection bag [1]. It is mostly seen in patients with chronic urinary catheterization, constipation, and urinary tract infection [2]. The purple color is thought to be caused by bacterial metabolization of dietary tryptophan into indigo and indirubin inside the urinary catheter system [3]. Here, we describe two illustrative cases.

2. Case 1

An 81-year-old man was admitted to the nephrology ward because of anorexia, weight loss, and acute on chronic renal failure. His past medical history was remarkable for atrophy of the left kidney, myocardial infarction, follicular type non-Hodgkin lymphoma treated with CHVmP/BV chemotherapy (19 years prior to the present admission), and prostate cancer treated with androgen deprivation (6 years prior to the present admission). The patient had a permanent suprapubic catheter that was changed at 6-weekly intervals. On admission, he was found to have extensive supra- and infradiaphragmatic lymphadenopathy, with encasement of the right ureter and hydronephrosis of the right kidney. An urgent nephrostomy had been performed. Biopsy of a palpable cervical lymph node later revealed diffuse large B-cell lymphoma.

During the hospitalization, a sudden purple discoloration of the suprapubic urine collection bag was noted (see Figure 1). The nephrostomy urine had a normal color. The patient had been constipated during the preceding days, for which he had been treated with macrogol laxatives. His other medications had not been changed and included enoxaparin, aspirin, bisoprolol, amlodipine, rosuvastatin, sertraline, and three-monthly injection of goserelin. The patient had no other complaints.

Vital parameters were normal. Physical exam showed right cervical lymphadenopathy and the presence of a nephrostomy with normal colored urine and a suprapubic catheter with obvious purple color of urine bag and tubing. Laboratory evaluation revealed renal insufficiency with creatinine of 1.49 mg/dL and blood urea nitrogen of 25 mg/dL (creatinine

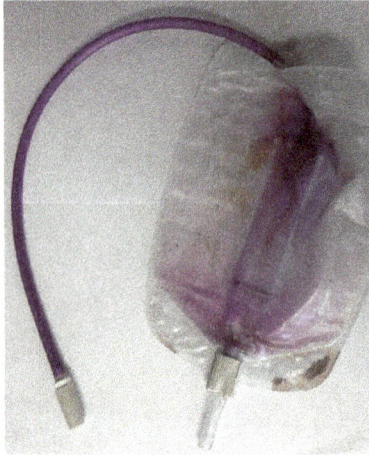

FIGURE 1: Purple discoloration of urine bag and tubing coming from suprapubic catheter. Note that the nephrostomy urine bag (not shown) had a normal color.

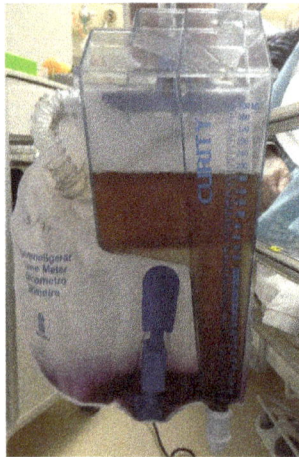

FIGURE 2: Purple color of the urine bag. Note that the color of the urine in the collection device before entering the bag is normal.

at admission, before the nephrostomy procedure, had been 6.36 mg/dL). Hemogram showed a mild normochromic normocytic anemia with hemoglobin of 10.5 g/dL; white blood cell differential count and platelets were normal. Liver function tests were within normal limits. Lactate dehydrogenase was elevated (505 U/L): this was attributed to the diffuse large B-cell lymphoma. The level of CRP was 25 mg/L (reference value < 5 mg/L). Analysis of the suprapubic catheter urine showed pyuria and trace hematuria. Urinary pH was 9.0. Urine culture came back positive for *Pseudomonas aeruginosa* and *Enterococcus faecalis*. Analysis of the nephrostomy catheter urine showed trace hematuria, with a pH of 6.0 and a negative culture. As the nephrostomy urine was sterile and the patient had no signs of urinary infection, no antibiotics were given. The purple discoloration gradually disappeared during the following week. At discharge, kidney function had improved back to baseline with creatinine of 1.20 mg/dL. The patient was subsequently treated with R-CVP chemotherapy, with remission after 6 cycles.

3. Case 2

An 80-year-old man was hospitalized because of heart failure with cardiorenal dilemma. His past medical history included coronary bypass surgery, ischemic cardiomyopathy, chronic kidney disease, chronic obstructive pulmonary disease, prostate cancer treated with total androgen deprivation, and type 2 diabetes, treated with diet only. His medication included pantoprazole, enoxaparin, aspirin, bumetanide, carvedilol, atorvastatin, bicalutamide, darbepoetin alfa, macrogol laxatives, and fluticasone, salmeterol, and tiotropium inhalation therapy. He had been admitted with pulmonary edema, for which continuous venovenous hemofiltration (CVVH) was started. Afterwards, he was transferred to the nephrology ward for continuation of chronic intermittent hemodialysis. He had a residual diuresis of 600 mL per 24 hours. An indwelling urinary catheter had been placed on the first day of hospitalization to monitor urinary output.

On the 13th day of hospitalization, the urine inside the urine bag suddenly turned purple (see Figure 2). The patient had a burning sensation in the lower abdomen. Vital parameters were unremarkable. Physical examination showed bilateral basal crepitations on auscultation, systolic cardiac murmur, mild peripheral edema, and indwelling urinary catheter with remarkable purple color of the collecting bag, while the urine in the tubing before the bag had a normal color. Laboratory assessment showed anemia (hemoglobin 8.9 g/dL) with mild macrocytosis, normal leukocyte count and differentiation, and platelets of 115×109/L. Creatinine before dialysis was 3.11 mg/dL and blood urea nitrogen was 48 mg/dL. Liver function tests were normal. CRP was 23 mg/L (reference value < 5 mg/L). Urine analysis showed pyuria and trace hematuria; urinary pH was 8.5. Culture was positive for *Escherichia coli*. The indwelling catheter was removed. The patient was treated with amoxicillin for 7 days. He was discharged in good health, with continuation of thrice-weekly hemodialysis. Shortly thereafter, the patient developed urinary obstruction for which a permanent suprapubic catheter was placed. The purple urine color never recurred.

4. Discussion

Purple urine bag syndrome is a rare condition that can seem alarming, but it is mostly benign. The syndrome was first described in 1978 [1]. Since then, less than 100 cases have been published. Most are institutionalized female patients with chronic indwelling urinary catheters. Purple urine bag syndrome is associated with urinary tract infection and with constipation [2].

The pathogenesis is controversial. According to the most popular hypothesis [3], dietary tryptophan is converted to indole by gut bacteria, which is further metabolized in the liver to indoxyl sulphate and then excreted in the urine. Constipation favors conversion of tryptophan to indole by gut bacteria.

Once excreted, indoxyl sulphate can be processed by bacteria colonizing the urinary catheter to indoxyl, which is further converted to indigo (blue) and indirubin (red). These pigments result in a deep purple color in interaction with the

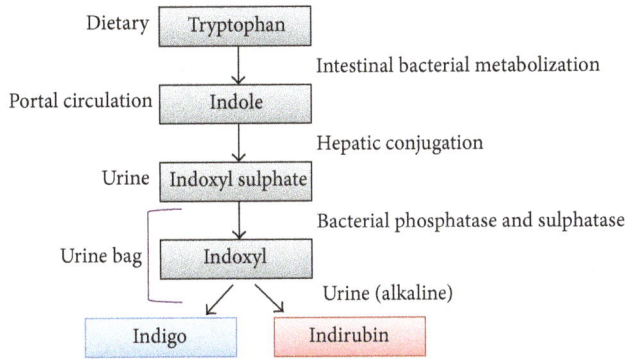

FIGURE 3: Pathogenesis of the purple urine bag syndrome (adapted from Hadano et al. [2]).

plastic tubing (see Figure 3). The most commonly involved bacteria are *Providencia stuartii*, *Providencia rettgeri*, *Escherichia coli*, *Klebsiella pneumoniae*, *Proteus mirabilis*, *Morganella morganii*, *Pseudomonas aeruginosa*, and *Enterococcus* species [4]. These bacteria produce indoxyl phosphatase and sulphatase enzymes. Although alkaline urine is an important risk factor, purple urine bag syndrome has been described in acidic urine as well [5].

Note that, in our first patient, only the suprapubic urine bag (with *Pseudomonas* colonization) turned purple, whereas the (sterile) nephrostomy bag did not. The second case shows that the discoloration only occurred after contact with the plastic bag.

Purple urine bag syndrome is a sign of colonization of the urinary catheter system. Antibiotic therapy is only indicated in patients with symptomatic urinary infection. For asymptomatic patients, treatment of underlying risk factors (e.g., constipation) might suffice [6]. The mainstay of preventing purple urine bag syndrome is the avoidance of chronic catheterization by prompt removal of urinary catheters once they are no longer needed.

Consent

Written informed consent was obtained from both patients for the publication of this case report and the accompanying images.

Conflict of Interests

The authors declare that there is no conflict of interests regarding the publication of this paper.

References

[1] G. B. Barlow and J. A. S. Dickson, "Purple urine bags," *The Lancet*, vol. 311, no. 8057, pp. 220–221, 1978.

[2] Y. Hadano, T. Shimizu, S. Takada, T. Inoue, and S. Sorano, "An update on purple urine bag syndrome," *International Journal of General Medicine*, vol. 5, pp. 707–710, 2012.

[3] S. F. Dealler, P. M. Hawkey, and M. R. Millar, "Enzymatic degradation of urinary indoxyl sulfate by *Providencia stuartii* and *Klebsiella pneumoniae* causes the purple urine bag syndrome,"
Journal of Clinical Microbiology, vol. 26, no. 10, pp. 2152–2156, 1988.

[4] F.-H. Su, S.-Y. Chung, M.-H. Chen et al., "Case analysis of purple urine-bag syndrome at a long-term care service in a community hospital," *Chang Gung Medical Journal*, vol. 28, no. 9, pp. 636–642, 2005.

[5] N. Mantani, H. Ochiai, N. Imanishi, T. Kogure, K. Terasawa, and J. Tamura, "A case-control study of purple urine bag syndrome in geriatric wards," *Journal of Infection and Chemotherapy*, vol. 9, no. 1, pp. 53–57, 2003.

[6] C.-H. Lin, H.-T. Huang, C.-C. Chien, D.-S. Tzeng, and F.-W. Lung, "Purple urine bag syndrome in nursing homes: ten elderly case reports and a literature review," *Clinical Interventions in Aging*, vol. 3, no. 4, pp. 729–734, 2008.

32

Acute Oxalate Nephropathy following Ingestion of *Averrhoa bilimbi* Juice

Sreeja Nair, Jacob George, Sajeev Kumar, and Noble Gracious

Department of Nephrology, Medical College, Thiruvananthapuram, Kerala 695011, India

Correspondence should be addressed to Sreeja Nair; sreejasnair82@gmail.com

Academic Editor: Anja Haase-Fielitz

Plant toxins are known to cause acute kidney injury in tropical countries. We report two cases of acute kidney injury with tubular oxalate deposition following ingestion of *Averrhoa bilimbi* fruit juice. Both patients had complete renal recovery though one required dialytic support.

1. Introduction

Plant toxins are an important cause of tropical acute kidney injury. Several plant parts are ingested for medicinal, cosmetic, and even suicidal purposes [1]. *Averrhoa bilimbi* (commonly known as bilimbi, cucumber tree, tree sorrel, Irumban Puli, or Chemmeen Puli) is a plant with several suggested medicinal properties. It, however, has a high content of oxalic acid which could contribute to nephrotoxicity [2]. We describe two cases of acute oxalate nephropathy following ingestion of *Averrhoa bilimbi* juice.

2. Case 1

A forty-five-year-old female presented to the nephrology outpatient clinic with history of bilateral pedal edema, facial puffiness, and abdominal distention of three-day duration. There was no history of oliguria, hematuria, or frothing of urine. She did not have fever, dysuria, shortness of breath, or haemoptysis. She was diagnosed with systemic hypertension 18 years back for which she was taking enalapril 2.5 mg once daily. She was detected to have dyslipidemia on routine evaluation 3 months back and was advised dietary modification and life style changes only. She was on regular follow-up and was documented to have normal renal function two months back. On probing for history of nephrotoxic drugs or alternative medicine intake, she gave history of intake of around 100 mL of undiluted juice made from fifteen

fruits of *Averrhoa bilimbi*, locally known as "Irumban Puli" (Figure 1), three days back, presuming that it would correct her dyslipidemia.

On examination, she was conscious and alert. She had bilateral periorbital puffiness along with pitting pedal edema extending up to one-third of both legs. Her blood pressure was 220/100 mm Hg in the right upper limb in sitting position. Abdominal examination revealed distension of abdomen with abdominal wall edema without evidence of free fluid in abdomen. The rest of clinical examination was within normal limits.

Laboratory investigations at time of admission are shown in Table 1. Her urine deposits showed plenty of oxalate crystals (Figure 2). Her 24-hour urinary oxalate done later was negative. Ultrasound abdomen revealed right kidney 10.0 × 5.4 cms and left kidney 10.5 × 4.5 cms with bilateral normal echogenicity and normal corticomedullary differentiation. There was no evidence of calculi or hydronephrosis. A renal biopsy was planned on the initial day of admission but was deferred due to high blood pressure. She was initiated on antihypertensive medications including nitroglycerine infusion. Her blood pressure was controlled on second day and renal biopsy was done which revealed nine glomeruli of which four were obsolescent. The obsolescent glomeruli were small and globally sclerotic. Viable glomeruli were near normal in size and cellularity. Peripheral capillary loops appeared delicate and one glomerulus revealed simplified tuft with wrinkled capillary loops. Tubules showed simplification

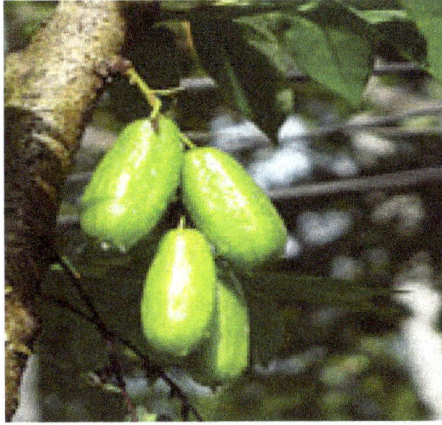

FIGURE 1: Picture of fruit of *Averrhoa bilimbi*.

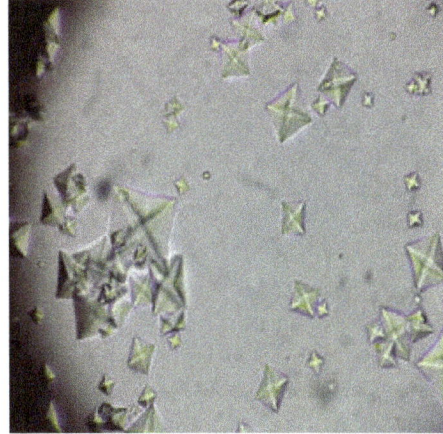

FIGURE 2: Calcium oxalate crystals in urine in high power view.

and vacuolation of epithelium and polarising crystals with fractured glass appearance in the lumen, morphology of which was suggestive of calcium oxalate (Figure 3(a)). Some of the tubules revealed epithelial calcification. There were thin strips of atrophic tubules amounted to around ten % of the cortex. Interstitium showed patchy edema and mild mononuclear infiltrate especially around the atrophic glomeruli and tubules. There was no significant interstitial fibrosis. Large calibre artery showed mild intimal fibroplasia. Interlobular artery revealed medial hypertrophy and arterioles showed hyperplastic change. Immunofluorescence studies were negative for IgG, IgA, IgM, C3, C1q, and both kappa and lambda light chains. A histological diagnosis of acute tubular injury associated with calcium oxalate crystals in a background of mild global glomerulosclerosis and hypertensive vascular changes was made. Patient was managed conservatively as she was nonoliguric. Her renal function initially showed progressive worsening and serum creatinine reached up to 4.9 mg %. She also had high blood pressure which required usage of multiple antihypertensive drugs including amlodipine, atenolol, clonidine, prazosin, telmisartan, minoxidil, and nitroglycerine. Her renal functions gradually improved and blood pressure improved. She was discharged ten days later with serum creatinine of 1.4 mg/dL and three antihypertensive drugs (amlodipine, atenolol, and clonidine).

3. Case 2

A forty-seven-year-old male presented with nausea, vomiting, and generalized edema of three-day duration. He had decreased urine output (<400 mL) for past four days. There was no previous history of systemic hypertension or diabetes mellitus. He was diagnosed with dyslipidemia recently. He gave history of ingestion of 150 mL undiluted juice of *Averrhoa bilimbi* for two consecutive days seven days back.

On examination, he had bilateral periorbital puffiness with bilateral pitting pedal edema. Blood pressure was 140/90 mm Hg in the right upper limb in sitting position. Abdominal examination revealed free fluid in abdomen. The rest of clinical examination was within normal limits.

Laboratory investigations at time of admission are shown in Table 1. Ultrasound abdomen revealed right kidney 10.5 × 5.0 cms and left kidney 10.6 × 4.5 cms with bilateral normal echogenicity and normal corticomedullary differentiation. There were no calculi or hydronephrosis. Renal biopsy done after two sessions of hemodialysis revealed six viable glomeruli with near normal size and cellularity. No endocapillary proliferation or crescents were seen. Tubules revealed marked simplification of epithelium and many refractile polarisable crystals with fractured glass appearance in the tubular lumen (Figures 3(b) and 4). Some of the tubules showed regenerative changes. No tubular atrophy or interstitial fibrosis was seen. Interstitium was edematous with patchy infiltration by lymphocytes, plasma cells, and a few eosinophils (Figure 5). Part of large calibre artery, interlobular artery, and arterioles appeared within normal limits. Immunofluorescence studies showed ten glomeruli with mesangial 1+ IgA and 1+ lambda light chain. IgG, IgM, C3, C1q, and kappa light chains were negative.

As he had severe renal failure with oliguria and features of fluid overload, he was taken for hemodialysis. He required 4 sessions of hemodialysis. In view of dialysis requiring renal failure with histological evidence of acute interstitial nephritis, he was given three daily pulses of methyl prednisolone followed by oral prednisolone. His blood pressure was controlled with amlodipine 5 mg twice daily. His urine output and renal function gradually improved. On discharge after sixteen days, his urine output had improved, blood pressure had normalised, and S. creatinine had decreased to 2.1 mg %. Steroids were tapered and antihypertensive drugs were stopped.

4. Discussion

Averrhoa bilimbi belongs to the family of Oxalidaceae. It is widely cultivated in the tropics and its origins are not yet clear. Nevertheless, Corrêa reported its presence in India in 1962 [2]. Bilimbi is a small tree 5–10 meters high. Fruits are fairly cylindrical with five broad rounded longitudinal lobes and produced in clusters. Bilimbi fruits are very sour

TABLE 1: Laboratory investigations at admission to hospital.

Urine	Case 1	Case 2
Protein	+	Trace
Deposits		
Red blood cells (RBCS)	0-1/hpf	0-1/hpf
White blood cells (WBCS)	5-6/hpf	1-2/hpf
Calcium oxalate crystals	Plenty	Nil
Blood		
Hemoglobin (Hb)	12.3 g%	12 g%
Total white blood cell count (TC)	9000 cells/mm^3	8300 cells/mm^3
Differential white blood cell count (DC)	P78 L15 E7	P73 L20 E7
Erythrocyte sedimentation rate (ESR)	17	18
Platelet count	2.7 lakhs/mm^3	2.18 lakhs/mm^3
Random blood sugar	70 mg%	106 mg%
Blood urea	74 mg%	142 mg%
Serum creatinine	4.4 mg%	10 mg%
Serum sodium	135 mg%	116 mg%
Serum potassium	4.3 mg%	4.6 mg%
Serum bilirubin total	1.2 mg%	0.7 mg%
Direct	0.8 mg%	0.2 mg%
Indirect	0.4 mg%	0.5 mg%
Serum alanine transaminase (ALT)	22 units	26 units
Serum aspartate transaminase (AST)	34 units	18 units
Total protein	7.5 g%	6 g%
Serum albumin	4.2 g%	4 g%
Serum alkaline phosphatase	69	58
Serum calcium	8.6 mg%	7.7 mg%
Serum phosphorus	4.5 mg%	5.7 mg%
Serum uric acid	9 mg%	10 mg%

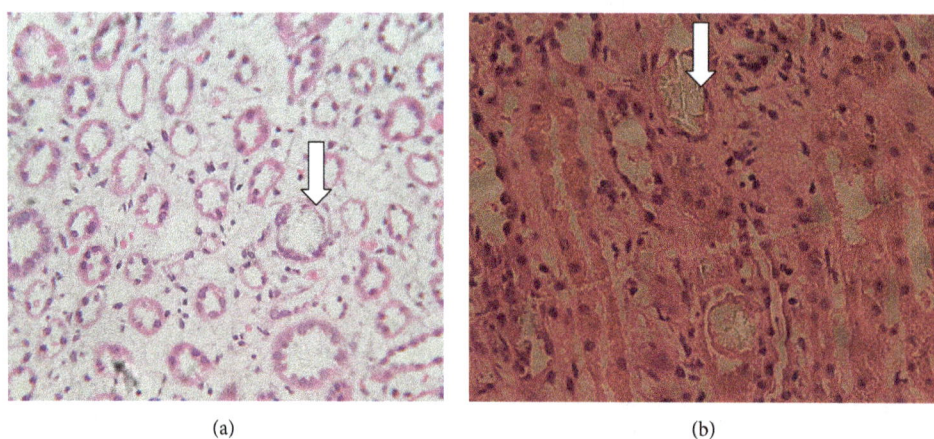

(a)   (b)

FIGURE 3: Renal biopsy specimen (40X) with arrow showing calcium oxalate crystals.

and are commonly used in the production of vinegar, wine, and pickles. It was considered to have medicinal properties and was an ingredient of mixtures against cough, mumps, rheumatism, pimples, and scurvy. The fruit juice has also been used to remove iron-rust stains from clothes and to impart shine to brassware [2].

Both our patients took *Averrhoa bilimbi* juice as a presumed treatment for dyslipidemia. Several studies suggest hypoglycemic, hypolipidemic, antioxidant, and antiatherogenic properties of *Averrhoa bilimbi*. There are reports on hypoglycemic and hypolipidemic effect of ethanolic extract of *Averrhoa bilimbi* leaves in streptozotocin diabetic rats

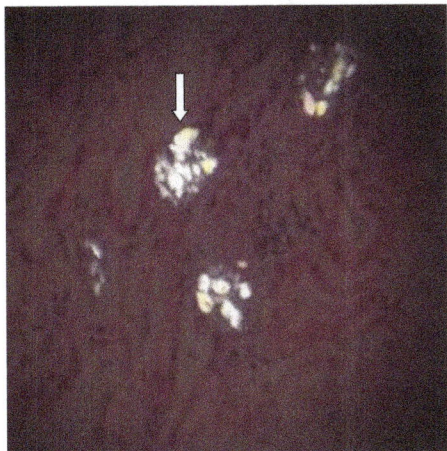

FIGURE 4: Renal biopsy specimen under polarizing microscope with arrow showing crystals of calcium oxalate.

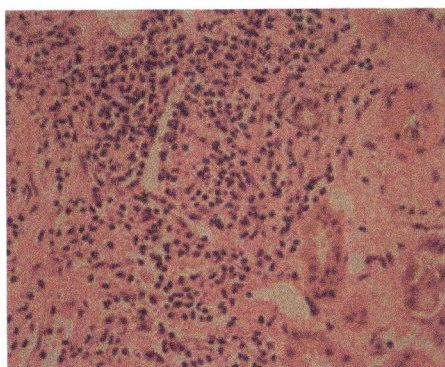

FIGURE 5: Acute interstitial nephritis.

[3]. Bilimbi extract significantly lowered blood glucose by 50% and blood triglyceride by 130% when compared with metformin and distilled water. Bilimbi extract has also been shown to significantly increase the HDL cholesterol concentrations and increases the antiatherogenic index. However, like metformin, bilimbi extract did not affect total cholesterol and LDL cholesterol concentrations, though it significantly reduced the kidney lipid peroxidation levels [3]. Using Triton-induced hypercholesterolemia in rats as a model, bilimbi fruit and its water extract showed remarkable antihypercholesterolemic activity [4]. Oxalic acid content of Averrhoa bilimbi fruit has been reported to range between 8.57 and 10.32 mg/g with highest levels seen in half ripe fruit in rainy season and lowest levels in ripe fruits in dry season (25.1 mg/100 g) [2]. The oxalate content of other fruits and vegetables is much less (e.g., cranberry 1.1 mg/100 g, grape 1.6 mg/100 g, tomato 5.5 mg/100 g, pineapple 7.3 mg/100 g, orange 2.2 mg/100 g, apple 0.5 mg/100 g, and banana 3.2 mg/100 g) [5]. Other foods that are rich in oxalate include beans (green and dried), beer, beets, berries, black tea, black pepper, celery, chocolates, cocoa, eggplant, figs (dried), greens (collard green, dandelion green, mustard green, and spinach), green peppers, lemon peel, orange peel, nuts, peanut butter, and okra [6].

There are several case reports of acute oxalate nephropathy due to several agents described in the literature. Bakul et al. had reported a series of cases from five hospitals in the state of Kerala who developed ARF due to acute oxalate nephropathy after consumption of Averrhoa bilimbi juice. In that series 7 out of 10 patients had dialysis requiring renal failure after intake of juice but fortunately all had renal recovery [5].

Though Averrhoa bilimbi is consumed in several ways, acute kidney injury is mostly seen when it is consumed as raw juice. It is possible that the concentration as well as total amount consumed may have a role to play in the pathogenesis of acute kidney injury. Whether cooking reduces the nephrotoxicity also needs to be studied as there are no reports on acute kidney injury following Averrhoa bilimbi pickle intake. Acute oxalate nephropathy has also been reported after ingestion of Averrhoa carambola commonly known as star fruit [7], though the oxalic acid content in Averrhoa carambola is lesser than Averrhoa bilimbi (0.8 to 7.3 mg/g) [2]. There are also case reports of acute oxalate nephropathy following ingestion of ethylene glycol and octreotide. Acute oxalate nephropathy is also described to be associated with chronic pancreatitis and following administration of octreotide and massive doses of ascorbic acid [8–12].

One of our patients had plenty of calcium oxalate crystals in the initial urine sample though her 24-hour urinary oxalate done later was negative. The other patient had no evidence of urinary oxalate excretion which may have been due to decreased excretion in view of severe renal dysfunction. Serum oxalate levels could not be assessed in both our patients as the facility was not available in our hospital. The first patient had very high blood pressure disproportionate to renal dysfunction. A possible toxic effect of Averrhoa bilimbi fruit may have contributed to that but this needs further evaluation.

Conflict of Interests

The authors declare that there is no conflict of interests regarding the publication of this paper.

References

[1] V. Jha and S. Parameswaran, "Community-acquired acute kidney injury in tropical countries," Nature Reviews Nephrology, vol. 9, no. 5, pp. 278–290, 2013.

[2] V. L. A. Galvão de lima, E. de Almeida Mélo, and L. dos Santos Lima, "Physicochemical characteristics of bilimbi (Averrhoa bilimbi)," Revista Brasileira de Fruticultura, vol. 23, no. 2, pp. 421–423, 2011.

[3] P. Pushparaj, C. H. Tan, and B. K. H. Tan, "Effects of Averrhoa bilimbi leaf extract on blood glucose and lipids in streptozotocin-diabetic rats," Journal of Ethnopharmacology, vol. 72, no. 1-2, pp. 69–76, 2000.

[4] S. Ambili, A. Subramoniam, and N. S. Nagarajan, "Studies on the antihyperlipidemic properties of Averrhoa bilimbi fruit in rats," Planta Medica, vol. 75, no. 1, pp. 55–58, 2009.

[5] G. Bakul, V. N. Unni, N. V. Seethaleksmy et al., "Acute oxalate nephropathy due to "*Averrhoa bilimbi*" fruit juice ingestion," *Indian Journal of Nephrology*, vol. 23, no. 4, pp. 297–300, 2013.

[6] D. A. Bushinsky, F. L. Coe, and O. W. Moe, *Brenner and Rectors Diseases of the Kidney*, 9th edition, 2012.

[7] C.-L. Chen, H.-C. Fang, K.-J. Chou, J.-S. Wang, and H.-M. Chung, "Acute oxalate nephropathy after ingestion of star fruit," *American Journal of Kidney Diseases*, vol. 37, no. 2, pp. 418–422, 2001.

[8] J. W. Seo, J.-H. Lee, I. S. Son et al., "Acute oxalate nephropathy caused by ethylene glycol poisoning," *Kidney Research and Clinical Practice*, vol. 31, no. 4, pp. 249–252, 2012.

[9] A. Singh, S. R. Sarkar, L. W. Gaber, and M. A. Perazella, "Acute oxalate nephropathy associated with orlistat, a gastrointestinal lipase inhibitor," *American Journal of Kidney Diseases*, vol. 49, no. 1, pp. 153–157, 2007.

[10] C. Cartery, S. Faguer, A. Karras et al., "Oxalate nephropathy associated with chronic pancreatitis," *Clinical Journal of the American Society of Nephrology*, vol. 6, no. 8, pp. 1895–1902, 2011.

[11] K. Gariani, S. de Seigneux, M. Courbebaisse, M. Lévy, S. Moll, and P.-Y. Martin, "Oxalate nephropathy induced by octreotide treatment for acromegaly," *Journal of Medical Case Reports*, vol. 6, article 215, 2012.

[12] J. M. Lawton, L. T. Conway, J. T. Crosson, C. L. Smith, and P. A. Abraham, "Acute oxalate nephropathy after massive ascorbic acid administration," *Archives of Internal Medicine*, vol. 145, no. 5, pp. 950–951, 1985.

33

Severe Hypocalcemia due to Denosumab in Metastatic Prostate Cancer

Mohammed Muqeet Adnan,[1] **Usman Bhutta,**[1,2] **Tanzeel Iqbal,**[1] **Sufyan AbdulMujeeb,**[3] **Lukas Haragsim,**[2] **and Syed Amer**[4]

[1] *Department of Internal Medicine, University of Oklahoma Health Sciences Center, Oklahoma City, OK 73117, USA*
[2] *Department of Nephrology, University of Oklahoma Health Sciences Center, Oklahoma City, OK 73117, USA*
[3] *University of Illinois at Chicago, Chicago, IL 60607, USA*
[4] *Department of Internal Medicine, Mayo Clinic Hospital, Phoenix, AZ 85054, USA*

Correspondence should be addressed to Mohammed Muqeet Adnan; mohammedabdul-muqeetadnan@ouhsc.edu

Academic Editor: Yoshihide Fujigaki

Denosumab is a monoclonal antibody used for prevention of skeletal-related events (SREs) in patients with bone metastases from solid tumors. Hypocalcemia is a rare and dangerous side effect of the drug Denosumab. We present a case of a patient with metastatic prostate cancer who developed severe hypocalcemia after the administration of the drug. The patient's vitamin D levels were low when checked after administration of the drug, which likely predisposed him to the development of hypocalcemia. He was placed on high doses of oral and intravenous (IV) calcium and vitamin D without any appreciable response in the serum calcium level. His ionized calcium remained below 0.71 mmol/L despite very high doses of oral and IV calcium supplements. During the hospital course, he developed hydronephrosis from the spread of a tumor and did not want to undergo percutaneous nephrostomy tube placement; therefore, it was decided to dialyse him for acute renal failure and to correct his hypocalcemia. Checking calcium and vitamin D levels prior to the administration of Denosumab is vital in preventing hypocalcemia. If hypocalcemia is severe and not responsive to high doses of vitamin D, oral and IV calcium, then hemodialysis with a high calcium bath can correct this electrolyte abnormality.

1. Case Report

A 45-year-old gentleman with a three-year history of metastatic (bone, liver, and lymph nodes) prostate cancer and hypertension presented to the hospital with worsening leg swelling and hematuria. He had been treated with androgen deprivation therapy in the past, along with three doses of zoledronic acid for bone metastases. The bone pain was not controlled with the above regimen and it was decided to switch him to Denosumab. He received the dose approximately 13 days prior to hospitalization. Vitals at admission were significant for a blood pressure (BP) of 160/90 mmHg. Pertinent findings on physical examination were the presence of bilateral lower extremity edema and negative Chvostek and Trousseau's signs. The electrocardiogram showed a prolonged QT interval. Laboratory studies on admission revealed sodium of 135 mEq/L, potassium of 4.9 mEq/L, chloride of 105 mEq/L, bicarbonate of 23 mEq/L, blood urea nitrogen (BUN) of 22 mg/dL, creatinine of 1.34 mg/dL, glucose of 133 mg/dL, and calcium of 4.5 mg/dL, with albumin being 2.5 g/dL at admission. Phosphorus level was 6.1 mg/dL. The ionized calcium level at admission was 0.58 mmol/L. Laboratory studies done 13 days prior, when the drug was given, showed serum calcium of 8.4 mg/dL with an albumin of 2.9 g/dL. His vitamin D levels had not been checked prior to the administration of Denosumab. After admission to the hospital, his vitamin D 25-OH level was low at 12.1 ng/mL and vitamin D 1,25 dihydroxy level was high at 95.4 pg/mL. His initial PTH level was high at 440.7 pg/mL.

He was started on 50,000 IU of ergocalciferol every 7 days, 2 mcg of calcitriol twice daily, and high doses of IV and oral calcium supplementation. Over the next 16 days, the patient

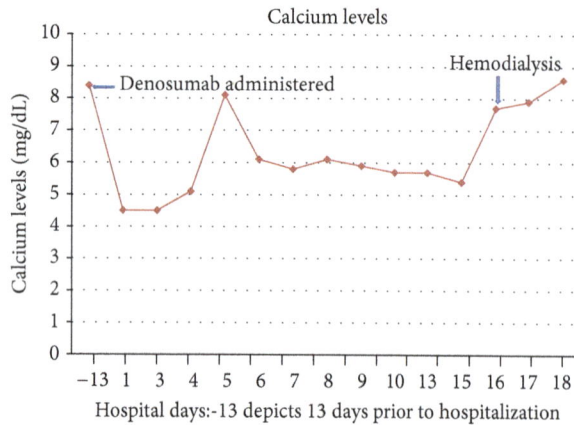

FIGURE 1: Calcium levels while in the hospital remaining low despite ergocalciferol, calcitriol, and high doses of IV and oral calcium supplementation.

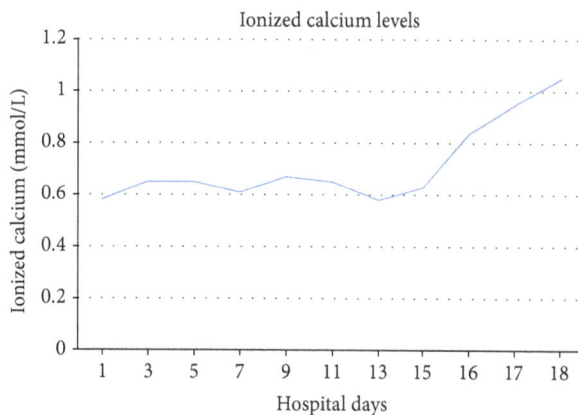

FIGURE 2: Ionized calcium levels during the hospital stay. Hemodialysis was initiated on day 16 due to worsening renal failure and persistent hypocalcemia.

received high doses of calcium carbonate; he was first started on 5 gm twice daily of calcium carbonate and 1337 mg of calcium acetate. Since the ionized calcium levels were consistently below 0.60 mmol/L, he was slowly increased to 10 gm twice daily of calcium carbonate and 3335 mg of calcium acetate thrice daily with meals. During the hospitalization, he received a total of 80 gm of IV calcium gluconate and 370 gm of oral calcium, but the highest ionized calcium level that could be achieved was 0.71 mmol/L. Figures 1 and 2 show the calcium and ionized calcium levels during the hospital while receiving oral and IV calcium supplementation.

He continued to have worsening lower-extremity edema, for which he was started on treatment with hydrochlorothiazide (HCTZ) to help with diuresis as well as with the hypocalcemia. His renal function kept worsening during his hospital stay and his creatinine reached 4.12 mg/dL. During workup for his renal failure, he was found to have hydronephrosis due to the spreading tumor. The options available were either placement of percutaneous nephrostomy tubes by

interventional radiology to relieve the hydronephrosis and continued attempts at correction of his electrolytes via medical management or placement of a tunneled dialysis catheter and starting hemodialysis. After a discussion of the risks and benefits of each procedure and the overall prognosis of his condition, the patient opted for hemodialysis. Hemodialysis was initiated on the sixteenth day of hospitalization. He was dialysed daily for the next nine days with a high calcium bath along with two- to three-liter ultrafiltration daily to help get fluid off. His edema improved significantly, his serum calcium levels came above 8 mg/dL, and his ionized calcium stayed above 1 mmol/L without any IV supplementation; however, the oral supplementation with calcium acetate and 10 gm of calcium carbonate twice daily was continued. Due to the poor prognosis of the underlying disease, it was decided to send him home on hospice after arrangement of outpatient hemodialysis to prevent further hypocalcemia and maintain euvolemia. He died approximately three weeks later.

2. Discussion

Denosumab is a fully human monoclonal antibody, administered subcutaneously, that inhibits osteoclast mediated bone resorption in bone metastases from solid tumors and multiple myeloma. It blocks the RANK ligand from activating the osteoclasts. Tumor cells secrete growth factors to stimulate osteoblasts to release RANK ligand. RANK ligand binds to RANK receptors on the osteoclasts and stimulates them to increase bone resorption. Denosumab blocks this action and hence a major part of calcium metabolism is blocked.

It has been approved by the US Food and Drug Administration (FDA) for use in postmenopausal women with risk of osteoporosis under the trade name Prolia and for the prevention of skeletal-related events in patients with bone metastases from solid tumors under the trade name XGEVA.

The recommended dose for XGEVA is 120 mg subcutaneously every four weeks, whereas for Prolia, it is 60 mg subcutaneous every six months.

The use of Denosumab is associated with a significantly increased risk of developing hypocalcemia [1, 2]. There have been very few case reports describing hypocalcemia to a great degree in patients who receive Denosumab [3]. One case report mentioned hypocalcemia in a dialysis patient after a single dose of Denosumab [3]. Patients are recommended to take 1000 mg oral calcium and 400 IU vitamin D daily in the insert for Prolia. The XGEVA insert recommends the administration of calcium and vitamin D as necessary to prevent hypocalcemia. None of the inserts recommend checking vitamin D levels prior to giving the drug or a certain vitamin D level below which the drug should not be administered.

We would like to emphasize the importance of checking and supplementing vitamin D levels prior to administration of this drug as well as checking serum calcium levels periodically after drug administration. Patients with low vitamin D levels can develop severe hypocalcemia that can be resistant to treatment. Patients might not always have symptoms of hypocalcemia until the serum calcium falls to dangerously low levels. Our patient did not have any of the classic symptoms of hypocalcemia (neuromuscular irritability, seizures, etc.) and presented to the hospital with worsening leg edema. The only manifestation of hypocalcemia that he had was a prolonged QT interval on electrocardiogram. Indeed, if he had not had leg swelling or hematuria, his hypocalcemia may not have been detected until he had a seizure or a fatal cardiac arrhythmia.

There are cases reported of hypocalcemia after administration of denosumab, but very few cases showing such resistant hypocalcemia. Since our patient was on very high doses of oral and IV calcium, discharge was virtually impossible. We elected to start the patient on hemodialysis for two reasons: firstly, his worsening acute renal failure due to hydronephrosis, as he did not want to undergo percutaneous nephrostomy tubes placed; and secondly, his resistant hypocalcemia. Even if the patient did not have renal failure, we may have resorted to hemodialysis just to treat his hypocalcemia since all our options for medically managing the patient were getting exhausted without any real increase in the serum calcium level.

In patients who are already on dialysis, the hypocalcemia can be treated with a high calcium bath in addition to vitamin D supplement. However, in patients with normal renal function, hypocalcemia can usually be treated with a combination of oral and IV calcium along with activated vitamin D. In rare cases like these, hemodialysis with a high calcium bath may be an option.

In conclusion, we would recommend checking vitamin D 25 OH and serum calcium levels prior to starting treatment with Denosumab. Baseline phosphorus, albumin, and parathyroid hormone should also be checked prior to administration. If vitamin D levels are low, they should be supplemented prior to starting treatment. If treatment cannot be delayed to bring the vitamin D level within the normal range, then vitamin D supplement should be provided along with starting the drug. In either case, the serum calcium level should be monitored periodically to ensure that it does not fall below the normal range. Patients should be maintained on low doses of oral calcium and vitamin D daily while getting Denosumab to prevent hypocalcemia. It has been reported that the prophylactic administration of calcium 500 mg a day and vitamin D 400 IU daily can decrease the risk of hypocalcemia induced by Denosumab [2, 4]. Prolia is not expected to cause such severe hypocalcemia due to the low dose at six-month intervals. XGEVA, on the other hand, might be expected to cause more hypocalcemia since it is given at a higher dose and more frequently.

Conflict of Interests

The authors declare that there is no conflict of interests regarding the publication of this paper.

References

[1] W.-X. Qi, F. Lin, A.-N. He, L.-N. Tang, Z. Shen, and Y. Yao, "Incidence and risk of denosumab-related hypocalcemia in cancer patients: a systematic review and pooled analysis of randomized controlled studies," *Current Medical Research and Opinion*, vol. 29, no. 9, pp. 1067–1073, 2013.

[2] Pharmaceuticals and Medical Devices Agency, http://www.info.pmda.go.jp/kinkyu_anzen/file/kinkyu20120911_1.pdf.

[3] B. B. Mccormick, J. Davis, and K. D. Burns, "Severe hypocalcemia following denosumab injection in a hemodialysis patient," *American Journal of Kidney Diseases*, vol. 60, no. 4, pp. 626–628, 2012.

[4] C. Buonerba, M. Caraglia, S. Malgieri et al., "Calcitriol: a better option than vitamin D in denosumab-treated patients with kidney failure?" *Expert Opinion on Biological Therapy*, vol. 13, no. 2, pp. 149–151, 2013.

34

An Unexpected Cause of Severe Hypokalemia

Fernando Caravaca-Fontan, Olga Martinez-Saez, Maria Delgado-Yague, Estefania Yerovi, and Fernando Liaño

Department of Nephrology, Hospital Universitario Ramón y Cajal, Carretera de Colmenar Viejo, Km. 9100, 28034 Madrid, Spain

Correspondence should be addressed to Fernando Caravaca-Fontan; fcaravacaf@gmail.com

Academic Editor: Helmut H. Schiffl

We describe an unusual case of severe hypokalemia with electrocardiographic changes, due to licorice consumption, in a 15-year-old female student with no previous medical history. Prompt replacement of potassium and cessation of licorice ingestion resulted in a favourable outcome. We also discuss the pathophysiology and diagnosis, emphasizing the importance of a detailed anamnesis to rule out an often forgotten cause of hypokalemia as the licorice poisoning.

1. Introduction

Hypokalemia is one of the most frequently encountered fluid and electrolyte abnormalities in clinical medicine. It can result from reduced potassium intake, transcellular potassium uptake, and extrarenal or renal potassium loss [1]. While underlying tubular disorders may be suspected in young patients, it is important to rule out secondary causes of hypokalemia, such as medications or herbal complexes [2]. Children and young adults tolerate hypokalemia better than elderly patients, although cardiac arrhythmia may occur in both cases. Prompt replacement of potassium to a safe level is mandatory.

2. Case Report

A 15-year-old female student with no relevant medical history was admitted to the emergency department with dizziness, nausea, and progressive weakness over the last 24 hours. She denied smoking, alcohol consumption, or diuretic use but recognized practicing aerobic exercise every day. Her familial medical history was unremarkable. She had not had dyspnoea, fever, vomiting, or diarrhea in the last days. Physical examination showed a blood pressure of 135/80 mmHg and heart rate of 75 beats per minute. Chest auscultation revealed regular heart sounds with no murmurs, and abdominal exam did not reveal tenderness, hepatomegaly, or masses.

In the electrocardiogram sinus rhythm was described, with prolonged QT interval of 600 milliseconds (Figure 1).

The initial laboratory data showed severe hypokalemia of 1.8 mmol/L and metabolic alkalosis with pH 7.6, pCO2 48 mmHg, and HCO3 47 mmol/L. Serum creatinine, sodium, calcium, phosphate, magnesium, and uric acid were within the normal range. Mild elevation of creatine kinase of 321 U/L was observed. A urine sample analysis showed urinary sodium of 50 mmol/L and potassium of 65 mmol/L, with a transtubular potassium gradient of 16.

Over the next six days, the patient received high doses of intravenous and oral potassium chloride, with slow progressive correction, and further studies were performed in order to exclude other potential causes. Low plasma renin concentration [<0.3 ng/mL/h (normal values 0.3–7 ng/mL/h)], low plasma aldosterone [3.4 ng/dL (normal 5–40 ng/dL)], normal cortisol concentration [10.5 mcg/dL (normal 3–20 mcg/dL)], and normal adrenocorticotropic hormone levels [15 pg/mL (normal 5–45 pg/mL)] were found on specific hormonal analysis. Abdominal computed-tomography findings were unremarkable. Although a primary hereditary tubular disorder was the first clinical suspicion, after detailed anamnesis the patient confessed regular consumption of licorice roots over the last two weeks. The clinical course was favourable and the patient was discharged ten days after, with complete correction of these biochemical abnormalities, correction of electrocardiographic changes, and a clear advice of not taking licorice again.

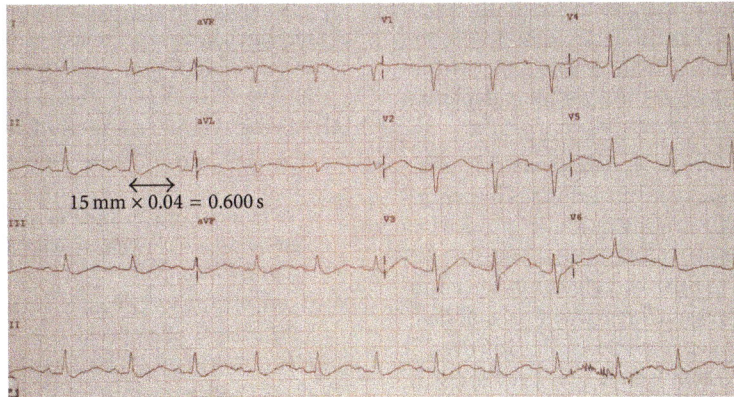

FIGURE 1: Electrocardiogram on admission shows sinus rhythm, mild increase in P waves, and mild depression of the ST segment. Note the prolonged QT interval of 600 milliseconds.

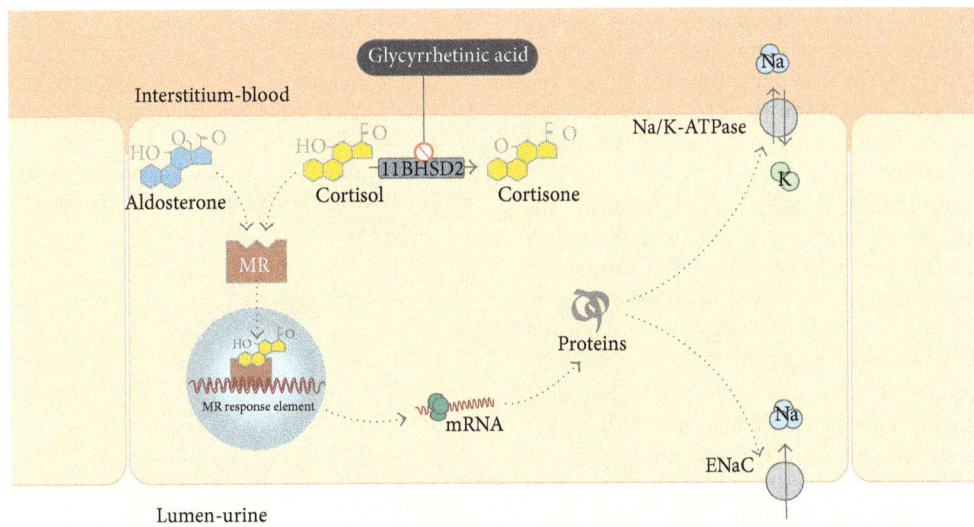

FIGURE 2: Aldosterone acts primarily in the distal nephron by diffusing into the tubular cell and attaching to specific mineralocorticoid receptor (MR). After that, the ligand-receptor complex migrates into the nucleus, where it interacts with specific sites and enhances messenger RNA (mRNA) and ribosomal RNA transcription. Aldosterone-induced proteins are synthesized, such as the apical epithelial sodium channel (ENaC) and basolateral Na/K-ATPase. *In vitro*, aldosterone and cortisol have similar affinity to the MR. The enzyme 11β-hydroxysteroid dehydrogenase type 2 (11BHSD2) converts cortisol to inactive cortisone, preventing cortisol from binding to the MR. Glycyrrhetinic acid inhibits 11BHSD2 leading to activation of MR by cortisol.

3. Discussion

This case highlights the potential toxicity of licorice in the development of severe hypokalemia with electrocardiographic changes, which could eventually lead to fatal arrhythmia in certain cases. Licorice contains glycyrrhizin and has been used in traditional Asian medicine for its anti-inflammatory properties [3]. On the other hand, licorice is present in the western world as a natural sweetener for foods and candies, as well as in natural roots. It has been reported that the concentration of glycyrrhetinic acid (GA) in licorice roots can vary up to 20% depending on the extraction process [4].

Under physiological conditions, aldosterone binds to the mineralocorticoid receptor (MR) in the principal cells of cortical collecting duct, resulting in signal transduction and subsequent expression of apical epithelial sodium channel and basolateral Na/K-ATPase. The net result is sodium reabsorption and potassium excretion [5]. The affinity of cortisol to MR is similar to that of aldosterone, but the presence of 11β-hydroxysteroid dehydrogenase type 2 (11BHSD2), an enzyme that converts cortisol to inactive cortisone, prevents cortisol from binding to the MR (Figure 2).

GA inhibits 11BHSD2 leading to activation of the MR by cortisol. Patients present with hypertension, hypokalemia, and metabolic alkalosis [6]. In most cases, potassium depletion develops slowly, and symptoms such as myalgia or cramps appear when serum potassium levels are severely low. Our patient needed high doses of potassium chloride, which may reflect a severe intracellular depletion of potassium.

Although hypokalemia is the most dangerous side effect of licorice consumption, the main adverse effect is hypertension. The USA Food and Drug Administration (FDA) advises avoiding eating large amounts of black licorice at one time [7]. An increase in extracellular volume and elevation of central systolic and diastolic blood pressure after two weeks of daily licorice consumption have been reported [8]. However, it has been suggested that individual factors may predispose to pseudoaldosteronism in certain patients, since some patients develop neither hypokalemia nor hypertension even after long time consuming licorice. In addition, some medications can interact with glycyrrhizin metabolism [3].

A precise diagnosis of hypokalemia secondary to licorice consumption requires a careful anamnesis, even though specific blood tests and urinalysis may give the definitive diagnosis. Urinalysis typically shows inappropriately elevated urinary potassium level, with a transtubular potassium gradient above 7, all of which with low plasma renin and aldosterone concentration [9].

A 24-hour urine collection may be necessary to rule out underlying tubular dysfunction. Decreased free urinary cortisone and an increased ratio of urinary free cortisol to urinary free cortisone are usually found in a 24-hour urine collection [9]. This may help make the diagnosis, but it is not required if a history of licorice ingestion has been obtained.

Other conditions to be included in the differential diagnosis of patients with hypokalemia, metabolic alkalosis, and hypertension are inherited disorders such as Liddle syndrome, apparent mineralocorticoid excess, and glucocorticoid-remediable aldosteronism [10]. These disorders are not correctable and patients usually need lifelong therapy with potassium supplements and potassium-sparing diuretics. In rare cases, incomplete phenotypes of tubular disorders become apparent after licorice ingestion.

In conclusion, it is important to keep in mind licorice abuse as a cause of symptomatic hypokalemia even in young patients. A careful anamnesis and a complete hormonal and urinary analysis are essential for diagnosis.

Conflict of Interests

The authors declare that there is no conflict of interests regarding the publication of this paper.

References

[1] R. J. Unwin, F. C. Luft, and D. G. Shirley, "Pathophysiology and management of hypokalemia: a clinical perspective," *Nature Reviews Nephrology*, vol. 7, no. 2, pp. 75–84, 2011.

[2] S. K. Haque, G. Ariceta, and D. Batlle, "Proximal renal tubular acidosis: a not so rare disorder of multiple etiologies," *Nephrology Dialysis Transplantation*, vol. 27, no. 12, pp. 4273–4287, 2012.

[3] T. Makino, "3-Monoglucuronyl glycyrrhretinic acid is a possible marker compound related to licorice-induced pseudoaldosteronism," *Biological and Pharmaceutical Bulletin*, vol. 37, no. 6, pp. 898–902, 2014.

[4] P. Ferrari, "Licorice: a sweet alternative to prevent hyperkalemia in dialysis patients?" *Kidney International*, vol. 76, no. 8, pp. 811–812, 2009.

[5] J. W. Funder, "11β-hydroxysteroid dehydrogenase: new answers, new questions," *European Journal of Endocrinology*, vol. 134, no. 3, pp. 267–268, 1996.

[6] C. van Noord, R. Zietse, M. A. van den Dorpel, and E. J. Hoorn, "The case: a 62-year-old man with severe alkalosis," *Kidney International*, vol. 81, no. 7, pp. 711–712, 2012.

[7] Black licorice: trick or treat?, Consumer Health Information, http://www.fda.gov/downloads/ForConsumers/ConsumerUpdates/UCM277166.pdf.

[8] M. H. Leskinen, E. J. Hautaniemi, A. M. Tahvanainen et al., "Daily liquorice consumption for two weeks increases augmentation index and central systolic and diastolic blood pressure," *PLoS ONE*, vol. 9, no. 8, Article ID e105607, 2014.

[9] R. V. Farese Jr., E. G. Biglieri, C. H. L. Shackleton, I. Irony, and R. Gomez-Fontes, "Licorice-induced hypermineralocorticoidism," *The New England Journal of Medicine*, vol. 325, no. 17, pp. 1223–1227, 1991.

[10] P. C. White, "Abnormalities of aldosterone synthesis and action in children," *Current Opinion in Pediatrics*, vol. 9, no. 4, pp. 424–430, 1997.

35

A Novel Technique for Laparoscopic Salvage of CAPD Catheter Malfunction and Migration: The Santosh-PGI Hanging Loop Technique

Santosh Kumar,[1] Shivanshu Singh,[1] Aditya Prakash Sharma,[1] and Manish Rathi[2]

[1]*Department of Urology, Postgraduate Institute of Medical Education and Research, Chandigarh 160012, India*
[2]*Department of Nephrology, Postgraduate Institute of Medical Education and Research, Chandigarh 160012, India*

Correspondence should be addressed to Santosh Kumar; santoshsp1967jaimatadi@yahoo.co.in

Academic Editor: Kostas C. Siamopoulos

CAPD catheter malfunction is a common problem. Obstruction due to wrapping by appendices epiploicae of sigmoid colon has been rarely reported in literature. We report a case of CAPD catheter malfunction caused by catheter tip migration and obstruction by appendices epiploicae that was successfully managed by laparoscopic hanging loop technique. This case report highlights the ease with which epiplopexy can be performed and catheter tip migration can be prevented by this innovative laparoscopic procedure.

1. Introduction

CAPD (Continuous Ambulatory Peritoneal Dialysis) is a prevalent mode of renal replacement therapy with nearly 197,000 ESRD patients using it globally [1]. One of the important aspects of CAPD catheter is its adequate function defined as one that allows adequate inflow and/or outflow of dialysate solution [2]. CAPD catheter malfunction is one of the major causes for its discontinuation. Catheter malfunction can result from its luminal occlusion due to omental or small bowel wrapping, malposition, or migration of catheter. Obstruction due to appendices epiploicae of the sigmoid colon is a rarely reported etiology [3]. Laparoscopic salvage of malfunctioning catheters helps in reducing patient's morbidity and need of intermediary hemodialysis. However, recurrent malfunction had motivated surgeons to innovate newer methods of laparoscopic CAPD catheter salvage. We report a case of CAPD catheter occlusion caused by wrapping of appendices epiploicae of sigmoid colon, a rare cause. Laparoscopic "Santosh-PGI Hanging Loop Technique," an innovative concept with multiple benefits, salvaged it.

2. Case Report

A 54-year-old gentleman having diabetes and hypertension was diagnosed as end-stage renal disease requiring renal replacement therapy. He opted for CAPD. His serum creatinine was 7.9 mg/dL. Straight Tenckhoff CAPD catheter insertion was done by standard open technique. Patient was discharged on postoperative day three. Two weeks after insertion, CAPD initiation was planned. However, there was slow inflow and a trickling outflow. Diagnosis of CAPD catheter malfunction was made. X-ray abdomen revealed malposition of CAPD catheter (Figure 1(a)). It was lying outside the pelvis in left lateral abdomen. Initial management with laxatives, bowel enema, failed with no improvement in dialysate flux. Repositioning of CAPD catheter was attempted under fluoroscopic guidance but it was unsuccessful. Keeping a diagnosis of CAPD catheter malposition with suspected omental wrapping, decision was made for diagnostic laparoscopy along with a salvage procedure as required.

Under general anesthesia, laparoscopy was performed with the patient in supine position with Trendelenburg tilt. Three ports were placed including one 12 mm camera and

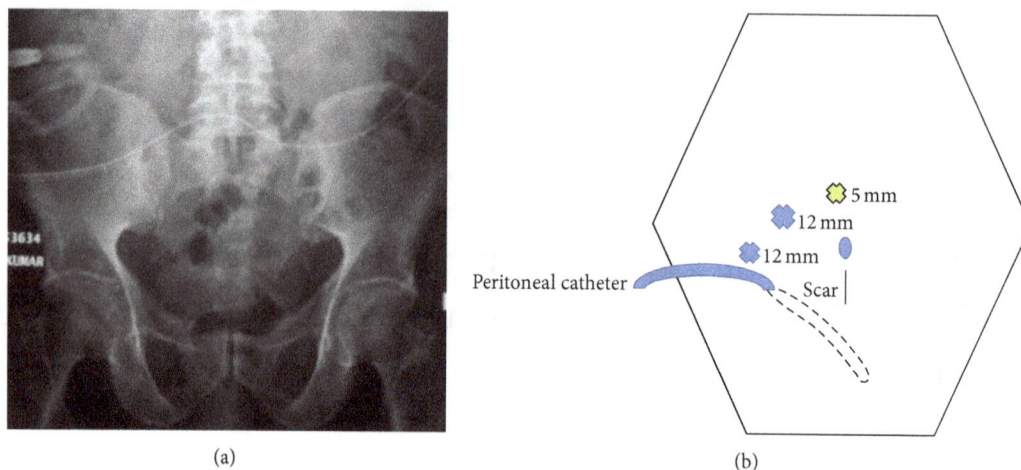

FIGURE 1: X-ray abdomen showing migrated CAPD catheter lying outside the pelvis (a). Illustration of laparoscopic port placement (b). The middle 12 mm blue cross is the camera port while the corners 12 mm and 5 mm are the working ports.

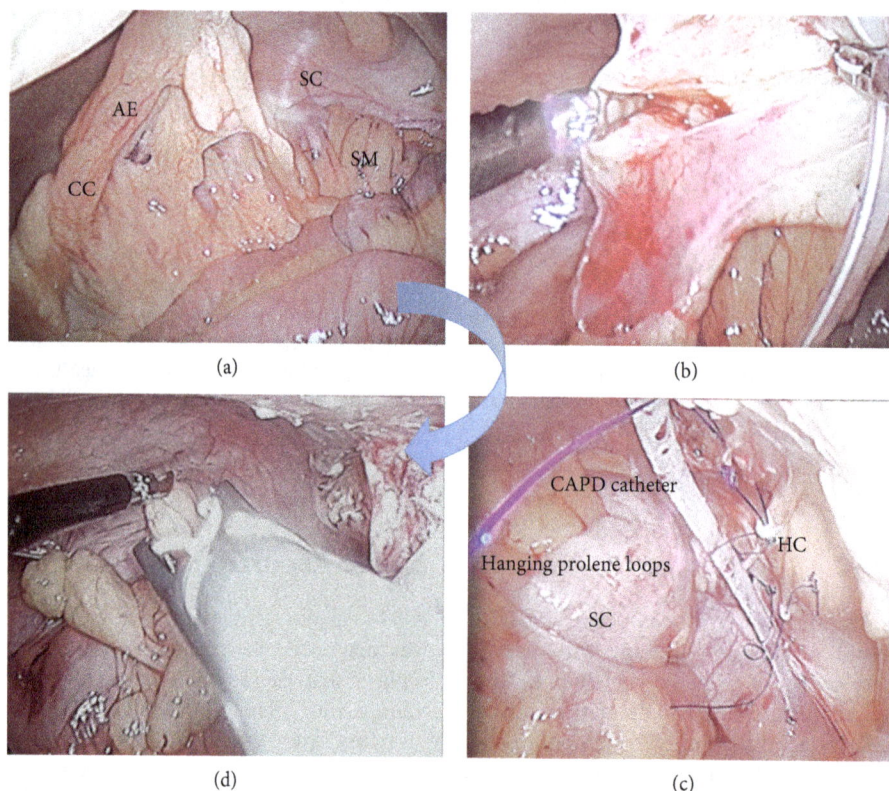

FIGURE 2: Laparoscopic view demonstrating wrapped-up CAPD catheter by appendices epiploicae of sigmoid colon (a). Dissection of the catheter from epiploicae using harmonic shear device (b). CAPD catheter hanging freely over prolene loops that are fixed to the pelvic parietal peritoneum using hemostatic clips (c). Epiplopexy using hemostatic clips (d) (AE = appendices epiploicae; CC = CAPD catheter; SC = sigmoid colon; SM = sigmoid mesocolon; HC = hemostatic clips).

two working ports (Figure 1(b)). To our surprise, the catheter was engulfed by appendices epiploicae of sigmoid colon (Figure 2). With the help of laparoscopic harmonic shear device, the catheter was completely dissected off from the appendices epiploicae. It was repositioned in the pelvis. Further, in an attempt to prevent recurrent CAPD catheter occlusion and migration, an innovative "Santosh-PGI Hanging

Loop Technique" was applied. In this, prolene 2-0 needleless suture was taken. Two knots were applied on it, one on each side. This suture was then passed into peritoneal cavity through one of the ports. A loop was made around the CAPD catheter and was fixed to the pelvic peritoneum with help of hemostatic clips. Similarly, two more loops were applied. In this way, the CAPD catheter was hanged freely underneath the pelvic peritoneum with the help of prolene suture. To prevent appendices epiploicae from falling back on the catheter, they were fixed to the left lower abdominal parietal peritoneum using hemostatic clips. On table catheter patency and position were confirmed. Postoperative period was uneventful. Low volume dialysis was started on 1st postoperative day. Normal volume dialysis was resumed by day 9. At 6-month follow-up his catheter is functioning well. Repeat X-ray imaging revealed its pelvic position.

3. Discussion

From 1997 to 2008, the number of peritoneal dialysis patients in developing countries increased by 24.9 patients per million population while in developed countries it increased by 21.8 per million population [1]. CAPD catheter malfunction is one of the major causes for discontinuation of this therapeutic modality. Incidence ranges from 12 to 73% [4]. Catheter malfunction accounts for 20% of patient transfers to hemodialysis [5]. Malfunction can result from occlusion of catheter by omental or small bowel wrapping with adhesions, fibrin clot, migration or malposition, and tunnel infections. Various series have reported omental wrapping and malposition to be the most common cause of malfunction [2, 6, 7]. Appendices epiploicae has been rarely reported as a cause of catheter occlusion [3]. CAPD catheter salvage instead of removal helps in functional rescue, thereby prolonging catheter life, decreasing patient morbidity, reducing financial burden, and allowing early institution of peritoneal dialysis, thereby decreasing dependence on intermediary hemodialysis [8]. Laparoscopic salvage of CAPD catheters has several reported advantages [8]. Laparoscopy provides a direct vision of the pathology, helps in diagnosis of other intra-abdominal pathologies, has lower incidence of postsurgical adhesions, incision related complications, postprocedure pain, thereby resulting in early ambulation, shorter hospital stay with quicker return to work. It allows early institution of peritoneal dialysis and better functional survival of catheter. Salvage procedures include laparoscopic unwrapping of omentum with omentectomy, omentopexy, [2] adhesiolysis, or laparoscopic milking of occluded catheters [9]. Laparoscopically salvaged catheters have been shown to have reasonably good period of catheter survival with a median of 163 days in some studies [7]. Initial success rates of as high as 100% have been reported [8] highlighting the usefulness of salvage procedures.

Catheter tip migration contributes to a substantial proportion of catheter malfunction. Those not corrected by conservative or stiff wire manipulation require surgical intervention. Laparoscopic salvage has definite advantages over open surgical procedures. Laparoscopic preperitoneal placement and pelvic fixation using extracorporeal knotting have been reported in an attempt to prevent catheter migration [10]. We report an innovative, easily performed technique of laparoscopic rescue of CAPD catheter malfunction due to wrapping by appendices epiploicae of sigmoid colon and catheter tip migration. In this, we first unwrapped the catheter from appendices epiploicae. The catheter was freely hanged underneath the pelvic peritoneum over prolene suture loops that

were fixed to the peritoneum with hemostatic clips using laparoscopic clip applicator. The tip of the catheter was in the pelvic cavity. This technique has several advantages. Suture fixation is easy with hemostatic clips. The catheter hangs freely in the loop thereby allowing easy removal or exchange in the future. No separate incisions are required for subcutaneous suture fixation as it is done intraperitoneally. In order to prevent appendices from falling back on catheter, it was fixed to left lateral wall with hemostatic clips. This technique highlights the simplicity with which the catheter migration and occlusion can be prevented.

4. Conclusion

CAPD catheter malfunction is a common problem. Laparoscopic salvage of such catheters decreases patient's morbidity. The laparoscopic hanging loop technique with epiplopexy using hemostatic clips helps in effectively preventing catheter tip migration out of pelvic cavity and rewrapping of catheter by appendices epiploicae.

Conflict of Interests

The authors report no conflict of interests.

References

[1] A. K. Jain, P. Blake, P. Cordy, and A. X. Garg, "Global trends in rates of peritoneal dialysis," *Journal of the American Society of Nephrology*, vol. 23, no. 3, pp. 533–544, 2012.

[2] H. M. Zakaria, "Laparoscopic management of malfunctioning peritoneal dialysis catheters," *Oman Medical Journal*, vol. 26, no. 3, pp. 171–174, 2011.

[3] J. H. Crabtree and A. Fishman, "Laparoscopic epiplopexy of the greater omentum and epiploic appendices in the salvaging of dysfunctional peritoneal dialysis catheters," *Surgical Laparoscopy, Endoscopy and Percutaneous Techniques*, vol. 6, no. 3, pp. 176–180, 1996.

[4] J. Bernardini, B. Piraino, J. L. Holley, J. R. Johnston, and R. Lutes, "A randomized trial of *Staphylococcus aureus* prophylaxis in peritoneal dialysis patients: mupirocin calcium ointment 2% applied to the exit site versus cyclic oral rifampin," *American Journal of Kidney Diseases*, vol. 27, no. 5, pp. 695–700, 1996.

[5] G. Ogunc, "Minilaparoscopic extraperitoneal tunneling with omentopexy: a new technique for CAPD catheter placement," *Peritoneal Dialysis International*, vol. 25, no. 6, pp. 551–555, 2005.

[6] G. Kazemzadeh, M.-H. S. Modaghegh, and A. Tavassoli, "Laparoscopic correction of peritoneal catheter dysfunction," *Indian Journal of Surgery*, vol. 70, no. 5, pp. 227–230, 2008.

[7] S. Santarelli, M. Zeiler, R. Marinelli, T. Monteburini, A. Federico, and E. Ceraudo, "Videolaparoscopy as rescue therapy and placement of peritoneal dialysis catheters: s thirty-two case single centre experience," *Nephrology Dialysis Transplantation*, vol. 21, no. 5, pp. 1348–1354, 2006.

[8] G. Ögünç, "Malfunctioning peritoneal dialysis catheter and accompanying surgical pathology repaired by laparoscopic surgery," *Peritoneal Dialysis International*, vol. 22, no. 4, pp. 454–462, 2002.

[9] C. Fourtounas, I. Maroulis, D. Karnabatidis, A. Hardalias, and J. G. Vlachojannis, "Salvage of a totally occluded peritoneal dialysis catheter by laparoscopic milking," *Seminars in Dialysis*, vol. 26, no. 1, pp. E8–E10, 2013.

[10] M. E. Gunes, G. Uzum, O. Koc et al., "A modified method in laparoscopic peritoneal catheter implantation: the combination of preperitoneal tunneling and pelvic fixation," *ISRN Surgery*, vol. 2013, Article ID 248126, 5 pages, 2013.

36

Solitary Crossed Renal Ectopia: Concurrence of Posterior Urethral Valve and Hypospadias

Amin Bagheri, Reza Khorramirouz, Sorena Keihani, Mehdi Fareghi, and Abdol-Mohammad Kajbafzadeh

Pediatric Urology Research Center, Pediatrics Center of Excellence, Children's Hospital Medical Center, Tehran University of Medical Sciences, Tehran 1419433151, Iran

Correspondence should be addressed to Abdol-Mohammad Kajbafzadeh; kajbafzd@sina.tums.ac.ir

Academic Editor: Neil Boudville

Solitary crossed renal ectopia (SCRE) represents an exceedingly rare congenital disorder. Although skeletal and genitourinary abnormalities most commonly accompany this condition, vesicoureteral reflux (VUR) has been described in only a few cases. Here, we present two unique cases of SCRE complicated by high-grade VUR concomitant with posterior urethral valve in one case and hypospadias in the other one. We also provide a brief review of the literature on this subject.

1. Introduction

Solitary crossed renal ectopia (SCRE) is a rare congenital anomaly with an estimated prevalence of 1 in 1,500,000 [1]. A combination of unilateral renal agenesis and contralateral renal ectopia that crosses the midline leads to SCRE. Mostly asymptomatic, SCRE often remains undiagnosed or presents a diagnostic challenge as an incidental finding during routine perinatal ultrasound, during screening imaging studies, or at autopsy [2].

Although several genitourinary and skeletal abnormalities may accompany SCRE, concomitant vesicoureteral reflux (VUR) is rarely reported [3, 4]. Moreover, the concurrence of posterior urethral valve (PUV) with these conditions has not been previously reported. Hypospadias is also rare in context of SCRE [4, 5]. Hereby, we report two unique cases of SCRE presenting with VUR complicated by hypospadias (Case 1) and PUV (Case 2) and also provide a brief literature review.

2. Case 1

A 3-month-old boy born with a single umbilical artery was referred with a penile hypospadias. Ultrasound revealed an empty left renal fossa suggesting renal agenesis and a hypertrophic kidney (2.5 × 7.0 cm) on the right side with normal renal parenchyma. Dimercaptosuccinic acid (DMSA) scan showed acceptable cortical function of the right kidney; no tracer uptake was visualized on the left one. Voiding cystourethrogram (VCUG) demonstrated grade III VUR into the left ureter, with a path crossing the midline and entering the right kidney (Figure 1). On cystoscopy, single ureteral orifice was located on the left side. Dextranomer/hyaluronic acid copolymer (Deflux) was injected at the left ureteral orifice to correct the high-grade VUR. The patient was discharged asymptomatically with the resolution of VUR and was scheduled for a hypospadias repair.

3. Case 2

A 9-day-old male neonate was referred with an antenatal ultrasound suggestive of solitary unilateral hydronephrosis. Postnatal ultrasound confirmed absence of the left kidney; a large right kidney with severe hydroureteronephrosis was reported. DMSA demonstrated absent activity on the left side and normal cortical function of the right kidney. Additionally, initial VCUG revealed VUR into the right kidney and a typical PUV. The patient underwent endoscopic valve ablation at day 15 after birth but the ureteral orifice was not found on the right side. Postoperative VCUG still showed grade IV VUR into the left ureter with a megaureter (diameter:

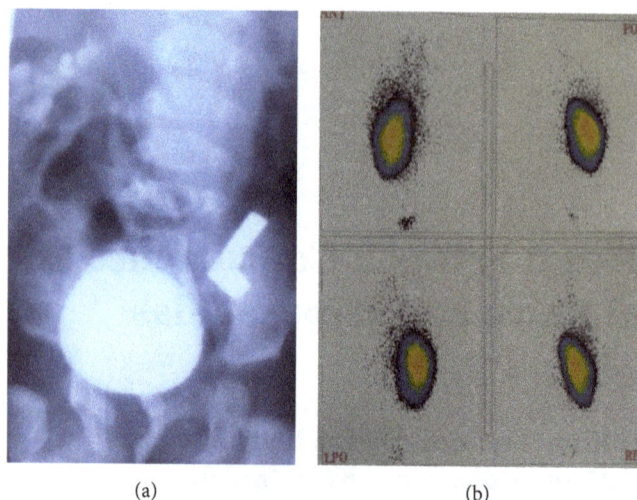

FIGURE 1: (a) VCUG, anteroposterior view showing VUR; ureter is seen crossing the midline from left to right side at the L5 level. (b) DMSA renal scan demonstrates absent activity in the left renal bed with acceptable cortical function of the right kidney.

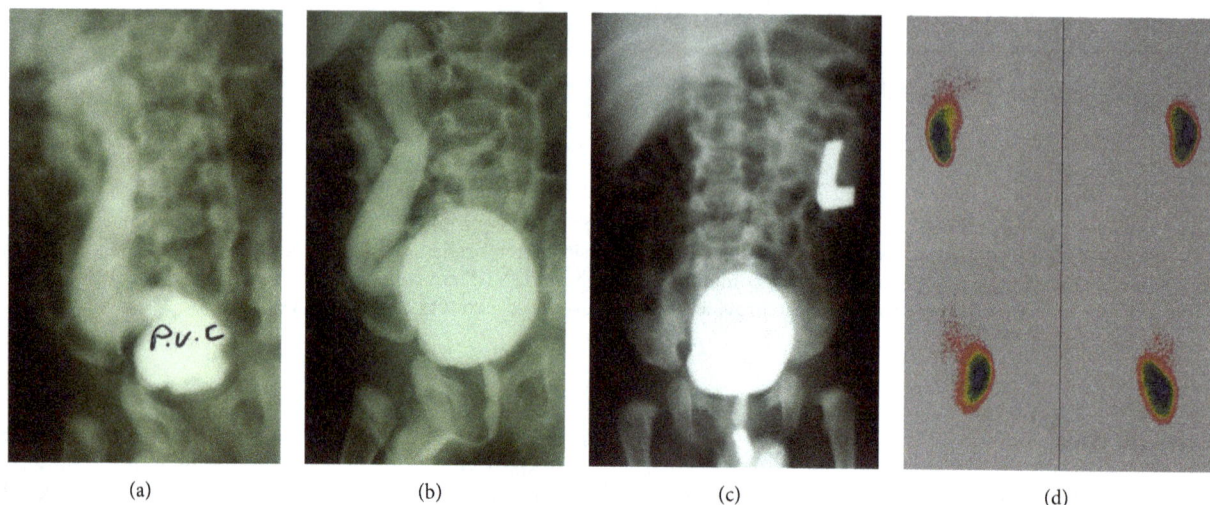

FIGURE 2: AP and oblique view VCUG showing left to right renal ectopia and high-grade left sided VUR that persisted after first valve ablation ((a), (b)) and resolution of VUR after second valve ablation (c). DMSA renal scan shows proper cortical function of the right kidney and nonvisualization of the left kidney (d).

7.0 mm) that crossed the midline and entered the right kidney. It also showed minimal posterior urethral dilation compatible with PUV remnants. Video urethrocystoscopy confirmed the presence of PUV remnants with a trabeculated bladder and absence of right ureteral orifice. Endoscopic PUV ablation was performed and VUR resolved subsequently in the follow-up VCUG at 6 months of age (Figure 2).

4. Discussion

Crossed renal ectopia defines a spectrum of congenital anomalies in which the kidney is located on one side, while the corresponding ureter enters the bladder in the contralateral side. In 1957, McDonald and McClellan [6] revised the categorization of crossed renal ectopia into 4 subtypes: (1) with fusion; (2) without fusion; (3) solitary crossed; and (4) bilateral crossed. Crossed renal ectopia with and without fusion constitutes more than 90% of all cases, whereas solitary crossed renal ectopia (SCRE) and bilateral crossed ectopia are exceedingly rare.

Unilateral renal agenesis accompanied by renal ectopia in the contralateral side results in SCRE. The exact embryologic mechanisms behind this anomaly remain widely unknown. Formation of metanephros begins when the ureteric buds meet the metanephric blastema early in development. Absence or incomplete development of a ureteric bud disrupts the association between collecting and excretory systems and precludes the development of a definitive kidney, being the embryologic basis behind renal agenesis [2]. However, little consensus exists on the exact cause of crossed renal ectopia. Wilmer [7] proposed that pressure from abnormally located umbilical arteries displaces the renal unit and facilitates its ascend to the opposite renal bed, where it faces lesser degrees of mechanical resistance. In another theory, a wandering ureteric bud is the main culprit that joins the contralateral metanephric blastema and continues to ascend in the wrong direction [8]. Ashley and Mostofi [9] also focused on the role of unknown signaling substances produced by contralateral metanephros that attract the developing ureteric bud deviating it from the normal path. Role of teratogens and also misalignment and rotation of medial axis during fetal development are among other theories proposed [2].

Most individuals with SCRE are male (ratio 2:1) and have left to right ectopia. SCRE has the highest rate of associated anomalies in crossed ectopia that may be more attributable to renal agenesis rather than crossed ectopia [2]. Absent vas deferens and cryptorchidism in males and vaginal atresia and uterine abnormalities in females are most frequent genitourinary anomalies in this group [2, 5]. Although concomitant VUR is reported in few cases [3, 4], the presence of PUV or hypospadias in SCRE complicated by VUR is exceedingly rare.

In most cases, SCRE remains asymptomatic and is diagnosed incidentally or on autopsy. Proper diagnosis needs a high degree of clinical suspicion and prompt attention to the accompanying abnormalities. Presence of cryptorchidism, vas anomalies, hypospadias, urethral valves, unilateral hydronephrosis, megaureter, or VUR can all signal to the underlying renal anomaly. Vague symptoms may develop later in life as hematuria, pyuria, or abdominal pain [2]. Urinary tract infection or renal calculi may be the only clue and may be attributable to abnormal kidney position or vascular supply that disrupts the normal drainage [2].

In modern medicine, ultrasonography and DMSA have largely replaced classic urography and retrograde pyelograms in diagnosis of SCRE. Although CT-scan and MRI can provide excellent information on urinary tract anatomy, their use is limited by radiation exposure and/or cost. In fact, most of the asymptomatic SCRE patients can be initially diagnosed by ultrasound and DMSA [2]. If needed, VCUG can provide extra information on bladder anatomy, presence of VUR and/or PUV, and path of the refluxing ureter. Cystoscopy also helps in assessing the urethral and bladder anatomy and position of the ureteral orifices or delivering treatment for PUV and VUR if needed. Taken together, ultrasound and DMSA are excellent diagnostic options for SCRE, with CT-scan and MRI reserved for selected cases or before extensive surgeries.

The overall prognosis of SCRE is excellent and most patients have a normal lifespan [2]. Morbidity may be due to associated anomalies needing prompt management. Although Grotas and Phillips [10] recently reported a rare case of renal cell carcinoma in SCRE and suggested an incidence of 1 in 22 million for this condition, even this value may be a large overestimation since they did not use the prevalence of "solitary" crossed renal ectopia in their calculation.

5. Summary

In conclusion, this study adds two new cases to the limited literature on SCRE. SCRE is a rare urinary tract disorder that may be asymptomatic or may be accompanied by other skeletal and genitourinary anomalies. Besides previously reported genitourinary comorbidities, hypospadias and PUV should also be regarded as associated anomalies in SCRE patients. It is intuitive to more thoroughly evaluate the urinary tract to find associated conditions when a congenital anomaly is diagnosed.

Conflict of Interests

The authors declare that there is no conflict of interests regarding the publication of this paper.

References

[1] L. J. Livermore and N. Thiruchelvam, "Whose side are you on? The diagnostic conundrum of solitary crossed renal ectopia," *Journal of Pediatric Urology*, vol. 6, no. 1, pp. 83–86, 2010.

[2] A. J. Wein, L. R. Kavoussi, and M. F. Campbell, *Campbell-Walsh Urology*, Elsevier Saunders, Philadelphia, Pa, USA, 2012.

[3] Z. Habib, J. Abudaia, F. Bamehriz, and S. Ahmed, "Fanconi's anemia with solitary crossed renal ectopia, vesicoureteric reflux, and genital abnormalities," *Pediatric Surgery International*, vol. 16, no. 1-2, pp. 136–137, 2000.

[4] K. Kesan, R. Gupta, A. Gupta et al., "Solitary crossed renal ectopia with vesicoureteric reflux presenting with impaired renal function in a neonate," *Journal of Clinical Neonatology*, vol. 2, no. 3, pp. 140–142, 2013.

[5] H. Kakei, A. Kondo, B. I. Ogisu, and H. Mitsuya, "Crossed ectopia of solitary kidney. A report of two cases and a review of the literature," *Urologia Internationalis*, vol. 31, no. 6, pp. 470–475, 1976.

[6] J. H. McDonald and D. S. McClellan, "Crossed renal ectopia," *The American Journal of Surgery*, vol. 93, no. 6, pp. 995–1002, 1957.

[7] H. A. Wilmer, "Unilateral fused kidney: a report of five cases and a review of the literature," *The Journal of Urology*, vol. 40, pp. 551–571, 1938.

[8] J. C. Alexander, K. B. King, and C. S. Fromm, "Congenital solitary kidney with crossed ureter," *The Journal of Urology*, vol. 64, no. 2, pp. 230–234, 1950.

[9] D. J. Ashley and F. K. Mostofi, "Renal agenesis and dysgenesis," *The Journal of Urology*, vol. 83, pp. 211–230, 1960.

[10] A. B. Grotas and J. L. Phillips, "Renal mass in solitary, crossed, ectopic pelvic kidney," *Urology*, vol. 73, no. 6, pp. 1223–1224, 2009.

37

Two Brothers with Bardet-Biedl Syndrome Presenting with Chronic Renal Failure

Cem Sahin,[1] **Bulent Huddam,**[2] **Gulhan Akbaba,**[3] **Hasan Tunca,**[1]
Emine Koca,[1] **and Mustafa Levent**[1]

[1]*Department of Internal Medicine, School of Medicine, Mugla Sıtkı Kocman University, Orhaniye Mahallesi İsmet Catak Caddesi, 48000 Mugla, Turkey*
[2]*Department of Nephrology, Mugla Sitki Kocman University Education and Research Hospital, 48000 Mugla, Turkey*
[3]*Department of Endocrinology, School of Medicine, Mugla Sıtkı Kocman University, 48000 Mugla, Turkey*

Correspondence should be addressed to Cem Sahin; cemsahin@mu.edu.tr

Academic Editor: Yoshihide Fujigaki

Bardet-Biedl Syndrome (BBS) is a rarely seen autosomal recessive transfer disease characterised by retinal dystrophy, obesity, extremity deformities, mental retardation, and renal and genital system anomalies. BBS shows heterogenic transfer. To date, 18 genes (BBS1–18) and 7 BBS proteins have been defined as related to BBS. All of the defined BBS genes have been shown to be related to the biogenesis or function of cilia. Renal failure accompanying the syndrome, especially in the advanced stages, is the most common cause of mortality. Therefore, as one of the major diagnostic criteria, renal damage is of great importance in early diagnosis. This paper presents the cases of two brothers with BBS who presented with chronic renal failure.

1. Introduction

Bardet-Biedl syndrome (BBS) is a genetic syndrome with autosomal recessive transfer, characterised by retinal dystrophy, obesity, extremity deformities, mental retardation, and renal and genital system anomalies. Apart from these typical findings, various anomalies such as speech defects, dental anomalies, anosmia, cardiac anomalies, diabetes mellitus, hepatic fibrosis, anal agenesis, Hirschsprung disease, and neurological involvement may be seen together with the syndrome. Renal failure accompanying the syndrome, especially in the advanced stages, is the most common cause of mortality. Therefore, as one of the major diagnostic criteria, renal damage is of great importance in early diagnosis. In this report, the typical findings of the disease considered in two brothers with BBS who presented with chronic renal failure and the importance of family scanning are emphasised.

2. Case Presentations

2.1. Case 1. A 41-year-old male applied to the emergency department with complaints of diarrhea, nausea, and vomiting (Figure 1(a)). From the tests done, as the kidney function test results were high, he was admitted with an initial diagnosis of acute kidney failure. However, following appropriate fluid replacement therapy there was no improvement apart from a relatively small drop in the kidney function tests. On the urinary system USG, the right kidney was calculated as 100×40 mm with parenchyma thickness of 10 mm and the left kidney as 110×51 mm with parenchyma thickness of 13 mm and GFR as 84 mL/min. Serum creatinine level was 1.67 mg/dL. Other biochemical markers were normal. The case was accepted as stage II chronic kidney failure.

The patient had height of 159 cm, body weight of 72.5 kg, and BMI of 28.5 and vital signs were normal. The physical examination revealed mental retardation, speech defects, apathetic facial appearance, corneal matte appearance, strabismus, central obesity, micropenis, syndactyly, and polydactyly. The HOMA index was calculated as normal (2.18) for the patient who had central obesity. No pathology was observed from tests in respect of hormonal parameters.

In respect to cardiac pathology, left ventricle function was evaluated as normal on the echocardiography. A moderate

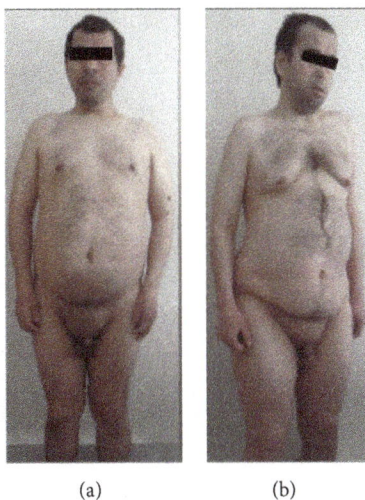

FIGURE 1: External appearance of the cases; (a) Case 1, (b) Case 2.

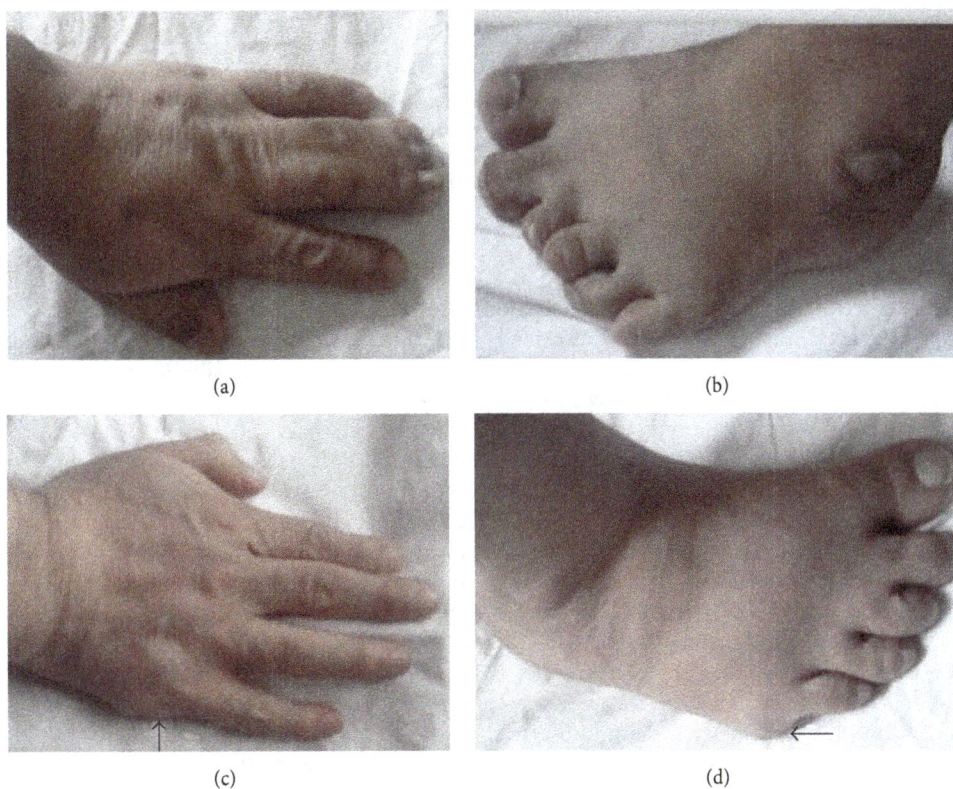

FIGURE 2: Extremities of the cases. (a) Polydactyly and syndactyly together in the left hand of Case 1, (b) polydactyly in the left foot of Case 1, and (c) and (d) right hand and foot of Case 2 (areas of previous surgery indicated by the arrow).

level of mental retardation (IQ: 35–49) was determined in the psychiatric evaluation. There was polydactyly in both hands and feet and syndactyly of fingers 3–5 on the left hand (Figure 2). The patient had total loss of vision and, in the ophthalmological examination, exotropia and mature cataracts were observed in both eyes. Fundus examination could not be conducted because of the cataracts. Following ERG, cataract surgery was recommended to the patient. On scrotal USG, the left testis could not be visualized (intra-abdominal ectopy?). As the patient had a micropenis and

undescended left testis (Figure 3(a)) in the sacral, pubic, and axillary hair areas, hormonal tests were performed and no findings of hypophyseal deficiency were observed. From all these findings, a diagnosis was made of BBS and renal failure. Questions were asked about similar anomalies in the family and the brother was called to the polyclinic for testing.

2.2. Case 2. The 38-year-old male had a height of 165 cm, a weight of 70 kg, and BMI of 25.7 and vital signs were normal

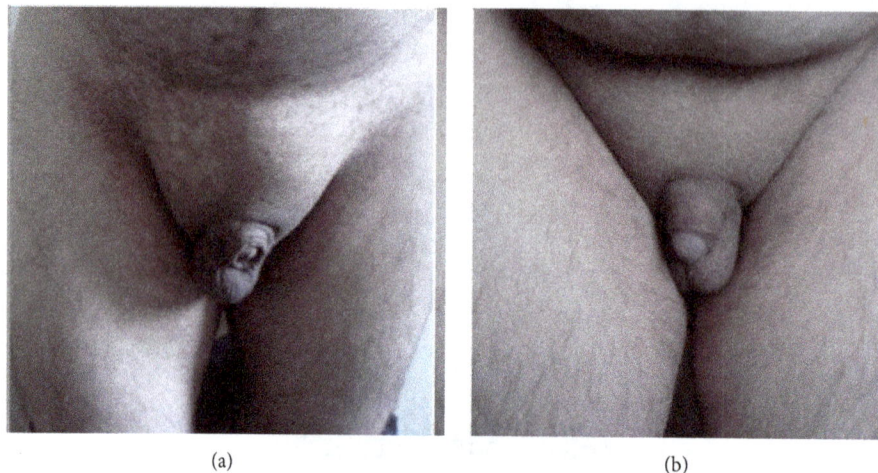

(a)   (b)

FIGURE 3: Hypogenitalism of the cases. (a) Micropenis and undescended left testis in Case 1. (b) Micropenis in Case 2.

(Figure 1(b)). The patient had mental retardation from birth and the physical examination determined speech defects, strabismus, loss of vision, gynecomastia, central obesity, and micropenis. The patient history revealed 6 fingers on both hands and feet from birth and the extra fingers had been surgically removed for cosmetic reasons during childhood.

In the hormonal tests done because of hypogenitalism (micropenis) (Figure 3(b)) in the sacral, pubic, and axillary hair areas, no findings of hypophyseal deficiency were observed. In the echocardiography applied in respect to cardiac pathology, the left ventricle function was evaluated as normal. Moderate level mental retardation (IQ, 35–49) was observed in the psychiatric evaluation and in the fundus of both eyes, and widespread bone spicules were determined. With these findings, the patient was diagnosed with retinitis pigmentosa and ERG was recommended. In kidney function tests applied 6 months previously, creatinine level had been observed to be high (4.98 mg/dL), but the patient had not been followed up by either the Nephrology or the Internal Medicine Department. On urinary USG, the right kidney was observed to be 92 mm in size with a parenchyma thickness of 6 mm and the left kidney was 76 mm in size with a parenchyma thickness of 6 mm. In addition, a 5 mm diameter stone was observed in the mid-section of the left kidney and simple cysts of maximum 10 mm diameter in both kidneys. With these findings and GFR calculated at 13 mL/min, the patient was diagnosed with BBS and end-stage kidney failure. The patient was referred to the Nephrology Department for renal replacement treatment.

3. Discussion

In Bardet-Biedl syndrome (BBS), apart from the major findings, different clinical effects can be observed evaluated under the heading of minor criteria, such as speech defects, dental anomalies, anosmia, ataxia, diabetes mellitus, and cardiac anomalies. Rod-cone dystrophy (90–100%), obesity (72–92%), polydactyly (63–81%), genital anomalies (59–98%), learning difficulties (50–61%), and renal anomalies (20–53%)

are the major components of BBS. Speech disorders (54–81%), developmental delay (50–91%), diabetes mellitus (6–48%), dental anomalies (51%), congenital heart disease (7%), brachydactyly/syndactyly (46–100%), ataxia/poor coordination (40–86%), cardiopathy (10%), deafness (11–12%), and anosmia/hyposmia (60%) are the minor components of BBS [1]. According to this, at least 4 major criteria or 3 major and 2 minor criteria together are sufficient for a diagnosis [1]. BBS, which is evaluated among the rarely seen genetic transfer diseases, shows autosomal recessive hereditary properties. While it is seen more often in isolated communities or those where there is widespread consanguinity (Kuwait 1 : 17,000 and Newfoundland 1 : 18,000), incidence in Europe and North America has been reported as 1 : 140,000–160,000 [1]. BBS shows a heterogeneous genetic transfer property. The latest update in 2014 related to the genetic characteristics of the syndrome reported that to date a relationship has been established between BBS and 18 genes (BBS 1–18) and 7 proteins (BBS 1, 2, 4, 5, 7, 8, and 9). Although the BBS mutation spectrum shows differences between populations, approximately 70–80% of the cases have been determined with BBS gene mutation [2]. Even though the results of some studies have reported a mild phenotypic correlation with BBS gene mutation, a clear and definitive relationship has not been shown between genotype and phenotype in BBS [3] and the correlation between the BBS genotype and phenotype varies among and within families. In the study of Shin et al., it was a genetically confirmed BBS case in a Korean family with a compound heterozygous mutation of the BBS7 gene [4].

While the underlying pathology of BBS clinical findings remains unknown, the study results of several subjects have suggested that the basic reason for this pleiotropic disease originates from basal body or cilia dysfunction [5]. Cilia are organelles resembling hairs which are found in nearly all cells of the body. Cilia are classified into two groups as motile or nonmotile (primary). Nonmotile cilia are thought to function as a sensory organelle in the regulation of signal transduction pathways. These primary cilia, which appear on the apical cell surface, mediate the transmission of mechanical and chemical stimuli through different signalling pathways [6].

Previous studies have shown a relationship of all known BBS genes with cilia biogenesis or function [7]. The defect occurring in nonmotile cilia has been shown to be clinically related to retinitis pigmentosa, polydactyly, situs inversus, learning difficulties, and cystic diseases of the kidney, liver, and pancreas [8].

BBS clinical characteristics generally start to be seen slowly in the first decade of life. Most cases are diagnosed in late childhood or early adolescence. Extremity anomalies determined at birth are one of the most important clinical signs for diagnosis. In terms of indicating diagnosis, extremity or renal anomalies at birth or in the intrauterine period are important. However, the variability which can be seen in these two characteristics and the late onset of other indications may be the reason for the diagnosis of the cases after childhood.

BBS is one of the most important causes of syndromic retinal dystrophy, which is seen with severe sight problems during preadolescence and with generally total loss of vision before the second decade [7]. Ophthalmological findings in BBS patients may be seen in various forms from iris coloboma, bilateral aniridia, cataracts, myopia, to anophthalmia. The classic form is retinitis pigmentosa. Different from classic retinitis pigmentosa which is not related to systemic diseases, in these patients macular degenerative changes are seen in the early stages and, in most cases, total loss of vision develops before the second decade. Different forms of retinal dystrophy have been defined, such as cone-rod dystrophy, rod-cone dystrophy, choroidal dystrophy, and global severe retinal dystrophy. Cone-rod dystrophy is known as progressive retinal degeneration and is characterised by reduced visual acuity and impaired colour vision. Ophthalmological findings are observed in 90–100% of BBS cases [7].

In BBS cases, obesity, especially central obesity, is the second major clinical finding in terms of significance and prevalence. Rates of obesity incidence have been reported as 72–92% in BBS cases. While birthweight is generally normal, 1 in 3 syndromic babies with normal birthweight becomes obese before the age of 1 year [9]. Obesity starts in early childhood and continues to increase over time. In some BBS cases, type II DM may develop related to the degree of obesity.

Extremity anomalies such as polydactyly and syndactyly as the earliest seen signs in BBS patients which are determined at birth are one of the most important clinical indicators for diagnosis. Typically, polydactyly is seen in 63–81% of BBS cases. As it is seen from birth onwards, it is the most important finding for suspicion of the syndrome [8]. Most commonly, postaxial polydactyly, polydactyly, and brachydactyly are seen in both hands and feet. Other extremity anomalies are often reported such as brachydactyly and syndactyly in both hands and feet.

Hypogonadism as another major criterion of the syndrome may be seen with delayed onset of puberty in both genders, hypogenitalism in males and genital anomalies in females. Gonadal dysfunction is seen more often in male patients than female patients. Small penis size and decreased testis volume are often seen in male patients and in female patients; there is often a delay in the onset of the menstrual cycle. In female patients, hypoplasia of the fallopian tubes, uterus, and ovaries, vaginal atresia, and genital malformations such as hematocolpos and vesicovaginal fistula may be seen.

Mental retardation, learning difficulties, speech defects, autism, and behavioural problems such as psychosis are neuropsychiatric impairments seen in BBS. Mental retardation is the fourth most important characteristic of the syndrome. Psychosocial development is retarded and IQ test scores are low. Cognitive dysfunction is noticed in most cases after they start school. It has been shown that primary cilia are one of the most important organelles in the human brain and are necessary for the hippocampal development stages. It has been shown in a study that the hippocampus volume of BBS cases is low in comparison with healthy individuals [10].

Urogenital system malformations are common in BBS and all cases should be routinely investigated for renal anomalies. The onset of renal dysfunction has not been evaluated as a major component of the syndrome. However, in the subsequent period, the observation of renal involvement in most cases and that it is the most common cause of mortality causes renal dysfunction to be defined as a major criterion of the syndrome [11].

Although a range of renal anomalies may be seen, the classic appearance is tubular disease and anatomic malformations. Renal symptoms are generally nonspecific. In approximately a third of cases, polyuria/polydipsia is seen to be associated with defective vasopressin-resistant urine concentration [9]. In patients who have not developed polyuria or where it has been ignored if present, the first renal sign may be chronic kidney disease or end-stage kidney disease [12].

The most commonly seen renal function impairment is impaired urine concentration capacity. In most cases of the urine concentration defect, no deterioration in renal function tests is observed [9, 13]. Hypertension may be seen in the early stages of life; two-thirds of all patients have hypertension with 30–50% of the patients aged below 34 years [14]. Hypertension in the absence of renal failure is not a commonly seen characteristic.

In kidney histology, chronic interstitial nephritis, mesangial proliferative glomerulopathy, and structural changes in the glomerular basal membrane may be observed. In some cases, advanced renal failure may develop due to cystic kidney disease. This may cause recurrent urinary system infections, chronic pyelonephritis, and kidney failure. As radiological findings in addition to renal function impairments in BBS patients, structural renal defects may be seen such as renal cysts, diverticulae, calyceal deformity, fetal lobulation, scars, and diffuse cortical loss.

An effective multidisciplinary approach is required to manage this pleiotropic situation. There is no definitive treatment method for BBS. Complications related to BBS should be treated symptomatically. There should be an awareness of complications for which BBS has laid the base and patients should be followed up in this respect. Effective weight management is necessary to prevent related morbidities such as metabolic syndrome. Patients with metabolic syndrome should be evaluated in respect to potential hypertension, diabetes mellitus, hyperlipidemia, and cardiovascular diseases. A detailed ophthalmological evaluation including electroretinogram (ERG) is required to determine the onset and extent of retinal dystrophy. Renal ultrasound should be applied to all patients at the time of diagnosis to discount renal malformation. Patients with findings of chronic renal failure should be referred to a nephrologist. Developmental and educational evaluations are necessary for all patients [8].

BBS generally shows autosomal recessive inheritance. Although triallelic inheritance has been reported in some cases, it is difficult to determine as it is seen in less than 10% of all cases. Information should be given about the heterogeneous nature of the patients and their relatives. In families who know the mutation causing the disease, there is the possibility of preimplantation genetic diagnosis or prenatal testing. In families at risk whom the mutation is unknown to, ultrasonography can be applied in the third trimester for the visualization of axial polydactyly and renal malformations [8].

4. Conclusion

For patients presenting with impaired kidney function accompanied by findings such as polydactyly, mental retardation, obesity, vision problems, or micropenis, BBS should certainly be considered.

However, the syndrome is rarely observed; kidney involvement is common.

When it is considered that renal failure is the most common cause of mortality, early diagnosis of renal damage is of great importance.

The syndrome and renal damage can be determined in early stages by family scanning.

Conflict of Interests

The authors declare that there is no conflict of interests regarding the publication of this paper.

References

[1] O. M'Hamdi, I. Ouertani, and H. Chaabouni-Bouhamed, "Update on the genetics of bardet-biedl syndrome," *Molecular Syndromology*, vol. 5, no. 2, pp. 51–56, 2014.

[2] O. M'hamdi, C. Redin, C. Stoetzel et al., "Clinical and genetic characterization of Bardet-Biedl syndrome in Tunisia: defining a strategy for molecular diagnosis," *Clinical Genetics*, vol. 85, no. 2, pp. 172–177, 2014.

[3] B. Pawlik, A. Mir, H. Iqbal et al., "A novel familial BBS12 mutation associated with a mild phenotype: implications for clinical and molecular diagnostic strategies," *Molecular Syndromology*, vol. 1, no. 1, pp. 27–34, 2010.

[4] S. J. Shin, M. Kim, H. Chae et al., "Identification of compound heterozygous mutations in the BBS7 Gene in a Korean family with Bardet-Biedl Syndrome," *Annals of Laboratory Medicine*, vol. 35, no. 1, pp. 181–184, 2015.

[5] M. V. Nachury, A. V. Loktev, Q. Zhang et al., "A core complex of BBS proteins cooperates with the GTPase Rab8 to promote ciliary membrane biogenesis," *Cell*, vol. 129, no. 6, pp. 1201–1213, 2007.

[6] S. Y. Wong and J. F. Reiter, "The primary cilium at the crossroads of mammalian hedgehog signaling," *Current Topics in Developmental Biology*, vol. 85, pp. 225–260, 2008.

[7] A. Mockel, Y. Perdomo, F. Stutzmann, J. Letsch, V. Marion, and H. Dollfus, "Retinal dystrophy in Bardet-Biedl syndrome and related syndromic ciliopathies," *Progress in Retinal and Eye Research*, vol. 30, no. 4, pp. 258–274, 2011.

[8] E. Forsythe and P. L. Beales, "Bardet-Biedl syndrome," *European Journal of Human Genetics*, vol. 21, no. 1, pp. 8–13, 2013.

[9] A. Putoux, T. Attie-Bitach, J. Martinovic, and M.-C. Gubler, "Phenotypic variability of Bardet-Biedl syndrome: focusing on the kidney," *Pediatric Nephrology*, vol. 27, no. 1, pp. 7–15, 2012.

[10] K. Baker, G. B. Northam, W. K. Chong, T. Banks, P. Beales, and T. Baldeweg, "Neocortical and hippocampal volume loss in a human ciliopathy: a quantitative MRI study in Bardet-Biedl syndrome," *American Journal of Medical Genetics Part A*, vol. 155, no. 1, pp. 1–8, 2011.

[11] B. Sowjanya, U. Sreenivasulu, J. N. Naidu, and N. Sivaranjani, "End stage renal disease, differential diagnosis, a rare genetic disorder: Bardet-Biedl syndrome: case report and review," *Indian Journal of Clinical Biochemistry*, vol. 26, no. 2, pp. 214–216, 2011.

[12] M. R. Ansari and A. M. Junejo, "Bardet-biedl syndrome presenting with end stage renal failure," *Journal of the College of Physicians and Surgeons Pakistan*, vol. 16, no. 7, pp. 487–488, 2006.

[13] M. K. Raychowdhury, A. J. Ramos, P. Zhang et al., "Vasopressin receptor-mediated functional signaling pathway in primary cilia of renal epithelial cells," *American Journal of Physiology—Renal Physiology*, vol. 296, no. 1, pp. F87–F97, 2009.

[14] O. Imhoff, V. Marion, C. Stoetzel et al., "Bardet-biedl syndrome: a study of the renal and cardiovascular phenotypes in a French cohort," *Clinical Journal of the American Society of Nephrology*, vol. 6, no. 1, pp. 22–29, 2011.

38

Chronic Renal Failure Presenting for the First Time as Pulmonary Mucormycosis with a Fatal Outcome

B. Jayakrishnan,[1] Jamal Al Aghbari,[1] Dawar Rizavi,[1] Sinnakirouchenan Srinivasan,[2] Ritu Lakhtakia,[3] and Dawood Al Riyami[1]

[1]*Department of Medicine, Sultan Qaboos University Hospital, 123 Muscat, Oman*
[2]*Department of Anaesthesia, Sultan Qaboos University Hospital, 123 Muscat, Oman*
[3]*Department of Pathology, College of Medicine and Health Sciences, Sultan Qaboos University, 123 Muscat, Oman*

Correspondence should be addressed to B. Jayakrishnan; drjayakrish@hotmail.com

Academic Editor: Phuong Chi Pham

Pulmonary mucormycosis is an uncommon, but important, opportunistic fungal pneumonia which is often diagnosed late. Renal failure as the predominant presenting feature is not common in mucormycosis. Moreover, sudden, massive hemoptysis is not a usual complication. In this report we describe fatal pulmonary mucormycosis in a young patient with a previously undiagnosed chronic renal failure.

1. Introduction

Mucormycosis, an uncommon invasive fungal infection, occurs predominantly in debilitated or immunosuppressed hosts. The conditions predisposing to mucormycosis include malignant hematological disease, prolonged and severe neutropenia, poorly controlled diabetes mellitus with or without diabetic ketoacidosis, iron overload, major trauma, prolonged use of corticosteroids, illicit intravenous drug use, neonatal prematurity and malnourishment, and chronic renal insufficiency [1]. However, mucormycosis has been described in previously healthy individuals as well [2, 3]. Pulmonary mucormycosis has been reported in renal failure, either as a part of chronic uremia or after transplantation [2, 3]. In a literature search spanning 30 years, 13% of the patients with pulmonary mucormycosis had renal disease of which 55% were posttransplant patients [3]. It almost always occurs in patients with an established renal disease. Renal involvement can also occur as a part of a disseminated disease. Mucormycosis has not been reported as the initial presentation of chronic renal failure. The mortality rate is often high, 65% with isolated pulmonary mucormycosis, 96% for those with disseminated disease, and 80% overall. Moreover, mucormycosis is an unusual cause of massive

hemoptysis [4, 5]. Here we report fatal pulmonary mucormycosis as the initial presentation of chronic renal failure.

2. Case Report

A 26-year-old male expatriate was brought to the emergency of Sultan Qaboos University Hospital, Muscat, Oman, in severe respiratory distress. He was having vomiting, shortness of breath, productive cough, and mild fever for almost a week. There was no history of any previous illness.

On arrival he was in severe distress with a respiratory rate of 44/minute, heart rate of 103/minute, and blood pressure of 148/97 mmHg. Arterial blood gas analysis while on oxygen showed severe metabolic acidosis {pH—6.9, PCO_2—12 mmHg, PO_2—600 mmHg, and HCO_3—4.4 mmol/L}. Creatinine and urea were very high and the hemoglobin was very low. The basic blood test results were as follows: fasting blood sugar—4.9 mmol/L; creatinine—1327 μmol/L; urea—46.8 mmol/L; bicarbonate—2 mmol/L; sodium—119 mmol/L; potassium—5.8 mmol/L; glomerular filtration rate—4 mL/min/1.73 m^2; anion gap—22 mmol/L; calcium—2.18 mmol/L; phosphate—3.98 mmol/L; lactate—0.7 mmol/L; hemoglobin—5.4 g/dL; white cell count—52 × 10^9/L; lactate dehydrogenase—378 U/L; creatine kinase—2548 U/L; INR—1.29; activated partial thromboplastin time—69.2 seconds.

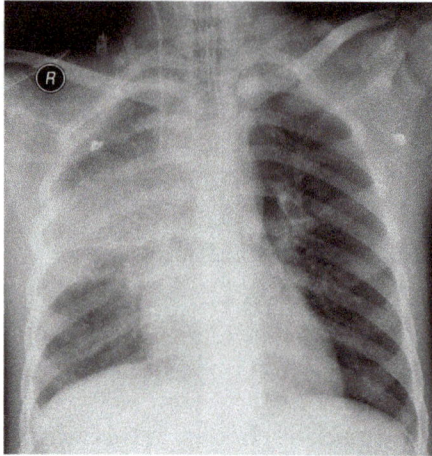

FIGURE 1: Chest radiograph showing a right mid zone consolidation and a slightly blunt right costophrenic angle.

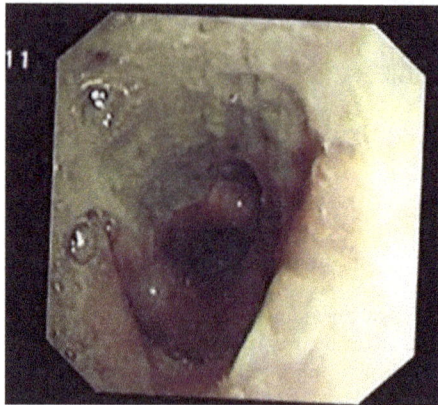

FIGURE 2: Bronchoscopy showing inflamed right bronchi and the subdivisions lined by a thick layer of yellow secretions.

Urine dipstick showed the presence of proteins, glucose, and red blood cells. Chest radiograph showed consolidation in the right mid zone and slight blunting of the right costophrenic angle (Figure 1).

The grossly elevated creatinine and urea, low hemoglobin, severe metabolic acidosis, bilateral small kidneys in ultrasound scan of the abdomen, and a high white cell count suggested a primary renal involvement complicated by a pneumonic illness and possibly sepsis. He deteriorated rapidly and was electively intubated and mechanical ventilation was initiated. He received supportive care, fluids, measures to reduce potassium, and broad spectrum antibiotics. Since the acidosis and the renal function did not show any improvement, he was taken up for dialysis later on the same day. Bronchoscopy showed inflamed right bronchi and the subdivisions lined by a thick layer of yellow secretions (Figure 2). The bronchial washings and brushings showed broad aseptate hyphae with right angled branching consistent with *Mucor* species (Figure 3).

Amphotericin (liposomal amphotericin B, 7 mg/kg/day) was added along with the broad spectrum antibiotics which he was receiving since admission. He continued to have dialysis on a regular schedule. Though there was mild improvement in the clinical and metabolic parameters, he continued to be critically ill. He was extubated on the seventh day of admission and was shifted to the ward once the vitals and the level of consciousness were stable. Two days later during dialysis he suddenly developed hypotension. The patient was conscious and communicating and the blood pressure picked up with inotropes. However, he suddenly developed massive hemoptysis. Though he was reintubated and cardiopulmonary resuscitation was initiated he could not be resuscitated.

3. Discussion

Mucormycosis is an invasive fungal infection caused by members of the family Mucoraceae and occurs predominantly in debilitated or immunosuppressed hosts. Mucormycosis is an uncommon disease, even in high-risk patients, and represents 8.3%–13% of all fungal infections encountered in such patients [1]. Six predominant clinical forms of the disease exist, which are, in decreasing frequency, rhinocerebral, pulmonary, disseminated, cutaneous, gastrointestinal, and uncommon rare forms [1].

Mucormycosis has been reported in patients of chronic renal failure on treatment as a complication or a terminal event. However, it is rare in an undiagnosed renal failure. Patients with chronic renal failure on maintenance hemodialysis and those receiving deferoxamine therapy for aluminum toxicity have been reported to be more susceptible to mucormycosis. Renal transplant recipients on conventional immunosuppressive therapy are also more prone to develop mucormycosis with an incidence varying from 0.4 to 2% [2, 6]. Mucormycosis usually occurs in the first year after renal transplant [2]. Isolated renal mucormycosis has occurred in intravenous drug users as well as renal transplant recipients in developing countries with warm climates such as India, Egypt, Saudi Arabia, Kuwait, and Singapore [1].

Studies have shown that renal failure portends a poor outcome, and neutropenia in patients with mucormycosis was clearly a predictor of death [3]. Renal involvement has been reported in up to 22% patients with disseminated mucormycosis, but isolated involvement is rare. In a review of 49 patients published in 1971, 10% had uremia. Renal failure is almost universal in patients with bilateral renal involvement [6]. Gupta et al. reported a patient presenting with renal failure and recent GI bleed who had disseminated disease including kidney involvement [7]. In a series of nine cases of fatal disseminated mucormycosis, four patients had chronic renal failure while five had acute renal failure: only two of the latter had proven renal involvement [8]. Primary mucormycosis of the renal allograft is a dreaded disease with a grave prognosis [9, 10]. Interestingly, our patient had features of renal failure and mucormycosis on first presentation.

An immunodeficient state in renal failure seems to be the major factor responsible for increased vulnerability to invasion by opportunistic infections. Decreased cell-mediated immunity and impaired neutrophil function have been documented in renal failure for a long time [11]. In addition,

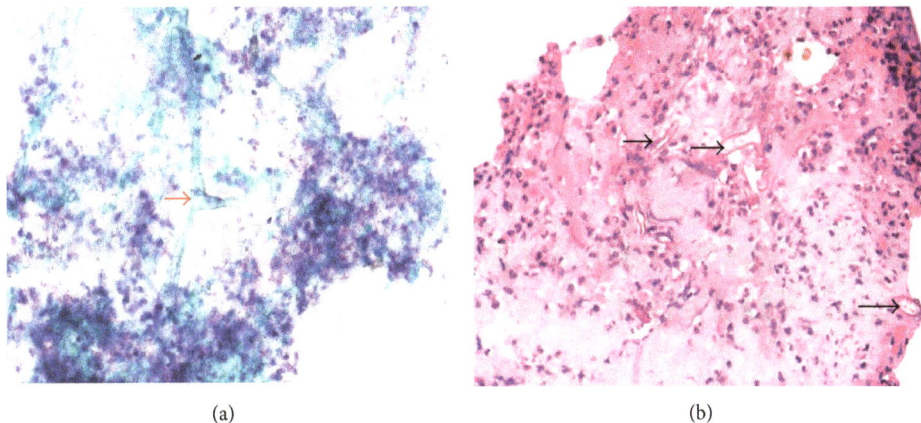

(a)   (b)

FIGURE 3: Bronchoalveolar lavage specimen showing broad, irregular, aseptate hyphae of *Mucor* with wide angled branching (arrow-heads) in a neutrophil-rich inflammatory background. (a) Papanicolaou (smear) ×600 and (b) haematoxylin and eosin (cell block) ×600.

the accompanying acidosis increases the susceptibility to mucormycosis since the iron required for hyphal growth is released from transferrin as the blood pH drops [12]. Specific host immune defects predispose to different forms of mucormycosis. Patients with diabetic ketoacidosis are prone to develop rhinocerebral form and pulmonary mucormycosis typically affects severely immunocompromised individuals.

A hallmark of mucormycosis is extensive angioinvasion with resultant vessel thrombosis and tissue necrosis. Interaction of Mucorales spores with endothelial cells appears to play a critical role in angioinvasion [13]. Sudden, massive hemoptysis is a common fatal complication [4, 5]. The most common causes of death are fungal sepsis (42%), respiratory insufficiency (27%), and hemoptysis (13%).

Our patient had no apparent previous illness. He thus presented for the first time with features of a pulmonary infection and advanced renal failure. This young patient's acute presentation and rapid deterioration are likely due to the pulmonary mucormycosis in the background of chronic renal failure. There was no evidence of renal mucormycosis or disseminated disease from the available evidence. It would be logical to conclude that he had chronic renal failure (undiagnosed/neglected) and the severe fungal infection brought him to the hospital. Tough, sudden, massive hemoptysis is not usual; it is a common cause of mortality in patients with pulmonary mucormycosis.

Conflict of Interests

The authors declare that there is no conflict of interests regarding the publication of this paper.

References

[1] G. Petrikkos, A. Skiada, O. Lortholary, E. Roilides, T. J. Walsh, and D. P. Kontoyiannis, "Epidemiology and clinical manifestations of mucormycosis," *Clinical Infectious Diseases*, vol. 54, supplement 1, pp. S23–S34, 2012.

[2] S. M. Godara, V. B. Kute, K. R. Goplani et al., "Mucormycosis in renal transplant recipients: predictors and outcome," *Saudi Journal of Kidney Diseases and Transplantation*, vol. 22, no. 4, pp. 751–756, 2011.

[3] F. Y. W. Lee, S. B. Mossad, and K. A. Adal, "Pulmonary mucormycosis: the last 30 years," *Archives of Internal Medicine*, vol. 159, no. 12, pp. 1301–1309, 1999.

[4] H. W. Murray, "Pulmonary mucormycosis with massive fatal hemoptysis," *Chest*, vol. 68, no. 1, pp. 65–68, 1975.

[5] S. Yagihashi, K. Watanabe, K. Nagai, and M. Okudaira, "Pulmonary mucormycosis presenting as massive fatal hemoptysis in a hemodialytic patient with chronic renal failure," *Klinische Wochenschrift*, vol. 69, no. 5, pp. 224–227, 1991.

[6] K. L. Gupta, "Fungal infections and the kidney," *Indian Journal of Nephrology*, vol. 11, pp. 147–154, 2001.

[7] K. L. Gupta, K. Joshi, B. J. G. Pereira, and K. Singh, "Disseminated mucormycosis presenting with acute renal failure," *Postgraduate Medical Journal*, vol. 63, no. 738, pp. 297–299, 1987.

[8] K. L. Gupta, B. D. Radotra, A. K. Banerjee, and K. S. Chugh, "Mucormycosis in patients with renal failure," *Renal Failure*, vol. 11, no. 4, pp. 195–199, 1989.

[9] C. T. Sajiv, B. Pawar, N. Calton et al., "Mucormycosis in the renal allograft: a case report," *Indian Journal of Nephrology*, vol. 13, pp. 38–39, 2012.

[10] N. Singh, T. Gayowski, J. Singh, and V. L. Yu, "Invasive gastrointestinal zygomycosis in a liver transplant recipient: case report and review of zygomycosis in solid-organ transplant recipients," *Clinical Infectious Diseases*, vol. 20, no. 3, pp. 617–620, 1995.

[11] J. Nelson, D. J. Ormrod, and T. E. Miller, "Host immune status in uraemia. VI. Leucocytic response to bacterial infection in chronic renal failure," *Nephron*, vol. 39, no. 1, pp. 21–25, 1985.

[12] A. N. Lestas, "The effect of pH upon human transferrin: selective labelling of the two iron binding sites," *British Journal of Haematology*, vol. 32, no. 3, pp. 341–350, 1976.

[13] G. Hamilos, G. Samonis, and D. P. Kontoyiannis, "Pulmonary mucormycosis," *Seminars in Respiratory and Critical Care Medicine*, vol. 32, no. 6, pp. 693–702, 2011.

39

Unexpected Abscess Localization of the Anterior Abdominal Wall in an ADPKD Patient Undergoing Hemodialysis

Nikos Sabanis,[1] **Eleni Paschou,**[2] **Eleni Gavriilaki,**[3] **Maria Mourounoglou,**[4] **and Sotirios Vasileiou**[1]

[1]*Department of Nephrology, General Hospital of Pella, 58200 Edessa, Greece*
[2]*Department of General Practice and Family Medicine, General Hospital of Pella, 58200 Edessa, Greece*
[3]*Medical School, Aristotle University of Thessaloniki, Thessaloniki, Greece*
[4]*Department of General Surgery, General Hospital of Pella, 58200 Edessa, Greece*

Correspondence should be addressed to Eleni Paschou; el_paschou@yahoo.gr

Academic Editor: Theodore I. Steinman

Autosomal Dominant Polycystic Kidney Disease (ADPKD) is one of the most common monogenic disorders and the leading inheritable cause of end-stage renal disease worldwide. Cystic and noncystic extrarenal manifestations are correlated with variable clinical presentations so that an inherited disorder is now considered a systemic disease. Kidney and liver cystic infections are the most common infectious complications in ADPKD patients. Furthermore, it is well known that ADPKD is commonly associated with colonic diverticular disease which recently has been reported to be linked to increased risk of infection on hemodialysis patients. Herein, we present a case of anterior abdominal wall abscess caused by *Enterococcus faecalis* in a patient with ADPKD undergoing hemodialysis. Although the precise pathway of infection remains uncertain, the previous medical history as well as the clinical course of our patient led us to hypothesize an alternative route of infection from the gastrointestinal tract through an aberrant intestinal barrier into the bloodstream and eventually to an atypical location.

1. Introduction

Autosomal Dominant Polycystic Kidney Disease (ADPKD) is the leading inheritable cause of end-stage renal disease affecting 1/500 to 1000 live births globally [1]. The progressive renal function impairment due to renal cyst formation is regarded as the cornerstone of the disease accounting for 5–10% of patients that require renal replacement therapy [2].

ADPKD is considered a systemic disease since not only are the kidneys affected but also multiorgan cystic and noncystic extrarenal features can occur [3]. Infectious complications in ADPKD patients, especially those undergoing hemodialysis, remain potential life-threatening consequences and tend to reoccur. Among extrarenal manifestations of polycystic kidney disease, colonic diverticulosis has been reported to be connected with infections in hemodialysis patients [4].

Herein, we present a case of an abscess located in the anterior abdominal wall, caused by *Enterococcus faecalis* in an ADPKD patient with colonic diverticular disease undergoing hemodialysis. We emphasize the importance of the predisposing factors in ADPKD patients that potentially promote bacterial migration from intestinal tract via the bloodstream to other tissues and organs.

To the best of our knowledge, this is the first report in the literature of an abscess of abdominal wall in an ADPKD patient receiving hemodialysis.

2. Case Presentation

A 67-year-old Caucasian male patient was admitted to emergency department due to abdominal pain lasting two days, accompanied with weakness, chills, and high-grade fever. He was a nonsmoker, retired state employee and drank alcohol only occasionally. He had not travelled abroad and no contact with domestic animals was mentioned on routine questioning. On physical examination, the patient was pale and confused and his temperature was 40.1°C. We observed tachypnea with respiratory rate 30/min and SpO_2 98% while lung auscultation was normal. Heart rate was 110 beats per minute and his blood pressure measured 100/60 mmHg. The remaining physical examination revealed signs of skin inflammation of the upper left abdominal quadrant including redness, smooth swelling, warmth, and tenderness. No inflammation signs of the arteriovenous fistula or skin wounds were observed. The liver was palpable 6 cm below the right costal margin. Digital rectal examination was negative. No other signs compatible with diverticulosis were recognized.

Initial laboratory examinations revealed leukocytosis (white blood cells $12.7 \times 10^3/\mu L$) and neutrophilia (87.3%), anemia (hematocrit 30.6%, hemoglobin 10 g/dL), and highly increased inflammation markers (C-reactive protein 55.1 mg/dL with normal range 0–0.5 mg/dL, and Erythrocyte Sedimentation Rate 98 mm/h).

The patient had a medical history of hypertension and ADPKD undergoing hemodialysis through arteriovenous fistula during the last 15 years and his father was also an ADPKD patient. In the past, the patient had experienced recurrent episodes of gross hematuria and nephrolithiasis complicated with urinary tract infections (UTI). Two months before, the patient had been hospitalized due to *Escherichia coli* UTI, without further imaging findings of cyst infection, receiving ciprofloxacin treatment based on antibiogram susceptibility. During the last month, he also encountered severe episodes of intradialytic hypotension that required reassessment of dry weight and discontinuation of antihypertensive therapy.

Abdominal Computed Tomography showed an extensive, well-limited abscess of the left anterior abdominal wall with dimensions 5.7×5.5 cm (Figure 1), splenomegaly, multiple kidney and liver cysts, and colonic diverticulosis with no evidence of active infection (Figure 2).

The patient underwent immediate surgical drainage and the cultures revealed non-vancomycin resistant *Enterococcus faecalis*. Blood and urine cultures were negative. Transthoracic echocardiography revealed no evidence of infective endocarditis. He received antibiotic treatment with linezolid in a dose of 600 mg twice daily and metronidazole 500 mg twice daily for 12 days in total. After surgical intervention, the patient's clinical course remained uneventful and he was discharged home on the 13th day.

3. Discussion

Autosomal Dominant Polycystic Kidney Disease is considered a systemic disease with diverse cystic and noncystic manifestations that can lead to increased morbidity and mortality [5]. Infectious complications are frequently related to cyst infections and remain potentially a life-threatening outcome [6]. In general, the route of renal and liver cyst infections in ADPKD patients remains questionable [7, 8] although the retrograde pathway from the bladder or the biliary tree prospectively has been proposed as a driving-force mechanism.

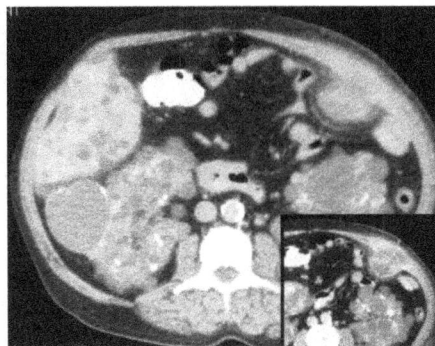

FIGURE 1: Abdominal Computed Tomography: abscess of the left anterior abdominal wall.

Moreover, ADPKD patients with increased intra-abdominal pressure due to kidneys and liver cystic enlargement are characterized by increased risk of cyst infections [9] possibly due to an additional reduction of venous return leading to impaired cardiac output and as a result of intestinal ischemia. Thus, intra-abdominal hypertension can significantly increase the intestinal mucosa permeability through reduction of microcirculation blood flow leading to bacterial or endotoxin translocation [10, 11]. Finally, essential alterations in the function and structure of intestinal smooth muscle cells as a direct effect of PKD1/PKD2 mutations may increase the incidence of bacterial translocation [12–14].

The key role of bacterial translocation as an alternative pathway related to infections has not been elucidated even though the colon diverticular disease has been correlated with increased risk [4]. In addition, recent studies have focused on the close relationship between the kidney and the gastrointestinal track, ordinarily referred to as "kidney-gut axis" [15]. Hence, bacterial translocation depicts the epiphenomenon of a complicated interplay between the human gut microflora via aberrant epithelial barrier and the uremic milieu [16].

The presence of end-stage renal disease (ESRD) has been correlated with structural and functional alterations of the intestinal mucosa barrier and important changes of gut microbiota composition and development [17]. As a result, intact bacteria or bacterial bioproducts migrate from the intestinal lumen into systemic circulation. In this regard, the appearance of unusual infections in remote locations could be related to bacterial translocation. In hemodialysis patients, the high risk of bacterial translocation has been associated with various predisposing factors such as the prolonged colonic transit time due to dietary restrictions and the epithelial wall edema due to heart failure [18]. The use of phosphate binders and wide range antibiotics deteriorates the reduced intestinal motility and worsens the vulnerable balance of the intestinal ecosystem, respectively [19]. In the same context, jeopardized perfusion during recurrent episodes of intradialytic hypotension alters the transepithelial resistance.

Our patient was an ADPKD patient with increased abdominal pressure due to enlarged kidney and liver cysts.

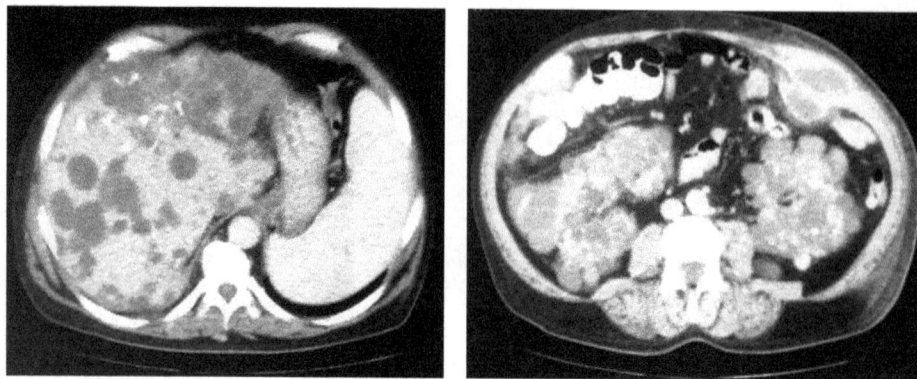

FIGURE 2: Abdominal Computed Tomography: diffuse involvement of polycystic disease in both kidneys, liver, and colon.

The coexistence of diverticular colon disease, persistent constipation, and the previous ciprofloxacin treatment that resulted in derangement of gut microflora in combination with recurrent episodes of intradialytic hypotension led us to assume that bacterial translocation could explain the uncommon abscess localization. The fact that no other inflammation outbreaks were recognized and especially the absence of diverticulitis could support our hypothesis.

4. Conclusion

Infectious complications in ADPKD patients are usually referred to hepatic or renal cystic infections and the retrograde path has been considered the leading pathophysiological mechanism. The potential role of bacterial translocation as an alternative pathway has only been described in ADPKD patient with diverticular disease. In our case, we focus on the coexistence of diverse predisposing factors that enhance bacterial translocation and may explain the unexpected localization of an abscess in the abdominal wall caused by a pathogen of intestinal microbiota.

Conflict of Interests

The authors declare that there is no conflict of interests regarding the publication of this paper.

References

[1] O. Z. Dalgaard and S. Norby, "Autosomal dominant polycystic kidney disease in the 1980's," *Clinical Genetics*, vol. 36, no. 5, pp. 320–325, 1989.

[2] E. M. Spithoven, A. Kramer, E. Meijer et al., "Renal replacement therapy for autosomal dominant polycystic kidney disease (ADPKD) in Europe: prevalence and survival—an analysis of data from the ERA-EDTA Registry," *Nephrology, Dialysis, Transplantation*, vol. 29, supplement 4, pp. iv15–iv25, 2014.

[3] R. Torra, "Autosomal dominant polycystic kidney disease, more than a renal disease," *Minerva Endocrinologica*, vol. 39, no. 2, pp. 79–87, 2014.

[4] Y. Pirson and N. Kanaan, "Infectious complications in autosomal dominant polycystic kidney disease," *Néphrologie & Thérapeutique*, vol. 11, no. 2, pp. 73–77, 2015.

[5] G. M. Fick, A. M. Johnson, W. S. Hammond, and P. A. Gabow, "Causes of death in autosomal dominant polycystic kidney disease," *Journal of the American Society of Nephrology*, vol. 5, no. 12, pp. 2048–2056, 1995.

[6] M. Sallée, C. Rafat, J.-R. Zahar et al., "Cyst infections in patients with autosomal dominant polycystic kidney disease," *Clinical Journal of the American Society of Nephrology*, vol. 4, no. 7, pp. 1183–1189, 2009.

[7] Y. Tsuchiya, Y. Ubara, T. Suwabe et al., "The renal cyst infection caused by *Salmonella enteritidis* in a patient with autosomal dominant polycystic kidney disease: how did this pathogen come into the renal cysts?" *Clinical and Experimental Nephrology*, vol. 15, no. 1, pp. 151–153, 2011.

[8] A. O. Tokat, S. Karasu, M. A. Barlas, and Y. A. Akgün, "Thoracic empyema due to bacterial translocation in acute appendicitis," *Tuberkuloz ve Toraks*, vol. 61, no. 1, pp. 54–56, 2013.

[9] T. Kaussen, P. K. Srinivasan, M. Afify et al., "Influence of two different levels of intra-abdominal hypertension on bacterial translocation in a porcine model," *Annals of Intensive Care*, vol. 2, supplement 1, article S17, 2012.

[10] J.-T. Cheng, G.-X. Xiao, P.-Y. Xia, J.-C. Yuan, and X.-J. Qin, "Influence of intra-abdominal hypertension on the intestinal permeability and endotoxin/bacteria translocation in rabbits," *Zhonghua Shao Shang Za Zhi*, vol. 19, no. 4, pp. 229–232, 2003.

[11] J. Cheng, Z. Wei, X. Liu et al., "The role of intestinal mucosa injury induced by intra-abdominal hypertension in the development of abdominal compartment syndrome and multiple organ dysfunction syndrome," *Critical Care*, vol. 17, no. 6, article R283, 2013.

[12] G. S. Markowitz, Y. Cai, L. Li et al., "Polycystin-2 expression is developmentally regulated," *The American Journal of Physiology—Renal Physiology*, vol. 277, no. 1, pp. F17–F25, 1999.

[13] Q. Qian, L. W. Hunter, M. Li et al., "Pkd2 haploinsufficiency alters intracellular calcium regulation in vascular smooth muscle cells," *Human Molecular Genetics*, vol. 12, no. 15, pp. 1875–1880, 2003.

[14] A. Sabatino, G. Regolisti, I. Brusasco, A. Cabassi, S. Morabito, and E. Fiaccadori, "Alterations of intestinal barrier and microbiota in chronic kidney disease," *Nephrology Dialysis Transplantation*, vol. 30, no. 6, pp. 924–933, 2015.

[15] N. D. Vaziri, J. Yuan, A. Rahimi, Z. Ni, H. Said, and V. S. Subramanian, "Disintegration of colonic epithelial tight junction in uremia: a likely cause of CKD-associated inflammation," *Nephrology Dialysis Transplantation*, vol. 27, no. 7, pp. 2686–2693, 2012.

[16] A. Ramezani and D. S. Raj, "The gut microbiome, kidney disease, and targeted interventions," *Journal of the American Society of Nephrology*, vol. 25, no. 4, pp. 657–670, 2014.

[17] G. P. Lambert, "Stress-induced gastrointestinal barrier dysfunction and its inflammatory effects," *Journal of Animal Science*, vol. 87, no. 14, supplement, pp. E101–E108, 2009.

[18] L.-A. Ding and J.-S. Li, "Gut in diseases: physiological elements and their clinical significance," *World Journal of Gastroenterology*, vol. 9, no. 11, pp. 2385–2389, 2003.

[19] B. E. P. Balbo, M. T. Sapienza, C. R. Ono et al., "Cyst infection in hospital-admitted autosomal dominant polycystic kidney disease patients is predominantly multifocal and associated with kidney and liver volume," *Brazilian Journal of Medical and Biological Research*, vol. 47, no. 7, pp. 584–593, 2014.

40

Severe Rhabdomyolysis Associated with Simvastatin and Role of Ciprofloxacin and Amlodipine Coadministration

Nicolas De Schryver,[1] Xavier Wittebole,[1] Peter Van den Bergh,[2] Vincent Haufroid,[3] Eric Goffin,[4] and Philippe Hantson[1,3]

[1]Department of Intensive Care, Cliniques Universitaires Saint-Luc, Université Catholique de Louvain, 1200 Brussels, Belgium
[2]Centre de Référence Neuromusculaire, Cliniques Universitaires Saint-Luc, Université Catholique de Louvain, 1200 Brussels, Belgium
[3]Louvain Centre for Toxicology and Applied Pharmacology, Cliniques Universitaires Saint-Luc, Université Catholique de Louvain, 1200 Brussels, Belgium
[4]Department of Nephrology, Cliniques Universitaires Saint-Luc, Université Catholique de Louvain, 1200 Brussels, Belgium

Correspondence should be addressed to Philippe Hantson; philippe.hantson@uclouvain.be

Academic Editor: Aikaterini Papagianni

Simvastatin is among the most commonly used prescription medications for cholesterol reduction and the most common statin-related adverse drug reaction is skeletal muscle toxicity. Multiple factors have been shown to influence simvastatin-induced myopathy. In addition to age, gender, ethnicity, genetic predisposition, and dose, drug-drug interactions play a major role. This is particularly true for drugs that are extensively metabolized by cytochrome P450 (CYP)3A4. We describe a particularly severe case of rhabdomyolysis after the introduction of ciprofloxacin, a weak CYP3A4 inhibitor, in a patient who previously tolerated the simvastatin-amlodipine combination.

1. Introduction

Extremely severe rhabdomyolysis with statin therapy remains rare, in comparison with myalgias or mild elevation of muscular enzymes. Among precipitating factors, drug-drug interactions are playing an important role and should be investigated in depth. We are reporting a case of impressive rhabdomyolysis occurring soon after the introduction of antimicrobial therapy in patient who acquired peritoneal dialysis-related peritonitis.

2. Case Report

A 41-year-old African woman presented to the hospital for diffuse myalgia and intense weakness developing over the last 3 days. Her previous medical history included systemic lupus erythematosus (SLE) complicated by severe glomerulonephritis. After progression of renal failure, she required peritoneal dialysis (PD) for the last 3 years. She was on automated PD with 3 exchanges of 1,800 mL during the night and fill volume of 1,500 mL with icodextrin during daytime. Current medications included furosemide 125 mg b.i.d., amlodipine 10 mg o.d., bisoprolol 10 mg o.d., irbesartan 300 mg o.d., mycophenolate mofetil 500 mg o.d., hydroxychloroquine 200 mg b.i.d., calcium carbonate 1 g b.i.d., colecalciferol 625 μg weekly, sevelamer 800 mg b.i.d., calcitriol 0.25 μg three times a week, and simvastatin 20 mg o.d. Adherence to treatment was good and no modification in type or doses of any of these medications was done since the last 12 months. The patient had a residual creatinine clearance of 5 mL/min. Nine days before admission, she was diagnosed with a peritoneal dialysis-related peritonitis (PDRP) based on the cloudy aspect of the peritoneal dialysis effluent (PDE) with 1,300 cells/μL and 47% neutrophils. She was at this time poorly symptomatic with no fever or abdominal discomfort and was given empiric antimicrobial therapy with vancomycin 2,000 mg/3d, ciprofloxacin 500 mg b.i.d., and a single dose of gentamicin 80 mg according to our protocol [1].

Four days later, culture of the PDE grew for *Corynebacterium striatum* and ciprofloxacin was withdrawn. The next day, she started to complain of diffuse severe muscle pain with intense weakness and the PDE color appeared reddish. The patient became also progressively anuric. On admission, laboratory investigations showed an impressive rhabdomyolysis with creatine kinase (CK) 540,000 IU/L ($N < 200$), lactate dehydrogenase (LDH) 19,200 IU/L ($N < 248$), and aspartate aminotransferase 1,700 IU/L ($N < 50$). Urine output before the incidence of rhabdomyolysis was 1,500 mL/day. Serum creatinine value peaked at 12.4 mg/dL (usual value was 9 mg/dL). Severe electrolyte disorders were observed with potassium 6.3 mmol/L, phosphorus 12.8 mg/dL, and ionized calcium 2.9 mg/dL. The patient denied any recent ingestion of a substance or drug other than the prescribed antimicrobial therapy and she reported no recent strenuous exercise. Urine toxicological analysis was negative for opioids and cocaine. No biological sign was consistent with a progression of SLE (anti-DNA antibodies 3.2 U/mL ($N < 8$), C3 and C4 complement components, respectively, 82 mg/dL (N: 85–193) and 38 mg/dL (N: 10–40)). Thyroid function tests were normal. Blood cultures remained sterile and Epstein-Barr virus, cytomegalovirus, human immunodeficiency virus, and influenza A and B serologies were negative.

She was admitted to the intensive care unit (ICU) for the correction of electrolyte disorders and fluid balance. Serum CK peaked at 816,000 IU/L on day 2 and then progressively decreased. Peritoneal dialysis therapy was maintained (3 exchanges/day) and PDE progressively cleared. Peritonitis also progressively resolved. Renal function recovered partially with spontaneous reapparition of dark tea-colored urine output (600 mL/d). A right vastus lateralis needle muscle biopsy was performed. The biopsy was of small size and was normal except for increased size and amount of lipid droplets. Serum carnitine and acylcarnitine levels were normal. Lymphocyte carnitine palmitoyl-CoA transferase 2 activity was increased.

Genetic analysis was performed to identify potential gene variants responsible for altered absorption, distribution, metabolism, and excretion of statins and/or for higher susceptibility to myopathy. The patient was cytochrome P-450 (CYP) 3A4*1/*1 (absence of reduced activity *22 allele), CYP3A5*1/*1 (absence of inactive *3 allele rendering the patient CYP3A5 expressor), influx transporter gene SLCO1B1*1b/*1b (absence of reduced activity *5 allele considered as the main genetic risk factor for developing myopathy after simvastatin intake), and efflux transporter gene ABCB1 heterozygote 3435CT. Electrolyte disorders were corrected and the patient left the ICU on day 3. At 3-month follow-up, serum creatinine returned to previous values, while the patient was still on PD and had a complete functional recovery.

3. Discussion

This patient developed a severe rhabdomyolysis soon after the introduction of an antimicrobial therapy for a PDRP. The pathogen that was identified, namely, *Corynebacterium striatum*, is not the most common one but was still found in 5% of culture positive PDRP [2]. It is usually transmitted from the skin following errors of manipulation by the patient. The paucity of symptoms and the poor neutrophilic response are frequent and consistent with the indolent pattern of this microorganism.

Among the main etiologies of rhabdomyolysis (traumatism, exertion, muscle hypoxia, genetic defects, infection, hypo- or hyperthermia, and metabolic and electrolyte disorders), drugs and toxins are playing a significant role [3, 4]. Among the latter, statins, fibrates, alcohol, heroin, and cocaine are the commonest agents.

Statins are widely prescribed in developed countries. Although generally safe, they can induce muscle disorders ranging from myalgias without any biologic abnormality to life-threatening rhabdomyolysis. Statin-related rhabdomyolysis (SRR), usually defined as CK levels exceeding 10 times the upper limit of normal range, is reported to be very infrequent (in comparison with myopathy or myalgias), with an incidence of 0.01% for five-year therapy [5], that is, 0.04–0.12 cases per million prescriptions [6]. A recent review of literature data (1990–2013) identified 112 cases classified as rhabdomyolysis, and simvastatin was frequently cited (55/112) [7]. In about half of the cases of SRR, rhabdomyolysis could be precipitated by an interaction between statin and a new prescribed drug that is believed to interfere with statin metabolism [6, 7].

Statins metabolism varies from one type to another. After passive absorption by the intestinal cells, simvastatin is transported from the portal blood to the hepatocytes by an influx pump, the organic anion-transporting polypeptide 1B1 (OATP1B1). Simvastatin is an inactive lactone that is then predominantly ($\geq$80%) metabolized by CYP3A4 and 3A5 with a little contribution of CYP2A8 ($\leq$20%) into β,δ-dihydroxy acid, its active metabolite [8]. The metabolism is almost complete after hepatic first pass. Drugs inhibiting CYP3A4 such as azole antifungals, HIV protease inhibitors, macrolides, cyclosporine, verapamil, diltiazem, amiodarone, and grapefruit juice may increase serum simvastatin level and its toxicity. Sensitivity to those interactions varies from one patient to another due to heterogeneous CYP3A4 activity among individuals [6]. Ciprofloxacin is a known weak inhibitor of CYP3A4 and may thus inhibit simvastatin metabolism, increasing its myotoxicity. Amlodipine has also been shown to competitively inhibit the metabolic activity of CYP3A4/5. A pharmacokinetic interaction model revealed that coadministration of simvastatin with 10 mg amlodipine could significantly increase simvastatin bioavailability and decrease simvastatin clearance, but also that these changes could be minimized by using a simvastatin dose lower than 24 mg [9, 10].

While an interaction between statins and other drugs on the CYP3A4 metabolic pathway is well known, the implication of other mechanisms has been suggested. Among these, glycoprotein P (P-gp) inhibition could play a role. P-gp is an active tissue-specific drug transporter belonging to the ATP-binding cassette superfamily. Acting as an efflux pump, it avoids cellular uptake of several drugs and toxins, preventing notably their absorption through the gastrointestinal tract.

As simvastatin is not only an inhibitor but also a substrate of the P-gp, inhibition of P-gp by other drugs may increase serum levels of simvastatin when coadministered [11]. If P-gp interaction between ciprofloxacin and simvastatin has been suggested in a similar case report, there is currently still controversy to whether ciprofloxacin could be a substrate of P-gp [12]. Additionally, amlodipine is devoid of P-gp inhibiting properties [10].

The multiple drug protein 2 (MRP2) is another membrane transport protein from the ABC superfamily excreting toxins into bile that could play a role in drug-drug interactions as simvastatin is also a substrate of this transporter [13].

Several genetic factors may predispose to statin-related toxicity [14]. If gene variants coding for CYP3A4/5, the mitochondrial enzyme GATM, the influx transporter OATP1B1 (encoded by *SLCO1B1*), and the efflux transporters P-gp (encoded by ABCB1) have a theoretical potential for affecting absorption, distribution, metabolism, and excretion of statins, only the *5 allele of *SLCO1B1* has been strongly identified to be clinically associated with statin induced myopathy, especially for simvastatin [14, 15]. The *SLCO1B1*5 allele disrupts the localization of the OATPB1 influx transporter reducing the hepatic uptake of statins and increasing their plasma level and so their toxicity. Our patient was not found to be carrier of this allele. Her 3435CT heterozygote status for ABCB1 could not be theoretically associated with a decreased P-gp activity.

To date, only two other cases of rhabdomyolysis after drug interaction between simvastatin and ciprofloxacin have been reported, but none with a simvastatin-amlodipine interaction [16, 17].

Several other risk factors for SRR could also have influenced the severity of the rhabdomyolysis in our patient. First, CK levels are known to be higher in black people [18]. Secondly, SLE may be associated with a certain degree of latent myositis, even if no sign of progression of SLE was found in our patient. Third, the patient had terminal renal failure requiring PD. However, if statin-induced myopathy has been reported to be slightly increased among patients with renal failure [15], simvastatin does not seem to increase muscle disorders in patients with chronic kidney disease, even requiring peritoneal dialysis [19, 20].

In conclusion, this case illustrates the potentially dangerous interactions of some statins (simvastatin) with drugs that are also metabolized by the CYP3A4/5 pathway, even in the absence of genetic predisposing factors. While the US Food and Drug Administration (FDA) has advised that the daily dose of simvastatin should not exceed 20 mg in patients taking amlodipine concomitantly, the introduction of a new drug, even considered as a weak CYP3A4 inhibitor like ciprofloxacin, could increase the risk of myotoxicity [21].

Consent

A written authorization was obtained from the patient for the publication.

Conflict of Interests

The authors declare that there is no conflict of interests regarding the publication of this paper.

References

[1] E. Goffin, L. Herbiet, D. Pouthier et al., "Vancomycin and ciprofloxacin: systemic antibiotic administration for peritoneal dialysis-associated peritonitis," *Peritoneal Dialysis International*, vol. 24, no. 5, pp. 433–439, 2004.

[2] D. P. Kofteridis, A. Valachis, K. Perakis, S. Maraki, E. Daphnis, and G. Samonis, "Peritoneal dialysis-associated peritonitis: clinical features and predictors of outcome," *International Journal of Infectious Diseases*, vol. 14, no. 6, pp. e489–e493, 2010.

[3] X. Bosch, E. Poch, and J. M. Grau, "Rhabdomyolysis and acute kidney injury," *The New England Journal of Medicine*, vol. 361, no. 1, pp. 62–72, 2009.

[4] R. Zutt, A. van der Kooi, G. Linthorst, R. Wanders, and M. de Visser, "Rhabdomyolysis: review of the literature," *Neuromuscular Disorders*, vol. 24, no. 8, pp. 651–659, 2014.

[5] C. Baigent, A. Keech, P. M. Kearney et al., "Efficacy and safety of cholesterol-lowering treatment: prospective meta-analysis of data from 90 056 participants in 14 randomised trials of statins," *The Lancet*, vol. 366, no. 9493, pp. 1267–1278, 2005.

[6] P. D. Thompson, P. Clarkson, and R. H. Karas, "Statin-associated myopathy," *The Journal of the American Medical Association*, vol. 289, no. 13, pp. 1681–1690, 2003.

[7] P. Mendes, P. G. Robles, and S. Mathur, "Statin-induced rhabdomyolysis: a comprehensive review of case reports," *Physiotherapy Canada*, vol. 66, no. 2, pp. 124–132, 2014.

[8] T. Prueksaritanont, B. Ma, and N. Yu, "The human hepatic metabolism of simvastatin hydroxy acid is mediated primarily by CYP3A, and not CYP2D6," *British Journal of Clinical Pharmacology*, vol. 56, no. 1, pp. 120–124, 2003.

[9] H. Son, D. Lee, L. A. Lim, S. B. Jang, H. Roh, and K. Park, "Development of a pharmacokinetic interaction model for co-administration of simvastatin and amlodipine," *Drug Metabolism and Pharmacokinetics*, vol. 29, no. 2, pp. 120–128, 2014.

[10] Y.-T. Zhou, L.-S. Yu, S. Zeng, Y.-W. Huang, H.-M. Xu, and Q. Zhou, "Pharmacokinetic drug-drug interactions between 1,4-dihydropyridine calcium channel blockers and statins: factors determining interaction strength and relevant clinical risk management," *Therapeutics and Clinical Risk Management*, vol. 10, no. 1, pp. 17–26, 2014.

[11] C. W. Holtzman, B. S. Wiggins, and S. A. Spinler, "Role of P-glycoprotein in statin drug interactions," *Pharmacotherapy*, vol. 26, no. 11, pp. 1601–1607, 2006.

[12] M. S. Park, H. Okochi, and L. Z. Benet, "Is ciprofloxacin a substrate of p-glycoprotein?" *Archives of Drug Information*, vol. 4, no. 1, pp. 1–9, 2011.

[13] L. C. J. Ellis, G. M. Hawksworth, and R. J. Weaver, "ATP-dependent transport of statins by human and rat MRP2/Mrp2," *Toxicology and Applied Pharmacology*, vol. 269, no. 2, pp. 187–194, 2013.

[14] W. J. Canestaro, M. A. Austin, and K. E. Thummel, "Genetic factors affecting statin concentrations and subsequent myopathy: a HuGENet systematic review," *Genetics in Medicine*, vol. 16, no. 11, pp. 810–819, 2014.

[15] E. Link, S. Parish, J. Armitage et al., "SLCO1B1 variants and statin-induced myopathy—a genomewide study," *The New England Journal of Medicine*, vol. 359, no. 8, pp. 789–799, 2008.

[16] R. D. Sawant, "Rhabdomyolysis due to an uncommon interaction of ciprofloxacin with simvastatin," *Canadian Journal of Clinical Pharmacology*, vol. 16, no. 1, pp. e78–e79, 2009.

[17] N. Fountoulakis, L. Khafizova, M. Logothetis, G. Fanti, and J. A. Papadakis, "Case report of rhabdomyolysis possibly associated to the interaction of ciprofloxacin with simvastatin," *Hellenic Journal of Atherosclerosis*, vol. 1, no. 1, pp. 65–67, 2013.

[18] H. Y. Meltzer and P. A. Holy, "Black-white differences in serum creatine phosphokinase (CPK) activity," *Clinica Chimica Acta*, vol. 54, no. 2, pp. 215–224, 1974.

[19] C. Baigent, M. J. Landray, C. Reith et al., "The effects of lowering LDL cholesterol with simvastatin plus ezetimibe in patients with chronic kidney disease (Study of Heart and Renal Protection): a randomised placebo-controlled trial," *The Lancet*, vol. 377, no. 9784, pp. 2181–2192, 2011.

[20] D. Saltissi, C. Morgan, R. J. Rigby, and J. Westhuyzen, "Safety and efficacy of simvastatin in hypercholesterolemic patients undergoing chronic renal dialysis," *The American Journal of Kidney Diseases*, vol. 39, no. 2, pp. 283–290, 2002.

[21] FDA Drug Safety Communication, *New Restrictions, Contraindications, and Dose Limitations for Zocor (Simvastatin) to Reduce the Risk of Muscle Injury*, US Food and Drug Administration, 2014, http://www.fda.gov/Drugs/DrugSafety/ucm256581.htm.

41

Minimal Change Disease as a Secondary and Reversible Event of a Renal Transplant Case with Systemic Lupus Erythematosus

Elena Gkrouzman,[1] Kyriakos A. Kirou,[2] Surya V. Seshan,[3] and James M. Chevalier[4]

[1]University of Connecticut Health Center, 263 Farmington Avenue, Farmington, CT 06030-1235, USA
[2]Division of Rheumatology, Hospital for Special Surgery, 535 East 70th Street, New York, NY 10021, USA
[3]New York-Presbyterian Hospital, 525 East 68th Street, Starr Pavilion 1009, New York, NY 10021, USA
[4]Rogosin Kidney Center, 505 East 70th Street, New York, NY 10021, USA

Correspondence should be addressed to Elena Gkrouzman; egkrouzman@gmail.com

Academic Editor: Yoshihide Fujigaki

Secondary causes of minimal change disease (MCD) account for a minority of cases compared to its primary or idiopathic form and provide ground for consideration of common mechanisms of pathogenesis. In this paper we report a case of a 27-year-old Latina woman, a renal transplant recipient with systemic lupus erythematosus (SLE), who developed nephrotic range proteinuria 6 months after transplantation. The patient had recurrent acute renal failure and multiple biopsies were consistent with MCD. However, she lacked any other features of the typical nephrotic syndrome. An angiogram revealed a right external iliac vein stenosis in the region of renal vein anastomosis, which when restored resulted in normalization of creatinine and relief from proteinuria. We report a rare case of MCD developing secondary to iliac vein stenosis in a renal transplant recipient with SLE. Additionally we suggest that, in the event of biopsy-proven MCD presenting as an atypical nephrotic syndrome, alternative or secondary, potentially reversible, causes should be considered and explored.

1. Introduction

Minimal change disease (MCD) is a disease of the podocyte that manifests with sudden onset nephrotic syndrome. Isolated diffuse effacement of the epithelial foot processes on electron microscopy is the defining feature of MCD. Clinically, it is characterized by the development of massive proteinuria, hypoalbuminemia, edema, and hyperlipidemia.

Although the majority of patients have idiopathic or primary MCD, some may exhibit MCD secondary to another disease process or exposure to drugs. Examining patients with secondary MCD allows us to investigate shared mechanisms of pathogenesis [1]. Herein, we report a lupus patient with a renal transplant who developed *de novo* MCD associated with right external iliac vein stenosis.

2. Case Presentation

A 27-year-old Latina woman received a living related transplant from her mother for end stage renal disease (ESRD) secondary to advanced lupus nephritis and presented with nephrotic range proteinuria 6 months after transplantation.

The patient was diagnosed with systemic lupus erythematosus (SLE) at age of 17. During the course of the disease she fulfilled the American College of Rheumatology (ACR) criteria including malar rash, arthritis, pericarditis, class IV/V lupus nephritis, leucopenia, lymphopenia, and positive antinuclear (ANA) and anti-double-stranded DNA (anti-dsDNA) antibodies. The patient's lupus nephritis was treated with glucocorticoids, multiple doses of cyclophosphamide, mycophenolate mofetil, and rituximab. Despite aggressive treatment, she progressed to ESRD and required renal transplantation. She received a kidney from her mother, which was donor/recipient CMV +/−. The patient has been negative for anti-Ro, anti-La, anti-Sm, anti-RNP, $\beta2$ glycoprotein I, and lupus anticoagulant. The anticardiolipin antibody (ACLA), although reported as positive at one occasion which prompted the use of aspirin for prophylaxis, has been consistently negative ever since. She also has a history of hypertension and hypothyroidism due to Hashimoto's thyroiditis.

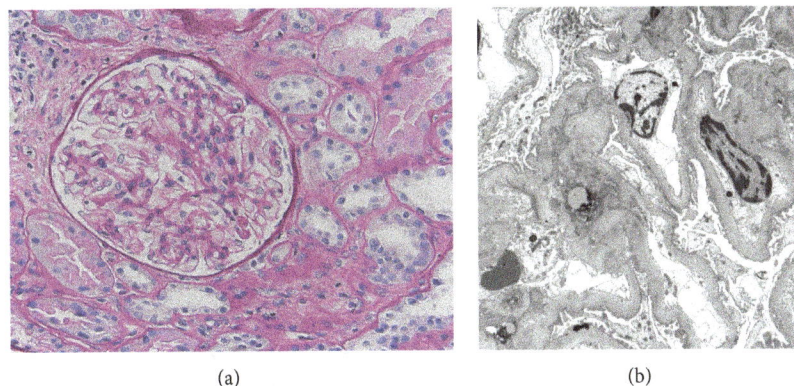

(a)   (b)

FIGURE 1: (a) Kidney biopsy with renal cortex showing a normal glomerulus with preserved architecture and mostly preserved tubules (×400, PAS stain). (b) Electron micrographs of glomerulus showing greater than 50% foot process effacement and normal thickness of capillary basement membranes without immune deposits (×6740).

The surgery and hospital course after transplantation were uneventful and the patient was discharged with excellent urine output and creatinine level of 1.0 mg/dL. Six months later she developed nephrotic range proteinuria at 4.6 mg/mg (Table 1) and her creatinine levels progressively rose to 2.5 mg/dL. However, she lacked edema, hypoalbuminemia, and hypercholesterolemia. Her medications at the time included tacrolimus, 4 mg in the morning and 3 mg in the evening, mycophenolate mofetil 500 mg bid, prednisone 5 mg/d, hydroxychloroquine 200 mg bid, enalapril 10 mg/d, aspirin 81 mg/d, trimethoprim-sulfamethoxazole 400–80 mg/d, valganciclovir HCl 450 mg/d, levothyroxine 0.15 mg/d, and omeprazole 20 mg/d. A kidney biopsy was performed that showed minimal glomerular change by light microscopy and diffuse podocyte foot process effacement by electron microscopy, consistent with MCD (Figures 1(a) and 1(b)). There was no evidence of acute cellular, antibody-mediated, or vascular rejection or immune-complex-mediated glomerulonephritis. In particular, immunofluorescence exam did not reveal significant glomerular staining for IgG, IgA, and C3. There was granular glomerular staining in mesangial regions and capillary loops for 1+ IgM while the tubulointerstitial compartment was negative for immunoglobulins or complement components. Arteries and arterioles stained 1+ for C3 but peritubular capillaries were negative for C3d and C4d. The serum C3 and C4 levels were within the normal range and anti-dsDNA antibody was 1+. Consequently, she received pulse methylprednisolone followed by oral prednisone to treat presumed MCD. She did not respond to treatment, while two additional subsequent renal biopsies were also consistent with MCD. In the following 12 months the patient developed several episodes of acute renal failure characterized by increasing proteinuria and creatinine levels that were attributed to dehydration. Her serum albumin levels decreased down to 2.7 g/dL secondary to ongoing protein loss in urine. However, this effect was transient and coincided with one of the peaks of her proteinuria (7.5 g). Otherwise, her albumin during this course usually ranged between 3 and 4 g/dL. Multiple ultrasounds of the kidney were performed. Initially they were normal showing patent renal artery and vein with good perfusion of the transplant on color and power Doppler. However, subsequently the studies exhibited mild hydronephrosis of the transplant kidney and turbulence in the right external iliac vein proximal to the attachment of the transplanted renal vein that was suggestive of narrowing. Eventually, because of worsening proteinuria and creatinine (9.7 mg/mg and 3.4 mg/dL, resp.), magnetic resonance imaging (MRI) of the pelvis without contrast was done for further investigation and revealed diminished signal intensity in the right iliac artery. A subsequent angiogram revealed a normal right iliac artery and renal transplant arterial anastomosis but outlined stenosis of the right external iliac vein adjacent to the transplant anastomosis with a pressure gradient of 7 mmHg between the common iliac vein and the external iliac vein. Balloon angioplasty of the right external iliac vein partially corrected the stenosis with a postangioplasty gradient of 2-3 mmHg. A few weeks later recurrent renal dysfunction necessitated a second venogram that showed restenosis and culminated in angioplasty and stent placement with pressure gradient improving from 10 mmHg to 0. After the stent deployment and dilation to 12–14 mm in diameter, a thrombus was identified within the stent which was aspirated. There was no thrombus seen prior to stenting which leads to the assumption that this was a procedure-related complication. Subsequently, the patient received one month of renally dosed enoxaparin as prophylaxis to decrease the possibility of in-stent thrombosis. Following the procedure, the proteinuria and creatinine levels steadily declined and reached her baseline of 300 mg/day and 1.5 mg/dL, respectively, at one-year follow-up (Figure 2).

3. Discussion

Our patient is a unique case of iliac vein stenosis mimicking a podocytopathy similar to *de novo* MCD. Her disease occurred 6 months after transplantation and was characterized by unresponsiveness to high-dose glucocorticoids but immediate and sustained remission of proteinuria and renal failure with restoration of normal venous blood flow at the anastomosis. We hypothesize that the mechanical forces

TABLE 1: Laboratory findings 6 months after renal transplantation, at the start of proteinuria and creatinine rise.

CBC	
Hemoglobin (g/dL)	11.9
Hematocrit (%)	36.8
WBC (10^9/L)	3.6
RBC (10^{12}/L)	4.37
PLT (10^9/L)	325
ANC (10^9/L)	2.9
ALC (10^9/L)	0.4
Metabolic panel	
Serum sodium (mmol/L)	136
Serum potassium (mmol/L)	4.3
Serum chloride (mmol/L)	107
Serum CO2 content (mmol/L)	20
Serum calcium (mg/dL)	9.3
Serum phosphorus (mmol/L)	3.5
Anion gap (mmol/L)	9
Serum creatinine (mg/dL)	1.48
Serum urea nitrogen (mg/dL)	22
Serum glucose (mg/dL)	86
Liver function tests	
Serum total protein (g/dL)	7
Serum albumin (g/dL)	4.4
Serum LDH (u/L)	178
Serum bilirubin total (mg/dL)	0.3
Serum bilirubin direct (mg/dL)	0.1
Serum ALP (u/L)	88
AST (u/L)	17
ALT (u/L)	12
INR	1
Prothrombin time (s)	10.3
Others	
Serum tacrolimus FK506 (ug/L)	7.7
Serum uric acid (mg/dL)	5.7
Creatine kinase (u/L)	143
SLE serology	
ANA by IF	Borderline
ANA titer/IF pattern	1 : 40/diffuse
Blood cultures	
Parvovirus B19	Not detected
Adenovirus Antibody	Not detected
BK virus PCR	Not detected
CMV virus PCR (copies/mL)	<200
EBV virus PCR (copies/mL)	<200
Urinalysis	
Urine color	Yellow
Urine appearance	Cloudy
Urine protein (mg/dL)	924
Urine creatinine (mg/dL)	202.8

TABLE 1: Continued.

RBCs	4–10
WBCs	10–25
Urine bacteria	Moderate
Urine blood	Negative
Urine ketones	Negative
Urine glucose	Negative
Urine pH	6
Urine bilirubin	Negative
Urine specific gravity	1.024
Urine nitrite	Negative
Urine leukocyte esterase	Negative
Urine culture	No growth of clean catch (<1,000 CFU/mL)

generated by the increase in venous blood pressure at the level of the glomerular tuft due to the iliac vein stenosis may have inflicted or predisposed the foot process effacement of the podocytes covering the glomerular basement membrane (GBM) and resulted in the appearance of MCD on renal biopsy and proteinuria. Our hypothesis may be supported by the fact that two doses of pulse methylprednisolone achieved only partial remission and a subsequent course of oral prednisone did not prevent the development of acute renal failure with persistently increased proteinuria and serum creatinine levels. Nevertheless, once the iliac vein stenosis was visualized and repaired, normal renal function was recovered.

Podocytes are highly specialized cells of epithelial origin that attach to the GBM through their foot processes. These foot processes interdigitate with one another and the filtration slits that are created between them are covered with an extracellular structure, the slit diaphragm [2]. The latter serves as a size- and charge-selective barrier of macromolecule filtration establishing selective permeability [3], while the foot processes with their contractile system stabilize the GBM and counteract local elastic distension caused by high capillary pressures [4]. Our hypothesis is based on observations suggesting that podocytes may respond to stress caused by increases in intracapillary pressures or exposure to toxins with foot process effacement and rearrangement of their actin cytoskeleton [5–7]. This process has been associated temporally with the emergence of proteinuria [8].

In order to explore the consequences of renal vein stenosis on the kidney and whether it has been previously associated with MCD in other instances, we examined cases of the "nutcracker syndrome." This syndrome is characterized by anatomical stenosis of the left renal vein inflicted by its compression between the aorta and proximal superior mesenteric artery. The left renal vein stenosis, which sometimes can be intermittent, causes congestion of the left kidney and leads to the formation of collateral veins. The clinical characteristics of this syndrome include flank pain, hematuria [9–11], and proteinuria [12–15], particularly of orthostatic type, on urine analysis. The onset of proteinuria in this syndrome may demonstrate a similar mechanism of mechanical forces

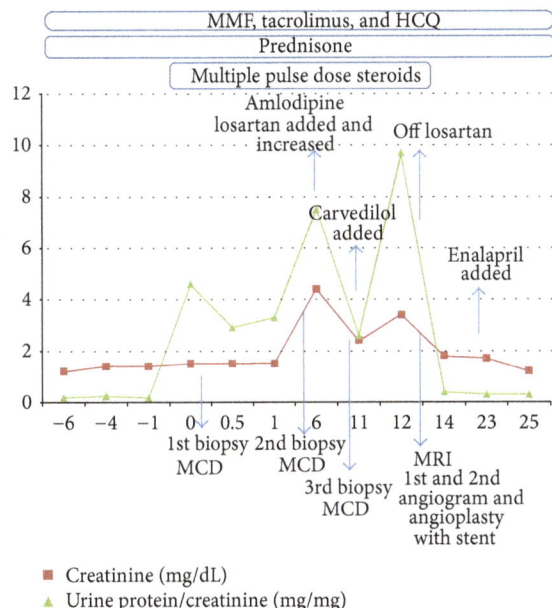

FIGURE 2: Serum creatinine and urine protein/creatinine ratio over time along with interventions and medical treatments. Time is noted in months where "0" indicates the onset of proteinuria and renal failure, which occurred approximately 6 months after renal transplantation. Patient's proteinuria improved significantly after the 2nd angioplasty (month 12) along with her serum creatinine. MMF: mycophenolate mofetil, HCQ: hydroxychloroquine, MCD: minimal change disease, and MRI: magnetic resonance imaging.

developing at the glomerulus due to renal or iliac vein stenosis in the posttransplant period that can act as a stress signal to the podocytes and cause foot process retraction in order to avoid further damage [6, 7]. Renal biopsy findings by electron microscopy in nutcracker syndrome complicated with proteinuria did not exhibit podocyte foot process effacement, although the small number of case reports with available electron microscopy reports and the intermittent nature of renal vein compression do not allow us to draw any definite conclusions [16, 17].

The exact pathogenesis of idiopathic MCD has not been fully elucidated. It has been suggested that a dysfunction of cell-mediated immunity, namely, an abnormal clone of T-cells, may result in the production of a cytokine or a circulating factor that alters the glomerular filtration barrier permeability and culminates in foot process effacement and proteinuria [18]. While the molecular structure of this factor remains yet to be discovered, additional data derived from case reports on the effectiveness of rituximab (a chimeric monoclonal antibody against CD20 on the surface of B cells) in steroid-dependent and recurrent cases of MCD may imply a role for humoral immunity in its pathogenesis or communication between B and T cells [19–21]. SLE is characterized by polyclonal B cell activation and hyperreactivity along with T helper cell expansion [22] that hypothetically could contribute to the production of a permeability factor. Furthermore, interferon alpha, which has been identified as a participant in the pathogenetic pathway of SLE [23],

when used as a treatment modality, has been reported in a few instances to be associated with MCD [24, 25]. Finally, complement-mediated injury, a major player in SLE disease, has been found able to disrupt the actin microfilament adhesion of podocytes to focal contacts and mediate their effacement [26]. In this context, the contribution of SLE in the development of MCD of this renal transplant with impaired venous outflow may also be interesting to explore.

Case reports or series have described the appearance of MCD in patients with a primary diagnosis of SLE. Dube et al. reported 7 cases of SLE patients with biopsy-proven MCD, of which 5 also exhibited mesangial electron-dense deposits with or without mesangial proliferation (lupus nephritis class II). All patients presented with nephrotic range proteinuria, peripheral edema, and hypoalbuminemia and responded to steroid therapy with rapid remission of their symptomatology. Three out of seven patients had a history of recent NSAID use [27]. Hertig et al. studied 11 SLE patients with nephrotic syndrome and a renal biopsy diagnosis of MCD in 4 patients or focal segmental glomerulosclerosis (FSGS) in 7 patients. None of the patients had a previous history or underlying lupus nephritis or triggers for secondary FSGS. Of interest was the fact that in nine out of eleven patients the development of nephrotic syndrome appeared at the time or shortly after SLE was diagnosed or coincided with a SLE flare of the disease. This observation led the authors to suggest that SLE could actively predispose to the development of nephrotic syndrome associated with MCD or FSGS [28]. We speculate that in our case iliac vein stenosis-induced increases of hydrostatic pressures, probably facilitated by a background of immune aberration, such as SLE, might have synergistically triggered the development of MCD.

De novo MCD in the posttransplantation period has been documented in the literature without, however, being attributed to any vascular complications of the graft. Although it has not been associated with any particular primary renal disease as a predisposing factor, it was observed in a case-series study that eight out of fourteen transplanted kidneys with *de novo* MCD originated from living donors, as seen in our patient. Moreover, most cases of posttransplantation nephrotic syndrome developed shortly after the surgery (within 4 months for 13/14 cases and at 24 months for one patient) and reached complete remission in 12/14 cases without adversely affecting in the long-term the kidney transplants [29].

Vascular complications after renal transplantation occur approximately in 2-3% of cases [30, 31]. The most common complication presented in large series of patients is renal artery stenosis whereas renal vein stenosis is fairly uncommon and mainly described in case reports [32–34] underlining the importance of recognizing such an entity in the clinical setting.

To our knowledge, this is a rare report of *de novo* MCD of a kidney transplant that is associated with iliac vein stenosis in the setting of SLE, which was reversible following stenting of the venous anastomosis. We suggest that in cases of nephrotic range proteinuria, especially with recurrent acute renal failure, without the other clinical features of the nephrotic syndrome, alternative causes of proteinuria, such as mechanical, should be considered, even with a biopsy-proven podocytopathy.

Consent

The patient has given her informed consent regarding this case report.

Conflict of Interests

The authors declare that there is no conflict of interests regarding the publication of this paper.

References

[1] R. J. Glassock, "Secondary minimal change disease," *Nephrology Dialysis Transplantation*, vol. 18, supplement 6, pp. vi52–vi58, 2003.

[2] P. Mundel and W. Kriz, "Structure and function of podocytes: an update," *Anatomy and Embryology*, vol. 192, no. 5, pp. 385–397, 1995.

[3] K. Tryggvason and J. Wartiovaara, "How does the kidney filter plasma?" *Physiology*, vol. 20, no. 2, pp. 96–101, 2005.

[4] W. Kriz, M. Elger, P. Mundel, and K. V. Lemley, "Structure-stabilizing forces in the glomerular tuft," *Journal of the American Society of Nephrology*, vol. 5, no. 10, pp. 1731–1739, 1995.

[5] C. Faul, K. Asanuma, E. Yanagida-Asanuma, K. Kim, and P. Mundel, "Actin up: regulation of podocyte structure and function by components of the actin cytoskeleton," *Trends in Cell Biology*, vol. 17, no. 9, pp. 428–437, 2007.

[6] W. Kriz, I. Shirato, M. Nagata, M. LeHir, and K. V. Lemley, "The podocyte's response to stress: the enigma of foot process effacement," *The American Journal of Physiology—Renal Physiology*, vol. 304, no. 4, pp. F333–F347, 2013.

[7] N. Endlich, K. R. Kress, J. Reiser et al., "Podocytes respond to mechanical stress in vitro," *Journal of the American Society of Nephrology*, vol. 12, no. 3, pp. 413–422, 2001.

[8] I. Shirato, "Podocyte process effacement in vivo," *Microscopy Research and Technique*, vol. 57, no. 4, pp. 241–246, 2002.

[9] H. E. Hanna, R. N. Santella, E. T. Zawada Jr., and T. E. Masterson, "Nutcracker syndrome: an underdiagnosed cause for hematuria?" *South Dakota Journal of Medicine*, vol. 50, no. 12, pp. 429–436, 1997.

[10] D. Russo, R. Minutolo, V. Iaccarino, M. Andreucci, A. Capuano, and F. A. Savino, "Gross hematuria of uncommon origin: the nutcracker syndrome," *American Journal of Kidney Diseases*, vol. 32, no. 3, article E3, 1998.

[11] H. Zhang, M. Li, W. Jin, P. San, P. Xu, and S. Pan, "The left renal entrapment syndrome: diagnosis and treatment," *Annals of Vascular Surgery*, vol. 21, no. 2, pp. 198–203, 2007.

[12] N. Shintaku, Y. Takahashi, K. Akaishi, A. Sano, and Y. Kuroda, "Entrapment of left renal vein in children with orthostatic proteinuria," *Pediatric Nephrology*, vol. 4, no. 4, pp. 324–327, 1990.

[13] Z. B. Özçakar, F. Yalçınkaya, S. Fitöz et al., "Nutcracker syndrome manifesting with severe proteinuria: a challenging scenario in asingle-kidney patient," *Pediatric Nephrology*, vol. 26, no. 6, pp. 987–990, 2011.

[14] S. J. Lee, E. S. You, J. E. Lee, and E. C. Chung, "Left renal vein entrapment syndrome in two girls with orthostatic proteinuria," *Pediatric Nephrology*, vol. 11, no. 2, pp. 218–220, 1997.

[15] M. Ekim, Z. B. Özçakar, S. Fitoz et al., "The 'nutcracker phenomenon'" with orthostatic proteinuria: case reports," *Clinical Nephrology*, vol. 65, no. 4, pp. 280–283, 2006.

[16] F. Şemsa Altugan, M. Ekim, S. Fitöz et al., "Nutcracker syndrome with urolithiasis," *Journal of Pediatric Urology*, vol. 6, no. 5, pp. 519–521, 2010.

[17] A. Basile, D. Tsetis, G. Calcara et al., "Nutcracker syndrome due to left renal vein compression by an aberrant right renal artery," *American Journal of Kidney Diseases*, vol. 50, no. 2, pp. 326–329, 2007.

[18] R. Shalhoub, "Pathogenesis of lipoid nephrosis: a disorder of T-cell function," *The Lancet*, vol. 2, no. 7880, pp. 556–560, 1974.

[19] V. Guigonis, A. Dallocchio, V. Baudouin et al., "Rituximab treatment for severe steroid- or cyclosporine-dependent nephrotic syndrome: a multicentric series of 22 cases," *Pediatric Nephrology*, vol. 23, no. 8, pp. 1269–1279, 2008.

[20] Y. Sawara, M. Itabashi, C. Kojima et al., "Successful therapeutic use of a single-dose of rituximab on relapse in adults with minimal change nephrotic syndrome," *Clinical Nephrology*, vol. 72, no. 1, pp. 69–72, 2009.

[21] A. Shahane, A. Khasnis, and C. Gota, "Rituximab-responsive nephrotic syndrome due to minimal change disease in systemic lupus erythematosus," *Journal of Clinical Rheumatology*, vol. 18, no. 4, pp. 199–202, 2012.

[22] C. C. Mok and C. S. Lau, "Pathogenesis of systemic lupus erythematosus," *Journal of Clinical Pathology*, vol. 56, no. 7, pp. 481–490, 2003.

[23] M. K. Crow and K. A. Kirou, "Interferon-α in systemic lupus erythematosus," *Current Opinion in Rheumatology*, vol. 16, no. 5, pp. 541–547, 2004.

[24] S. D. Averbuch, H. A. Austin III, S. A. Sherwin, T. Antonovych, P. A. Bunn Jr., and D. L. Longo, "Acute interstitial nephritis with the nephrotic syndrome following recombinant leukocyte A interferon therapy for mycosis fungoides," *The New England Journal of Medicine*, vol. 310, no. 1, pp. 32–35, 1984.

[25] A. Traynor, T. Kuzel, E. Samuelson, and Y. Kanwar, "Minimal-change glomerulopathy and glomerular visceral epithelial hyperplasia associated with alpha-interferon therapy for cutaneous T-cell lymphoma," *Nephron*, vol. 67, no. 1, pp. 94–100, 1994.

[26] P. S. Topham, S. A. Haydar, R. Kuphal, J. D. Lightfoot, and D. J. Salant, "Complement-mediated injury reversibly disrupts glomerular epithelial cell actin microfilaments and focal adhesions," *Kidney International*, vol. 55, no. 5, pp. 1763–1775, 1999.

[27] G. K. Dube, G. S. Markowitz, J. Radhakrishnan, G. B. Appel, and V. D. D'Agati, "Minimal change disease in systemic lupus erythematosus," *Clinical Nephrology*, vol. 57, no. 2, pp. 120–126, 2002.

[28] A. Hertig, D. Droz, P. Lesavre, J.-P. Grünfeld, and P. Rieu, "SLE and idiopathic nephrotic syndrome: coincidence or not?" *American Journal of Kidney Diseases*, vol. 40, no. 6, pp. 1179–1184, 2002.

[29] A. A. Zafarmand, E. Baranowska-Daca, P. D. C. Ly et al., "De novo minimal change disease associated with reversible posttransplant nephrotic syndrome. A report of five cases and review of literature," *Clinical Transplantation*, vol. 16, no. 5, pp. 350–361, 2002.

[30] S. Aktas, F. Boyvat, S. Sevmis, G. Moray, H. Karakayali, and M. Haberal, "Analysis of vascular complications after renal transplantation," *Transplantation Proceedings*, vol. 43, no. 2, pp. 557–561, 2011.

[31] P. Eufrásio, B. Parada, P. Moreira et al., "Surgical complications in 2000 renal transplants," *Transplantation Proceedings*, vol. 43, no. 1, pp. 142–144, 2011.

[32] S. Olliff, R. Negus, C. Deane, and H. Walters, "Renal transplant vein stenosis: demonstration and percutaneous venoplasty of a new vascular complication in the transplant kidney," *Clinical Radiology*, vol. 43, no. 1, pp. 42–46, 1991.

[33] J. P. Cercueil, D. Chevet, C. Mousson, E. Tatou, D. Krause, and G. Rifle, "Acquired vein stenosis of renal allograft—percutaneous treatment with self-expanding metallic stent," *Nephrology Dialysis Transplantation*, vol. 12, no. 4, pp. 825–826, 1997.

[34] A. Obed, D. C. Uihlein, N. Zorger et al., "Severe renal vein stenosis of a kidney transplant with beneficial clinical course after successful percutaneous stenting," *American Journal of Transplantation*, vol. 8, no. 10, pp. 2173–2176, 2008.

42

A Case of Newly Diagnosed Klippel Trenaunay Weber Syndrome Presenting with Nephrotic Syndrome

Egemen Cebeci,[1] Secil Demir,[2] Meltem Gursu,[1]
Abdullah Sumnu,[1] Mehmet Yamak,[2] Barış Doner,[1] Serhat Karadag,[1]
Sami Uzun,[1] Ahmet Behlul,[1] Oktay Ozkan,[1] and Savas Ozturk[1]

[1]*Department of Nephrology, Haseki Training and Research Hospital, 34087 Istanbul, Turkey*
[2]*Department of Internal Medicine, Haseki Training and Research Hospital, 34087 Istanbul, Turkey*

Correspondence should be addressed to Egemen Cebeci; egemencebeci@hotmail.com

Academic Editor: John A. Sayer

Klippel Trenaunay Weber syndrome (KTWS) is a rare disease characterized by hemihypertrophy, variceal enlargement of the veins, and arteriovenous (AV) malformations. Renal involvement in KTWS is not known except in rare case reports. Herein, we present a case of KTWS with nephrotic syndrome. A 52-year-old male was admitted due to dyspnea and swelling of the body for the last three months. The pathological physical findings were diffuse edema, decreased lung sounds at the right basal site, increased diameter and decreased length of the left leg compared with the right one, diffuse variceal enlargements, and a few hemangiomatous lesions on the left leg. The pathological laboratory findings were hypoalbuminemia, hyperlipidemia, increased creatinine level (1.23 mg/dL), and proteinuria (7.6 g/day). Radiographic pathological findings were cystic lesions in the liver, spleen, and kidneys, splenomegaly, AV malformation on the left posterolateral thigh, and hypertrophy of the soft tissues of the proximal left leg. He was diagnosed to have KTWS with these findings. Renal biopsy was performed to determine the cause of nephrotic syndrome. The pathologic examination was consistent with focal segmental sclerosis (FSGS). He was started on oral methylprednisolone at the dosage of 1 mg/kg and began to be followedup in the nephrology outpatient clinic.

1. Introduction

Klippel Trenaunay Weber syndrome (KTWS) is a rare idiopathic disease characterized by hemihypertrophy of the bones and soft tissues, variceal enlargement of the veins in the involved extremity, and arteriovenous (AV) malformations. The disease was first described by Klippel and Trenaunay as Klippel Trenaunay syndrome (KTS) which included hemihypertrophy and varices in 1900 after which Weber called the disease Klippel Trenaunay Weber syndrome with the addition of AV malformations in 1907 [1, 2]. The pathogenetic mechanism of the increased angiogenesis is thought to be mutations in the angiogenic factor (VG5Q) gene via transcription and increased activity [3]. VG5Q gene has been identified in blood vessels, is secreted during angiogenesis, and increases endothelial cell proliferation. The involvement is unilateral typically, of the lower extremity in 95%, upper extremity in

5%, and both lower and upper extremities in 15% of the cases [4]. Capillary lesions are associated with soft tissue swelling and bone hypertrophy. Patients with this syndrome have a wide spectrum of presentation from asymptomatic disease to life-threatening bleeding and embolism.

The symptoms appear before the age of ten in about 75% of cases in this congenital disease [5]. Although the treatment strategy is conservative unless complicated, patients need close orthopedic follow-up since the length of lower extremities differs frequently [6]. The differential diagnosis of KTWS includes KTS, Maffucci syndrome, Proteus syndrome, and other capillary malformations not associated with any syndrome [7].

Renal involvement in KTWS is not known except in rare case reports. Herein, we present a case of KTWS diagnosed at the age of 52 together with nephrotic syndrome.

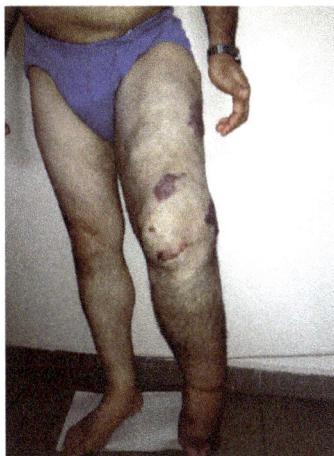

FIGURE 1: The appearance of the lower extremities of the patient showing shortness and thickness of the left leg with variceal enlargement of the veins and hemangiomas.

Key Message. The diagnosis of Klippel Trenaunay Weber syndrome may be delayed into adulthood and FSGS may coexist with this syndrome.

2. Case Presentation

A 52-year-old male was admitted to the outpatient clinic of the department of internal medicine with the complaints of progressively increasing dyspnea and swelling of the body during the last three months. The patient had variceal enlargements of the veins from the time of birth and his left leg was thicker than the right one, but he did not have a certain diagnosis. The family history was negative. The pathological findings on physical examination at the time of diagnosis were diffuse edema in the body, decreased lung sounds at the right basal site, increased diameter and decreased length of the left leg compared with the right one, diffuse variceal enlargements, and a few hemangiomatosis lesions on the left leg (Figure 1). The pathological laboratory findings were as follows: serum albumin: 2.2 g/dL, total cholesterol: 216 mg/dL, LDL cholesterol: 152 mg/dL, creatinine: 1.23 mg/dL, and proteinuria: 7.6 g/day. Urine sediment was inactive. The abdominal ultrasonography revealed a cystic lesion of 7 × 4.5 cm diameters in the liver with thin septations and dense content in some areas; splenomegaly (133 mm), a solid lesion resembling hemangioma measured 3 × 2.5 cm at the lower pole of the spleen; and multiple anechoic cysts measured at most 2 cm at the upper pole of the spleen. The sizes of the kidneys were normal, while the echogenicity was increased. There were one cortical cyst (2.5 cm) in the upper pole of the right kidney and two cysts (the bigger one measured 6 cm in diameter) in the upper pole of the left kidney. Dynamic magnetic resonance imaging of the abdomen with intravenous contrast material showed a cystic lesion measured 53 × 47 mm with peripheral capsular contrast involvement in the segment 4a-7 of the liver and nodular lesions consistent with hemangiomas in segments 7-8 and 4A of the liver. There were also splenomegaly (136 mm),

heterogeneity of the splenic parenchyma, and multiple lesions resembling hemangiomas measuring 25 mm at most in the spleen. There were simple cortical cysts in the kidneys, one in the upper pole of the right kidney (27 mm) and two in the upper pole of the left kidney (the bigger one measuring 6 mm). The radiologists reported bilateral pleural effusion reaching 15 mm of thickness on the right side and AV malformation on the left posterolateral thigh that fills the mesorectum and hypertrophy of the soft tissues of the proximal left lower extremity.

He was diagnosed to have KTWS putting together the hemihypertrophy, diffuse variceal enlargements of the veins, and AV malformations detected radiologically. Gastroscopic examination was normal, while colonoscopy revealed diffuse blue-purple variceal enlargements on the rectal mucosa (hemangioma) and a polyp in the rectum with a diameter of 1 cm. The rectal mucosa was bluish purple from the 10th cm to 20th cm (hemangioma) (Figure 2).

He was transferred to the nephrology clinic for evaluation of the cause of nephrotic syndrome. Paleness of the temporal regions and increased deepness of the optic hollow were detected at eye examination. Hepatitis serology, antineutrophil cytoplasmic antibody, and antinuclear antibody were negative. Complement levels were within normal limits. Renal biopsy was performed to determine the cause of nephrotic syndrome. Of the 13 glomeruli detected, five were globally sclerotic while another five had segmental sclerosis. There was prominent mesangial enlargement in other glomeruli together with patchy atrophy of tubuli, interstitial fibrosis, mild mononuclear cellular infiltration, and thickened arteriolar walls (Figure 3). No accumulation was detected with examination by immune fluorescence techniques. Electron microscopic examination was not available. With these findings, he was diagnosed as focal segmental sclerosis (FSGS). He was started on oral methylprednisolone at the dosage of 1 mg/kg and began to be followed up in the nephrology outpatient clinic. It was learned that he was admitted to the emergency clinic of another hospital due to profuse rectal bleeding at the end of the third week of steroid treatment. The steroid treatment was terminated at that time. Proteinuria was measured as 5.2 g/day and serum creatinine was 2.1 mg/dL. He is still under follow-up with conservative treatment.

3. Discussion

Klippel Trenaunay Weber syndrome is a rare vascular abnormality characterized by hemihypertrophy, variceal veins, and AV malformations. It is usually sporadic as in our case, although few familial cases have been reported [8]. It is a congenital disease diagnosed usually in childhood, but it should be kept in mind that there may be cases undiagnosed until adulthood as in our case.

The disease involves usually the lower extremity like our case although the trunk or face may be affected unilaterally. Hemangiomas may be limited to the skin or may be seen in bones, muscles, and solid organs. The patient we present had hemangiomas in the liver, spleen, and rectum besides

(a)   (b)

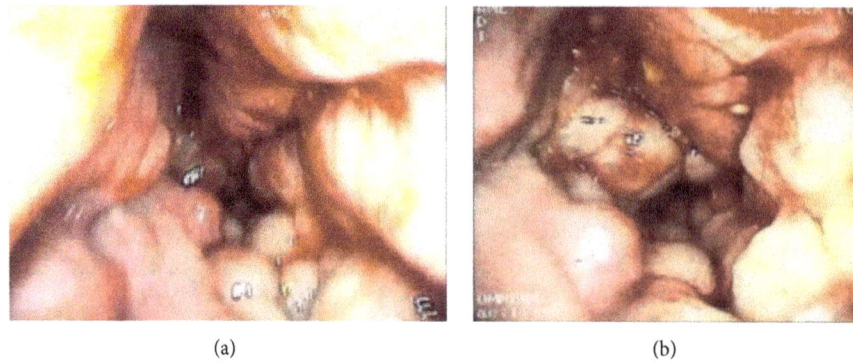

FIGURE 2: Colonoscopic findings. Diffuse blue-purple variceal enlargements on the rectal mucosa (hemangioma) and a polyp in the rectum with a diameter of 1 cm (a). The rectal mucosa was bluish purple from the 10th cm to 20th cm (hemangioma) (b).

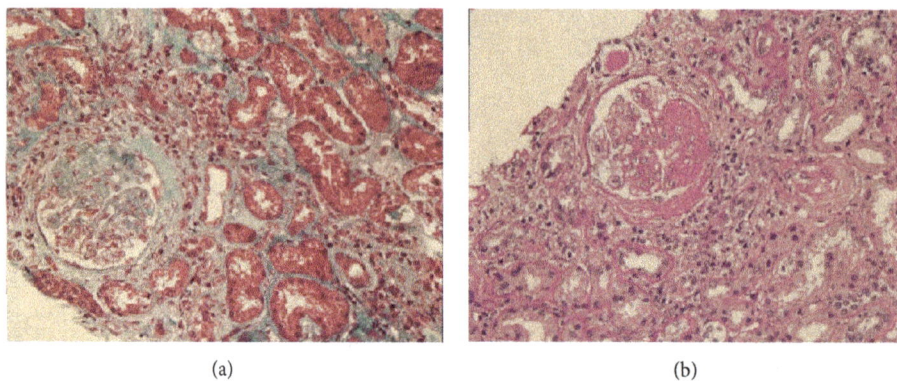

(a)   (b)

FIGURE 3: Segmental sclerotic lesion in the glomerulus. (a) Masson trichrome. (b) Periodic acid Schiff staining.

the lower extremity. Variceal veins appear in the first years of life and increase in dimensions until adolescence [7]. They may cause pain, lymphedema, thrombophlebitis, and skin ulcerations. Hemihypertrophy presents either as increased length of the bones or as increased diameter due to soft tissue involvement. Hemihypertrophy is present at birth and progresses until adolescence at which time it ceases to progress. The presented case had hypertrophy of both bone and soft tissue. There may be eye abnormalities in KTWS including vascular pathologies of optic nerve, iris, choroid, retina, and orbit. The pathological findings detected at the examination of the presented case were thought to be related with KTWS.

Renal involvement in KTWS was presented as case reports of aneurysm of the renal artery, renal hemangiomas, and hydronephrosis [9–12]. A case with KTWS and renal failure was reported of which the renal biopsy showed abnormal accumulation in the mesangial tissue [13]. One case with KTWB and proteinuria was reported [14], but no data has been found in the literature about the coexistence of KTWS and FSGS.

FSGS, although usually primary, may develop as secondary due to various reasons. Among the secondary reasons, hemodynamic factors, hyperfiltration, and renal vasodilation are the major ones. The presence of acute or subacute nephrotic syndrome together with hypoalbuminemia

is consistent with primary FSGS. Secondary FSGS is usually characterized by low grade proteinuria and normal serum albumin levels [15, 16]. Regarding these clinical differences between primary and secondary FSGS, the presented case was thought to be primary due to acute onset, nephrotic range proteinuria, and hypoalbuminemia. So he was started on steroid treatment. Otherwise, it was not possible to make a pathophysiological link between KTWS and FSGS present in this case.

Consent

The patient described in the case report had given informed consent for the case report to be published.

Conflict of Interests

The authors declare that there is no conflict of interests regarding the publication of this paper.

References

[1] M. Klippel and P. Trenaunay, "Du noevus variqueux osteo-hypertrphique," *Archives Générals de Médecine*, vol. 185, p. 641, 1900.

[2] F. P. Weber, "Angioma formation in connection with hypertrophy of limbs and hemihypertrophy," *British Journal of Dermatology*, vol. 19, article 231, 1907.

[3] X.-L. Tian, R. Kadaba, S.-A. You et al., "Identification of an angiogenic factor that when mutated causes susceptibility to Klippel-Trenaunay syndrome," *Nature*, vol. 427, no. 6975, pp. 640–645, 2004.

[4] M. A. Dohil, W. P. Baugh, and L. F. Eichenfield, "Vascular and pigmented birthmarks," *Pediatric Clinics of North America*, vol. 47, no. 4, pp. 783–812, 2000.

[5] L. A. Favorito, "Vesical hemangioma in patient with Klippel-Trenaunay-Weber syndrome," *International Braz J Urol*, vol. 29, no. 2, pp. 149–150, 2003.

[6] O. Enjolras and J. B. Mulliken, "The current management of vascular birthmarks," *Pediatric Dermatology*, vol. 10, no. 4, pp. 311–333, 1993.

[7] M. C. Garzon, J. T. Huang, O. Enjolras, and I. J. Frieden, "Vascular malformations/part II: associated syndromes," *Journal of the American Academy of Dermatology*, vol. 56, no. 4, pp. 541–564, 2007.

[8] G. E. Aelvoet, P. G. Jorens, and L. M. Roelen, "Genetic aspects of the Klippel-Trenaunay syndrome," *British Journal of Dermatology*, vol. 126, no. 6, pp. 603–607, 1992.

[9] S. Pourhassan, D. Grotemeyer, V. Klar, and W. Sandmann, "The Klippel-Trenaunay syndrom associated with multiple visceral arteries aneurysms," *Vasa*, vol. 36, no. 2, pp. 124–129, 2007.

[10] J. M. Campistol, C. Agusti, A. Torras, E. Campo, C. Abad, and L. Revert, "Renal hemangioma and renal artery aneurysm in the Klippel-Trenaunay syndrome," *Journal of Urology*, vol. 140, no. 1, pp. 134–136, 1988.

[11] Ç. Ecevit, T. Kavaklı, and A. Öztürk, "Klippel-Trenaunay sendromu tanılı bir olgu," in *50 Milli Pediatri Kongresi*, p. 182, Antalya, Turkey, November 2006.

[12] N. C. Ören, S. Vurucu, B. Karaman, and F. Örs, "Renal agenesis in a child with ipsilateral hemihypertrophy," *Pediatric Nephrology*, vol. 25, no. 9, pp. 1751–1754, 2010.

[13] R. D. Brod, J. A. Shields, C. L. Shields, O. R. Oberkircher, and L. J. Sabol, "Unusual retinal and renal vascular lesions in the Klippel-Trenaunay-Weber syndrome," *Retina*, vol. 12, no. 4, pp. 355–358, 1992.

[14] O. I. Iaroshevskaia, E. A. Kharina, and A. V. Brydun, "Hormone-sensitive nephrotic syndrome in a child with Klippel-Trenaunay syndrome," *Pediatriia*, no. 8, pp. 85–88, 1988.

[15] M. Praga, E. Morales, J. C. Herrero et al., "Absence of hypoalbuminemia despite massive proteinuria in focal segmental glomerulosclerosis secondary to hyperfiltration," *The American Journal of Kidney Diseases*, vol. 33, no. 1, pp. 52–58, 1999.

[16] M. Praga, E. Hernández, E. Morales et al., "Clinical features and long-term outcome of obesity-associated focal segmental glomerulosclerosis," *Nephrology Dialysis Transplantation*, vol. 16, no. 9, pp. 1790–1798, 2001.

43

Successful Treatment of Infectious Endocarditis Associated Glomerulonephritis Mimicking C3 Glomerulonephritis in a Case with No Previous Cardiac Disease

Yosuke Kawamorita,[1] Yoshihide Fujigaki,[1] Atsuko Imase,[1]
Shigeyuki Arai,[1] Yoshifuru Tamura,[1] Masayuki Tanemoto,[1] Hiroshi Uozaki,[2]
Yutaka Yamaguchi,[3] and Shunya Uchida[1]

[1] *Department of Internal Medicine, Teikyo University School of Medicine, 2-11-1 Kaga, Itabashi-ku, Tokyo 173-8605, Japan*
[2] *Department of Pathology, Teikyo University School of Medicine, 2-11-1 Kaga, Itabashi-ku, Tokyo 173-8605, Japan*
[3] *Yamaguchi's Pathology Laboratory, 20-31-1 Minoridai, Matsudo-shi, Chiba 270-2231, Japan*

Correspondence should be addressed to Yoshihide Fujigaki; fujigakiyoshihide@gmail.com

Academic Editor: Kouichi Hirayama

We report a 42-year-old man with subacute infectious endocarditis (IE) with septic pulmonary embolism, presenting rapidly progressive glomerulonephritis and positive proteinase 3-anti-neutrophil cytoplasmic antibody (PR3-ANCA). He had no previous history of heart disease. Renal histology revealed diffuse endocapillary proliferative glomerulonephritis with complement 3- (C3-) dominant staining and subendothelial electron dense deposit, mimicking C3 glomerulonephritis. Successful treatment of IE with valve plastic surgery gradually ameliorated hypocomplementemia and renal failure; thus C3 glomerulonephritis-like lesion in this case was classified as postinfectious glomerulonephritis. IE associated glomerulonephritis is relatively rare, especially in cases with no previous history of valvular disease of the heart like our case. This case also reemphasizes the broad differential diagnosis of renal involvement in IE.

1. Introduction

Infectious endocarditis (IE) has various renal histologies, including renal infarction due to septic emboli, acute postinfectious glomerulonephritis, membranoproliferative glomerulonephritis, immune or pauci-immune crescentic glomerulonephritis, and acute interstitial nephritis [1–3]. Some patients with IE show vasculitis-like general symptoms, renal failure, and positive PR3-ANCA with or without ANCA-related vasculitis. Thus, it is important to evaluate renal histopathology in patients with IE-related renal involvement to determine whether immunosuppressive therapy should be introduced.

The term C3 glomerulopathy is recently defined by the pathological findings of complement 3 (C3) which is deposited within the glomerulus in the absence of substantial immunoglobulin, and there may remain much room for discussion. Dysregulation of the alternative pathway of complement is brought by genetic and/or acquired defects, with interindividual variability giving rise to two broad subtypes of C3 glomerulopathy-membranoproliferative glomerulonephritis (dense deposit disease) and C3 glomerulonephritis [4]. It is known that C3 glomerulopathy may present following an infectious episode. It is not uncommon that typical cases of postinfectious glomerulonephritis show deposition of C3 without immunoglobulin [5]. In these cases, distinction of C3 glomerulopathy will depend on the absence of atypical features on light microscopy and electron microscopy and also on a typical clinical course with resolution [6].

Here we describe a case with no previous history of heart disease, presenting subacute IE associated with septic pulmonary embolism, rapidly progressive glomerulonephritis, and positive PR3-ANCA. Differential diagnosis by renal histopathology could not initially rule out C3 glomerulonephritis, but the case was classified as postinfectious

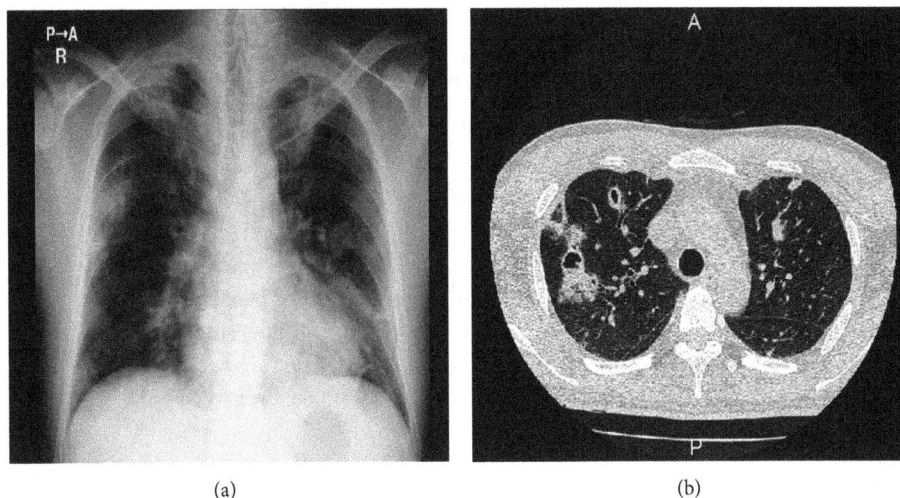

(a)   (b)

FIGURE 1: (a) Chest X-ray showing multiple bilateral nodular densities. (b) CT of the chest demonstrating bilateral multiple lung nodules, some of which are cavitated.

glomerulonephritis because the complement and renal dysfunction were recovered after treatment of IE.

2. Case Presentation

A 42-year-old Japanese man was referred to our hospital because of fever, appetite loss, myalgia, pain, and swelling of the left foot, leg edema, decreased renal function, and multiple nodules and cavities in bilateral lungs on computed tomography (CT) scan. The patient had been well until 6 weeks earlier, when he went to orthopedics about lumbago and dry cough. He consulted a doctor about leg edema 5 days ago and appetite loss and pain and swelling on the left foot 2 weeks ago. He was referred to local hospital and then transferred to our hospital on the same day because his laboratory data showed Hb of 8.8 g/dL, serum creatinine (Cr) of 3.87 mg/dL, and C-reactive protein of 32.0 mg/dL and multiple pulmonary nodules and cavities on CT scan.

Physical examination on admission showed the temperature 38.2°C, the blood pressure 106/64 mm Hg, the pulse 112 beats per minute, the respiratory rate 26 breaths per minute, and the oxygen saturation 100%. He had dry tongue, pain, redness, and swelling at the left dorsum of the foot and pitting edema on both legs. He had no symptom or sign of vasculitis on eyes, ears, and upper respiratory tract.

Laboratory-test results are shown in the Table 1, indicating anemia, hypoalbuminemia, renal failure with proteinuria and pyuria, and positive inflammatory signs. Saline and ceftriaxone (CTRX) were infused intravenously for dehydration and cellulitis at the left dorsum of the foot, respectively.

3 days after hydration, serum Cr level was decreased from 6.11 mg/dL to 3.69 mg/dL but was sustained around 2 to 3 mg/dL. Urinalysis began to show significant hematuria. PR3-ANCA was revealed to be positive. Thus, the findings of general symptom, rapidly progressive glomerulonephritis, positive PR3-ANCA, nodules on chest X-ray (Figure 1(a)), and multiple cavities on chest CT scan (Figure 1(b)), raised suspicion of granulomatosis with polyangiitis with renal

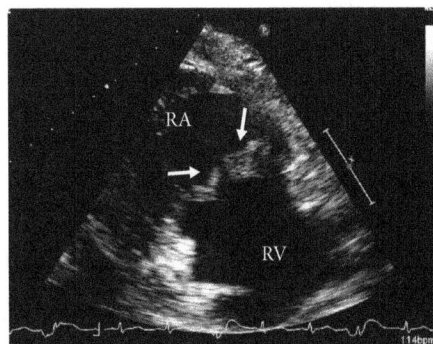

FIGURE 2: Transthoracic echocardiograph. Extensive bacterial vegetations are observed on the tricuspid (arrows) valves. RA: right atrium, RV: right ventricle.

involvement. Although the patient had no previous history of cardiac disease, echo cardiography showed tricuspid valve regurgitation with vegetation 17 mm × 11 mm in diameter (Figure 2). Blood culture revealed positive methicillin-susceptible *Staphylococcus aureus*; thus the patient was diagnosed to be subacute IE. Cellulitis may be a cause of IE in this case. Pulmonary multiple cavities should be caused by septic pulmonary embolism. Methicillin-susceptible *Staphylococcus aureus* was sensitive to cefmetazole (CEZ) and CEZ was started as substitute for CTRX.

Renal biopsy 2 weeks after CEZ treatment showed no global sclerosis out of 12 obtained glomeruli. Each glomerulus revealed no crescent formation but diffuse endocapillary proliferative glomerulonephritis (Figure 3(a)) with starry sky pattern of significant C3 deposition (Figure 3(b)) and minimal to absent immunoglobulins by immunofluorescence. Electron microscopy showed polymorphonuclear cells and monocytes infiltration in glomerular capillaries (Figure 3(c)) and the electron dense deposits in the subendothelial areas but no hump formation (Figure 3(d)). Our patient had IE associated with septic pulmonary embolism, and it is reported that some of glomerulonephritis associated with

TABLE 1: Laboratory data at the time of admission.

Blood		Urine	
Blood count		Dipstick test	
White blood cell	13,400/mm^3	Protein	1+
Eosinophil	0%	Glucose	(−)
Red blood cell	295 × 10^4/mm^3	Occult blood	(±)
Hemoglobin	8.7 g/dL	Sediment	
Hematocrit	24.7%	Leukocyte	10–19/HPF
Platelet	5.0 × 10^4/mm^3	Red blood cell	1–4/HPF
Biochemical tests		Epithelial cell	0-1/HPF
Total protein	6.4 g/dL	Red blood cell cast	0-1/HPF
Albumin	1.5 g/dL	Biochemical analysis	
Aspartate-aminotransferase	24 IU	Urine protein	0.61 g/gCr
Alanine-aminotransferase	22 IU	N-Acetyl-β-D-glucosaminidase	52.3 U/mL
Lactate dehydrogenase	220 IU	β2-Microglobulin	3,720 μg/L
Blood urea nitrogen	97.5 mg/dL	α1-Microglobulin	180 mg/L
Cr	6.11 mg/dL		
Uric acid	14.5 mg/dL		
Sodium	134 mEq/L		
Potassium	4.5 mEq/L		
Chloride	94 mEq/L		
Calcium	7.6 mg/dL		
Phosphate	5.5 mg/dL		
Creatine kinase	43 IU/L		
Fasting blood glucose	111 mg/dL		
HbA1c	5.8%		
eGFR	9.2 mL/min/1.73 m^2		
Immunology			
C-reactive protein	27.84 mg/dL		
Procalcitonin	4.0 ng/mL		
Immunoglobulin G	2,190 mg/dL		
Immunoglobulin A	364 mg/dL		
Immunoglobulin M	87 mg/dL		
Complement 3	142 mg/dL (65–135)		
Complement 4	30 mg/dL (13–35)		
CH50	52 U/mL (22–58)		
Anti-streptolysin O	37.6 U/mL		
Hepatitis B surface antigen	(−)		
Hepatitis C virus antibody	(−)		
Human immunodeficiency virus antibody	(−)		
RF	10.0 U/mL		
Antinuclear antibody	(−)		
MPO-ANCA	1.0 U/mL (<3.5)		
PR3-ANCA	21.3 U/mL (<3.5)		
Cryoglobulin	(−)		

Creatinine: Cr; MPO-ANCA: myeloperoxidase-anti-neutrophil cytoplasmic antibody; PR3-ANCA: proteinase 3-anti-neutrophil cytoplasmic antibody. The figure in the parenthesis shows the normal range.

IE and glomerulonephritis associated with visceral infection also show the glomerular lesions with dominant C3 deposition [7] similar to that in our case. Glomerulonephritis with dominant C3 deposition in our patient could not rule out C3 glomerulonephritis at the time of renal biopsy based on C3 glomerulopathy: consensus report [6]. Renal infarction and abscess were not found in the renal specimens and were not suggested by echo and CT scan.

Clinical course after admission was shown in Figure 4 C3 was found to be decreased at the time of renal biopsy.

(a)

(b)

(c)

(d)

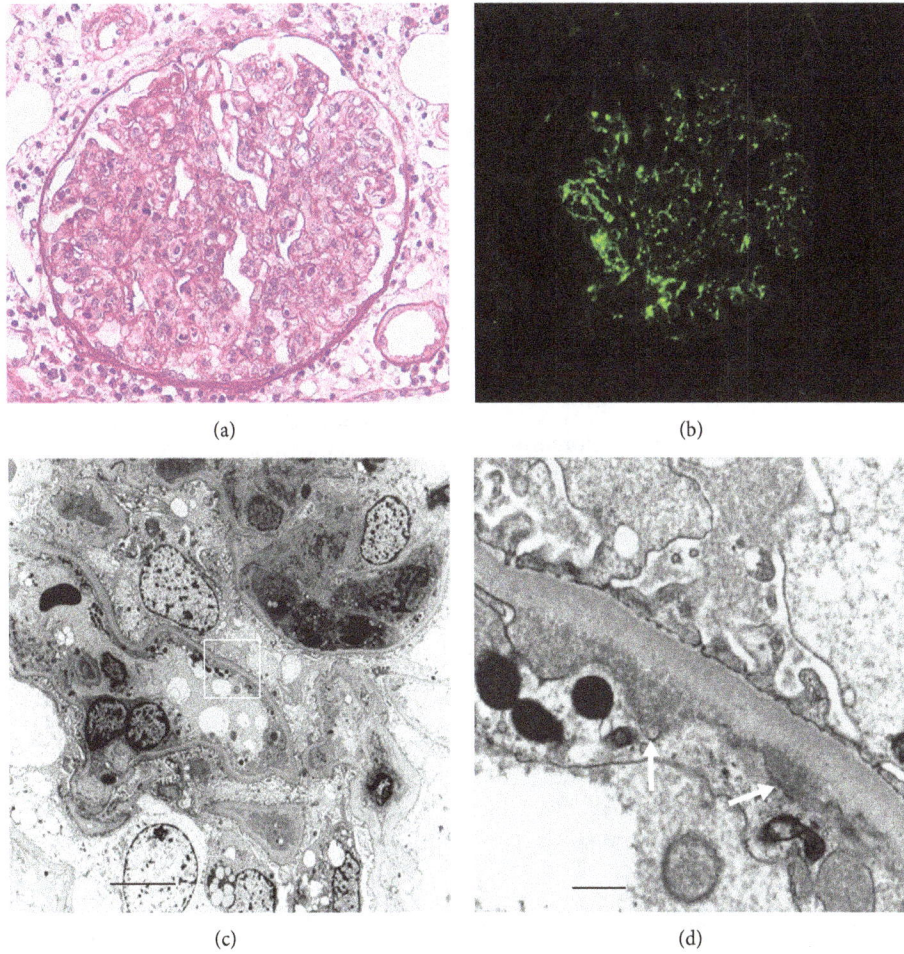

FIGURE 3: Photomicrographs of renal tissue. (a) Light microscopy shows a diffuse endocapillary proliferative glomerulonephritis with lobular formation. PAS staining. Original magnification ×400. (b) Bright C3 staining along capillary walls by immunofluorescence. (c) Electron microscopy shows polymorphonuclear cells and monocyte infiltration in the capillary wall. Bar = 2.0 μm. (d) The area of the square in Figure 3(c) shows subendothelial deposits (arrows). Bar = 0.2 μm.

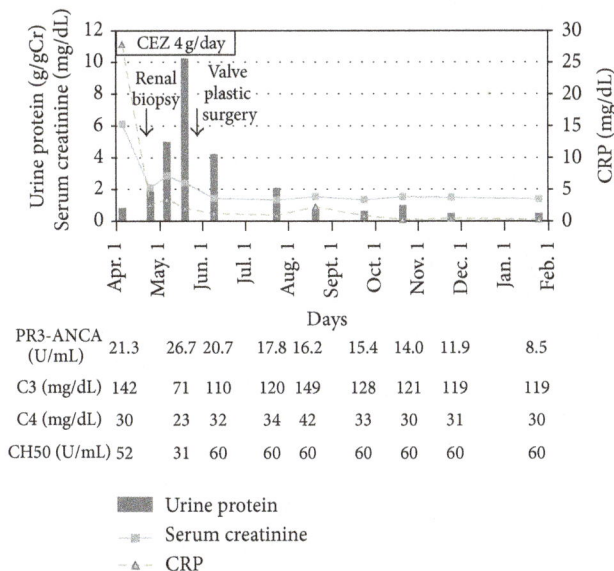

FIGURE 4: Clinical course after admission.

Although treatment with CEZ 4 g/day brought negative blood culture and partially ameliorated renal function, proteinuria began to increase and peaked 10 g/gCr 6 weeks after CEZ administration. Since vegetation grew to 27 mm × 15 mm in diameter at tricuspid valve, tricuspid valve plastic surgery was performed. Additional 6 weeks of treatment with CEZ after the operation got IE cured. Successful treatment of IE ameliorated hypocomplementemia and renal failure with active urinalysis. The titer of PR3-ANCA was gradually decreased and nodular lesions on chest X-ray disappeared after recovery from subacute IE. Ten months after the operation, the patient is well with proteinuria of 0.16 g/gCr, Cr of 1.32 mg/dL, C3 of 115 mg/dL, and PR3-ANCA of 8.9 U/mL.

3. Discussion

It is reported that around 75% of patients with IE have an underlying structural heart disease at the time when IE is diagnosed [8]. Glomerulonephritis associated with IE shows various renal lesions and is relatively rare, especially in cases with no previous heart disease like our case. ANCA, including PR3- and MPO-ANCA, occurs in a substantial proportion of IE cases with or without renal vasculitis. It is reported that, among 109 IE cases, 18% had cytoplasmic and/or perinuclear ANCA and 8% had PR3-ANCA or MPO-ANCA [9]. IE cases could present clinical manifestations that mimic a primary systemic vasculitis. Among IE cases with ANCA-positivity, some cases may develop vasculitis with crescentic glomerulonephritis [3, 9]. Thus, differential diagnosis of renal involvement of IE is important to make a decision on whether immunosuppressive therapy should be introduced. Our case did not show ANCA-associated glomerulonephritis. The PR3-ANCA in this case seemed to be just the epiphenomenon of the systemic infection.

Our case revealed diffuse endocapillary glomerulonephritis with C3-dominant immunofluorescence staining with minimal immunoglobulins. There were only subendothelial electron dense deposits without hump formation. It is rare, but a similar electron microscopic finding of glomerular lesion was reported in some cases with acute glomerulonephritis caused by staphylococcal [10] or streptococcal [11] infection. It is reported that glomerulonephritis associated with IE and glomerulonephritis associated with visceral infection especially secondary to staphylococcal infection include the glomerular lesions with dominant C3 deposition [7]. Sethi et al. reported that there were patients who show an underlying abnormality of the alternative pathway of complement among patients with persistent hematuria and proteinuria even after resolution of the infection, diagnosed with postinfectious glomerulonephritis [5]. They called them "atypical" postinfectious glomerulonephritis, showing the diffuse (endocapillary) proliferative pattern of glomerulonephritis and the possible presence of immunoglobulins and numerous subepithelial humps with mesangial and subendothelial deposits. They speculated that there might be an infectious trigger, which is the underlying abnormality of the alternative pathway that drives the disease process. It is known that C3 glomerulopathy often shows membranoproliferative glomerulonephritis but also several other renal histologies [12]. Some C3 glomerulonephritis was reported to be masqueraded as acute postinfectious glomerulonephritis [13]. Therefore, C3 glomerulonephritis was not pathologically excluded in our patient [6]. However, successful treatment of IE ameliorated renal failure with active urinalysis and hypocomplementemia. Thus, renal pathology of dominant C3 deposition in our case was classified as postinfectious glomerulonephritis [6].

Our case showed normocomplementemia on admission but exhibited transient low grade hypocomplementemia with decreased C3 during active IE. As several complement proteins, including C3 and C4, behave as acute phase proteins, an increased synthesis may mask accelerated catabolism. Therefore, the assessment of complement protein levels is often inadequate to detect complement activation. In addition, the range of normal complement protein concentrations is wide, thus low levels may be related to deficiency state [14].

PR-3 ANCA associated with IE was reported to be positive for several months to years after IE was cured [1, 15]. In accordance with the report, our case sustained low titer PR3-ANCA 3 to 4 months after IE was cured (stopping antibiotics) and then PR3-ANCA was declined in one half.

In summary, IE associated glomerulonephritis is relatively rare, especially in cases with no previous history of heart disease like our case. Successful treatment of IE ameliorated hypocomplementemia and renal failure; thus C3 glomerulonephritis-like lesion in our case was classified as postinfectious glomerulonephritis. The present case highlights the broad differential diagnosis of renal involvement in IE, including C3 glomerulonephritis triggered by IE.

Conflict of Interests

The authors declare that there is no conflict of interests regarding the publication of this paper.

References

[1] J. Neugarten and D. S. Baldwin, "Glomerulonephritis in bacterial endocarditis," *The American Journal of Medicine*, vol. 77, no. 2, pp. 297–304, 1984.

[2] A. Majumdar, S. Chowdhary, M. A. Ferreira et al., "Renal pathological findings in infective endocarditis," *Nephrology Dialysis Transplantation*, vol. 15, no. 11, pp. 1782–1787, 2000.

[3] H. Peng, W.-F. Chen, C. Wu et al., "Culture-negative subacute bacterial endocarditis masquerades as granulomatosis with polyangiitis (Wegener's granulomatosis) involving both the kidney and lung," *BMC Nephrology*, vol. 13, article 174, 2012.

[4] F. Fakhouri, V. Frémeaux-Bacchi, L.-H. Noël, H. T. Cook, and M. C. Pickering, "C3 glomerulopathy: a new classification," *Nature Reviews Nephrology*, vol. 6, no. 8, pp. 494–499, 2010.

[5] S. Sethi, F. C. Fervenza, Y. Zhang et al., "Atypical postinfectious glomerulonephritis is associated with abnormalities in the alternative pathway of complement," *Kidney International*, vol. 83, no. 2, pp. 293–299, 2013.

[6] M. C. Pickering, V. D. D'agati, C. M. Nester et al., "C3 glomerulopathy: consensus report," *Kidney International*, vol. 84, no. 6, pp. 1079–1089, 2013.

[7] T. Nadasdy and F. G. Silva, "Acute postinfectious glomerulonephritis and glomerulonephritis caused by persistent bacterial infection," in *Heptinstall's Pathology of the Kidney*, J. C. Jemmette, J. L. Olspn, M. M. Schwartz, and F. G. Silva, Eds., pp. 321–396, Lippincott Williams and Wilkins, Philadelphia, Pa, USA, 6th edition, 2007.

[8] D. S. McKinsey, T. E. Ratts, and A. L. Bisno, "Underlying cardiac lesions in adults with infective endocarditis. The changing spectrum," *The American Journal of Medicine*, vol. 82, no. 4, pp. 681–688, 1987.

[9] A. Mahr, F. Batteux, S. Tubiana et al., "Brief report: prevalence of antineutrophil cytoplasmic antibodies in infective endocarditis," *Arthritis and Rheumatology*, vol. 66, no. 6, pp. 1672–1677, 2014.

[10] J. A. Long and W. J. Cook, "IgA deposits and acute glomerulonephritis in a patient with staphylococcal infection," *American Journal of Kidney Diseases*, vol. 48, no. 5, pp. 851–855, 2006.

[11] T. Uchida, T. Oda, A. Watanabe et al., "Clinical and histologic resolution of poststreptococcal glomerulonephritis with large subendothelial deposits and kidney failure," *American Journal of Kidney Diseases*, vol. 58, no. 1, pp. 113–117, 2011.

[12] C. Rabasco-Ruiz, A. Huerta-Arroyo, J. Caro-Espada, E. Gutiérrez-Martínez, and M. Praga-Terente, "C3 glomerulopathies. A new perspective on glomerular diseases," *Nefrologia*, vol. 33, no. 2, pp. 164–170, 2013.

[13] G. Sandhu, A. Bansal, A. Ranade, J. Jones, S. Cortell, and G. S. Markowitz, "C3 glomerulopathy masquerading as acute postinfectious glomerulonephritis," *The American Journal of Kidney Diseases*, vol. 60, no. 6, pp. 1039–1043, 2012.

[14] I. J. Messias-Reason, S. Y. Hayashi, R. M. Nisihara, and M. Kirschfink, "Complement activation in infective endocarditis: correlation with extracardiac manifestations and prognosis," *Clinical and Experimental Immunology*, vol. 127, no. 2, pp. 310–315, 2002.

[15] L. Morel-Maroger, J. D. Sraer, G. Herreman, and P. Godeau, "Kidney in subacute endocarditis. Pathological and immunofluorescence findings," *Archives of Pathology*, vol. 94, no. 3, pp. 205–213, 1972.

44

Granulomatous Interstitial Nephritis Presenting as Hypercalcemia and Nephrolithiasis

Saika Sharmeen,[1] **Esra Kalkan,**[1] **Chunhui Yi,**[2] **and Steven D. Smith**[3]

[1]Department of Medicine, Mount Sinai St. Luke's-Roosevelt Hospital Center, New York, NY 10025, USA
[2]Department of Pathology, Mount Sinai St. Luke's-Roosevelt Hospital Center, New York, NY 10025, USA
[3]Department of Medicine, Division of Nephrology, Mount Sinai St. Luke's-Roosevelt Hospital Center, New York, NY 10025, USA

Correspondence should be addressed to Saika Sharmeen; ssharmeen@chpnet.org

Academic Editor: Ze'ev Korzets

We report a case of acute kidney injury as the initial manifestation of sarcoidosis. A 55-year-old male was sent from his primary care physician's office with incidental lab findings significant for hypercalcemia and acute kidney injury with past medical history significant for nephrolithiasis. Initial treatment with intravenous hydration did not improve his condition. The renal biopsy subsequently revealed granulomatous interstitial nephritis (GIN). Treatment with the appropriate dose of glucocorticoids improved both the hypercalcemia and renal function. Our case demonstrates that renal limited GIN due to sarcoidosis, although a rare entity, can cause severe acute kidney injury and progressive renal failure unless promptly diagnosed and treated.

1. Background

Granulomatous interstitial nephritis (GIN) is a rare cause of acute kidney injury (AKI). Causes of GIN include sarcoidosis, drugs (NSAIDs, antibiotics), and infections (mycobacterial, fungal, bacterial, and viral). Renal involvement as an initial manifestation of sarcoidosis is another rare entity. Renal failure commonly ranges from 0.7% to 4.3% in cases series of patients with previously identified sarcoidosis [1]. The majority of sarcoid related renal failure in these cases is due to two pathologic processes: (1) nephrocalcinosis with or without nephrolithiasis and (2) interstitial nephritis with or without granulomas. We report a case of GIN causing acute kidney injury as the initial presentation of sarcoidosis.

2. Clinical Case

A 55-year-old man was sent from his primary care physician's office with incidental findings of severe hypercalcemia and acute kidney injury (AKI). His medical history was significant for nephrolithiasis and ureteral stone removal one year prior to presentation at which time the serum creatinine was 2.05 mg/dL with a calcium of 10.5 mg/dL. No further

work-up was performed at that time. On presentation he was not taking any medications or using alcohol, tobacco, or illicit drugs. He had no prior surgeries. He denied cough, shortness of breath, polyuria, polydipsia, bone pain, and abdominal pain but complained of chronic low back pain and a 20 lb weight loss over the previous several months. The blood pressure was 165/102 mmHg, heart rate was 80, and he was afebrile. Physical exam was otherwise unremarkable with a clear chest, no peripheral lymphadenopathy, no rash, and no edema. Laboratories (Table 1) were remarkable for Ca 13.5 mg/dL, creatinine 7.6 mg/dL, and phosphorus 7.4 mg/dL. Urinalysis showed calcium-oxalate crystals with 4–10 RBCs/HPF with normal morphology and the urine albumin/creatinine ratio was normal at 24 mg/g. Evaluation of the hypercalcemia revealed the following: PTH < 3 (11–67 pg/mL), 25-hydroxyvitamin D 23.8 (30–95 ng/mL), 1,25-dihydroxyvitamin D 79 (18–72 pg/mL), and angiotensin converting enzyme (ACE) level 82 (9–67 U/L) (Table 2). Serum and urine immunofixations did not detect a monoclonal protein. A skeletal survey showed no lytic or blastic osseous lesions. Thyroid function tests were normal. His chest X-ray was negative and PFTs (pulmonary function tests) were normal but a computed tomography (CT) scan

TABLE 1: Lab values during hospitalization and after discharge.

Variable	Baseline labs, 6 months before admission	Hospital day 1	Hospital day 2	Hospital day 6	Hospital day 12,1 time dexamethasone was given	Hospital Day 16 (prednisone 60 mg Qd started)	Day 18 (discharge day)	15 days after discharge	Reference range
Sodium	139	135	134	136	138	138	135	139	136–146 mmol/L
Potassium	4.4	5.3	5.3	4.9	5.2	5.1	4.3	4.9	3.5–5.1 mmol/L
Chloride	104	101	106	112	104	110	111	104	96–107 mmol/L
Carbon dioxide	25	21	17	18	16	17	17	19	22–30 mmol/L
Blood urea nitrogen	23	57	57	40	57	65	67	68	8–24 mmol/dl
Creatinine	1.79	7.59	7.6	6.49	6.79	4.98	4.52	2.89	0.66–1.25 mg/dL
Glucose	137	167	148	99	106	216	145	94	74–106 mg/dL
eGFR	40	8	7	9	9	12	14	23	>90
Calcium	10.5	13.5	12.9	10.9	13.1	9.3	8.1	9.6	8.4–10.3 mg/dL
Corrected calcium*	10.4	Unable to calculate	13.4	11.8	13.2	10.3	Unable to calculate	9.8	8.5–10.5 mg/dL
Ionized Ca	Not checked	Not checked	1.7	Not checked	Not checked	Not checked	Not checked	Not checked	1.16–1.32 mmol/L
Phosphorus, inorganic	Not checked	7.4	6.1	4.7	7.5	Not checked	Not checked	3.4	2.5–4.5 mg/dL
Protein, total	7.3	Not checked	6	5.5	7.2	5.3	Not checked	6.2	6.3–8.2 g/dL
Albumin	4.1	Not checked	3.4	2.9	3.9	2.8	Not checked	3.7	3.5–5 g/dL
Bilirubin, total	0.6	Not checked	0.6	0.3	0.5	0.3	Not checked	0.4	0.2–1.3 mg/dL
Bilirubin, direct	0.1	Not checked	Not checked	Not checked	Not checked	0.2	Not checked	0.3	0.0–0.4 mg/dL
ALP	68	Not checked	43	42	113	66	Not checked	67	38–126 U/L
AST	26	Not checked	22	21	23	28	Not checked	20	15–46 U/L
ALT	24	Not checked	23	28	39	52	Not checked	25	13–69 U/L
WBC	12.8	12.8	13.2	8.6	10.8	18.7	13.1	14.8	3.4–11 k/μL
Hemoglobin	13	13	11.2	10.6	12.1	10.3	9.9	12.4	13.0–17 g/dL
Hct	39.2	39.2	33.6	33.1	37.2	32.1	31.8	37	38–51%
Platelet	386	386	302	298	295	306	105	300	150–450 k/μL
MCV	83.2	83.3	84.1	85.9	85.3	85.9	85.5	87.6	80–100 fL
Eosinophils (%)	5.2	5.2	3.9	6.7	7.1	0.4	Not checked	2.1	0.0–0.6%
Neutrophil (%)	77.6	77.6	77.8	70	69	91.1	Not checked	91	40–74%
Lymphocytes (%)	9	9	10	12.7	13.6	4.8	Not checked	4.3	18–44
Monocytes (%)	7.7	7.7	7.9	10.1	10.1	3.7	Not checked	2.4	4.7–12.0%
Basophil (%)	0.3	0.5	0.4	0.5	0.2	0	Not checked	0.2	0.1–1.4%

*The normal albumin level is defaulted to 4.

TABLE 2: Lab values.

Variable	Measurement	Reference range
LDH	478	313–618 U/L
Creatinine kinase	40	55–170
Cholesterol, total	187	<200 mg/dL
HDL	28	>40 mg/dL
LDL	87	<130 mg/dL
Cholesterol/HDL ratio	6.7	0.0–4.9
Triglycerides	362	<151 mg/dL
ESR	26	1–13 mm/hr
CRP	Not checked	
ACE, before steroid treatment	82	9–67 U/L
ACE, after steroid treatment	24	9–67 U/L
Vit D, 25 hydroxy	27.8	30–95 bng/mL
Vit D, 1,25 hydroxy, before steroid treatment	79	18–72 pg/mL
Vit D, 1,25 hydroxy, after steroid treatment	19	18–72 pg/mL
PTH, intact	3.72	11–67 pg/mL
ANA	Negative	Negative
Immunofixation, serum	Polyclonal pattern	
IgG, serum	1330	700–1600 mg/dL
IgA, serum	187	70–400 mg/dL
IgM, serum	44	40–230 mg/dL
Immunofixatin elec., urine	Polyclonal IGG and polyclonal light chains	
Protein, random urine	10	mg/dL
C3	119	90–180 mg/dL
C4	22	10–40 mg/dL
Quantiferon-Tb gold	Indeterminate	
Mitogen-nil	0.16	IU/ML
NIL	0.03	IU/ML
TB Ag-nil	0	IU/ML
ASO Ab	46	>200 IU/ML
ANCA vasculitides		
Proteinase 3 Ab	<1.0	<1.0
Myeloperoxidase Ab	<1.0	<1.0
Hep A Ab, IgM	Nonreactive	Nonreactive
Hep A Ab, total	Reactive	Nonreactive
Hep B sAg	Negative	Negative
Hep B Core Ab, total	Reactive	Nonreactive
Hep BS ab	Reactive	Nonreactive
HepC Ab	Negative	Negative
HIV 1/2 Ab screen, rapid	Nonreactive	Nonreactive
HgbA1c	6.9	4.2–5.9%
Urine culture	Negative	Negative
Urine chemistry		
Protein, random urine	21	mg/dL
Microalbumin, random, urine	2.4	mg/dL
Sodium, random, urine	105	30–90 mmol/L
Potassium, random, urine	14.9	mmol/L
Calcium, random, urine	11.4	mg/dL
Thyroxine, free	0.61	0.8–1.5 ng/dL
TSH	1.038	0.4–4.2 μIU/mL
PSA free	0.9	ng/mL
PSA percent free	43	>25%
Total PSA	2.1	≤4.0

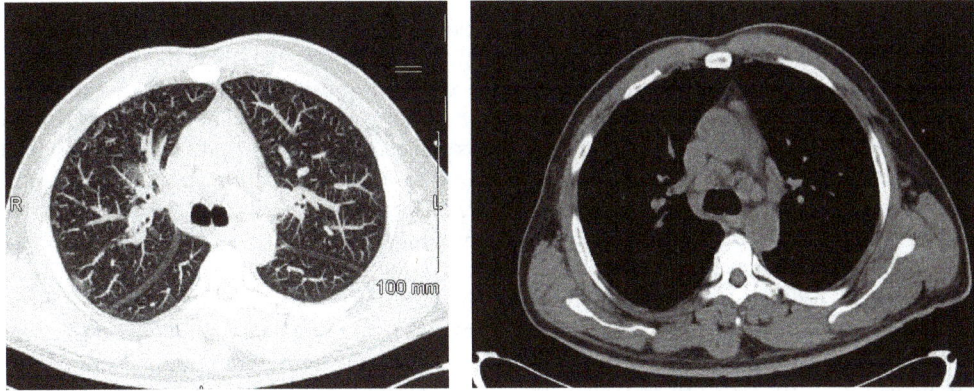

FIGURE 1: CT chest without IV contrast. Computed tomography without intravenous contrast showing mediastinal and hilar adenopathy.

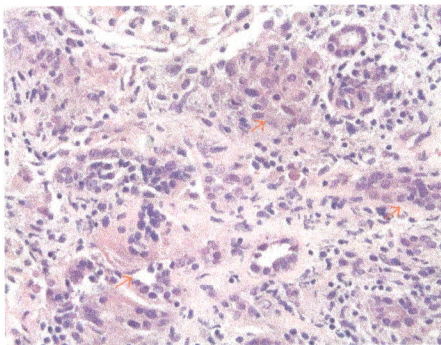

FIGURE 2: Renal Biopsy. Noncaseating granulomatous inflammation. Aggregation of epithelioid histiocytes aggregation (arrows), mixed with lymphocytes, forming granuloma. Hematoxylin and eosin (HE) stain 400x.

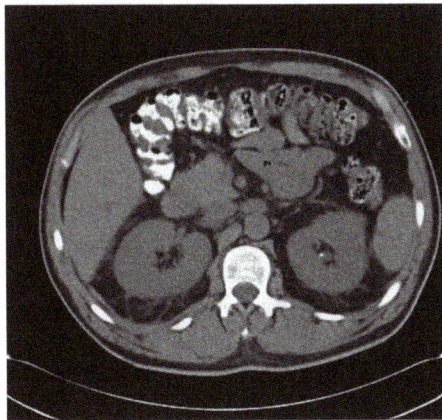

FIGURE 3: CT of abdomen and pelvis without IV contrast. CT of abdomen and pelvis without IV contrast showing a 3 mm nonobstructing left renal calculus with normal size kidneys and no nephrocalcinosis.

of the chest without contras showed mediastinal and hilar lymphadenopathy (Figure 1). An abdominal and pelvic CT showed a 3 mm nonobstructing left renal calculus with normal size kidneys and no nephrocalcinosis (Figure 3). Renal biopsy (Figure 2) showed granulomatous interstitial nephritis

with diffuse interstitial inflammation with focal noncaseating granulomas. Acid-Fast Bacillus (AFB) and Grocott-Gomori's stain were negative for mycobacteria or fungal elements. Immunofluorescent microscopy demonstrated no significant staining for IgG, IgA, IgM, C3, C1q, kappa, lambda light chains, or fibrinogen. A diagnosis of sarcoid was made. The patient was initially treated with intravenous normal saline with improvement in serum calcium but no improvement in his serum creatinine. His calcium rebounded. There was suspicion for intrinsic renal disease as opposed to renal failure based on these findings. The patient was then started on prednisone 40 mg/day and the decision was made to obtain renal biopsy for definitive diagnosis. Once the renal biopsy results showed GIN, the patient was started on IV methylprednisone 60 mg/d for three days after which oral prednisone was continued at 1 mg/kg/day with slow taper planned over 12–18 months. With the addition of the higher dose of steroids his calcium normalized to 8.6 mg/dL and the creatinine decreased to 4.5 mg/dL on discharge. Six months after discharge his creatinine improved to 2.55 mg/dL and has remained stable with a normal serum calcium. With steroid treatment the 1,25-dihydroxyvitamin D level decreased to 19 (18–72 pg/mL) and ACE level normalized at 24 (9–67 U/L).

3. Discussion

Sarcoidosis is a systemic disease of unknown cause that is characterized by the formation of immune granulomas in various organs, mainly the lungs and the lymphatic system [2]. Sarcoidosis can involve any organ but in more than 90 percent of patients it manifests with pulmonary involvement. Respiratory symptoms include cough, shortness of breath, and chest discomfort [3]. Most patients with GIN due to sarcoidosis present with extrarenal manifestations such as pulmonary, skin, or eye involvement [4, 5]. However, there are a few series reporting sarcoid GIN without extrarenal involvement [6–8]. Our patient did not have any respiratory symptoms and had a normal chest X-ray in addition to normal PFTs. His chest CT showed asymptomatic mediastinal and hilar lymphadenopathy. Renal failure commonly ranges from 0.7% to 4.3% of cases in previous reported clinical series of patients with sarcoidosis but renal failure from GIN itself is rare [1, 9]. A previous study found that 46 of 9,779 (0.5%) renal biopsy specimens had GIN [10]. The pathology contributing to AKI from GIN in sarcoidosis is thought to be due to noncaseating granulomatous inflammation, which is composed of a central follicle of macrophages, epithelioid cells, and multinucleated giant cells [9, 11, 12].

Hypercalcemia, a well-known metabolic complication of sarcoidosis, is only found in 10–20 percent of patients and can directly cause acute kidney injury from renal vasoconstriction and volume depletion as a result of nephrogenic diabetes insipidus [13]. Hypercalcemia is due to overproduction of 1,25-dihydroxy vitamin D. The normal conversion of 25-hydroxyvitamin D to 1,25-dihydroxyvitamin D (calcitriol) occurs in the kidney through 1-α hydroxylase, a cytochrome p 450 enzyme [9, 14]. In sarcoidosis and other granulomatous diseases pulmonary macrophages express 1-α hydroxylase, which is often resistant to negative feedback mechanisms causing overproduction of l,25-(OH)2-D3 [9, 15] leading to increased calcium uptake by the gut. Adams et al. demonstrated that l,25-(OH)2-D3 is the hypercalcemia-causing factor in sarcoidosis and that macrophages from patients with sarcoidosis are the synthetic source of hormone in the disease. Mason et al. identified a similar metabolite in preparations of sarcoid granulomas incubated with 25-OH-D [11, 16, 17]. In patients with sarcoid, hypercalciuria is three times more common than hypercalcemia [11, 18] with a frequency in some studies as high as 60% [19]. Both can lead to acute and chronic kidney injury in sarcoidosis by causing nephrolithiasis and nephrocalcinosis. Hypercalcemia and hypercalciuria contribute to the formation of calcium oxalate crystals which was likely the cause of nephrolithiasis in our patient. Interstitial calcium oxalate deposition is also seen in association with granulomas in sarcoidosis [20].

The differential diagnosis of hypercalcemia was initially broad for our patient and included hyperparathyroidism, malignancy related (multiple myeloma, lymphoma, PTHrp associated malignancy, and metastatic bone disease), infections such as tuberculosis, sarcoid, and vitamin D intoxication. Laboratory assessment narrowed the differential with an appropriately suppressed PTH and a low 25-hydroxyvitamin D level. The negative serum and urine immunofixations and absence of lytic or blastic lesions on a skeletal survey made malignancy less likely. The elevated ACE and 1,25-dihydroxyvitamin D level made sarcoid a strong possibility but lymphomas can also cause increased production of 1,25-D. Intrinsic renal disease was higher on the differential rather than renal failure from nephrocalcinosis based on the following reasons: (1) while the hypercalcemia was slowly improving with intravenous hydration, the serum creatinine did not improve. (2) the CT of the abdomen and pelvis showed a 3 mm nonobstructing left renal calculus with normal size kidneys and no nephrocalcinosis (Figure 3). Moreover, the renal biopsy was required for definitive diagnosis. In sarcoidosis, with the exception of Löfgren's syndrome, all other suspected cases require a biopsy specimen to establish diagnosis from the involved organ that is most easily accessed [21]. In our patient, the involved organ was the kidney. Since the patient had renal symptoms and no pulmonary symptoms (PFTs were normal and there were no clinical pulmonary symptoms) or skin involvement, the decision was made to proceed with a renal biopsy. It was ultimately the renal biopsy which demonstrated GIN in the absence of another cause that led to a diagnosis and an effective treatment plan.

The primary treatment option for GIN due to sarcoidosis is glucocorticoid therapy. Renal limited sarcoidosis with GIN is a rare occurrence but several case reports suggest that these patients do well with corticosteroid treatment [22–24] although Ikeda et al. report a case of GIN due to sarcoidosis requiring dialysis [25]. Early diagnosis and treatment may be necessary to prevent progression. Robson et al. hypothesized that idiopathic granulomatous interstitial nephritis may actually represent a renal-limited form of sarcoid. It may be associated with hypercalcemia and an elevated serum angiotensin-converting enzyme and usually responds to treatment with corticosteroids. They describe a number of patients with biopsy proven GIN without extrarenal sarcoid who also presented with hypercalcemia and renal failure all of whom responded well to steroids [26]. Hilderson et al. present a detailed overview of current treatment options for renal sarcoid with hypercalcemia. They highlight the fact that treatment guidelines are lacking and that a uniform approach is needed in treating these patients. Variation exists between the treatment of hypercalcemia in sarcoidosis and GIN sarcoidosis. Hypercalcemia in sarcoidosis is initially treated with IV saline hydration followed by prednisone at a dose of 0.3–0.5 mg/kg once daily with a maintenance dose of 5–10 mg/day and the total duration of treatment being at least 12 months. However, for GIN sarcoidosis, they suggest three days of intravenous methylprednisolone followed by oral prednisone 1 mg/kg/d in patients with major organ impairment. The dose of steroids may vary depending on severity of disease with total duration of treatment being 18–24 months including a steroid taper. In cases of glucocorticoid failure or contraindications, immunosuppressive agents such as azathioprine or mycophenolate mofetil have been used. In cases of steroid resistant sarcoidosis and when at least one other immunosuppressive agent has been tried, TNF-alpha inhibitors have shown promise [27, 28]. Our patient was initially started on prednisone 40 mg per day while awaiting the results of the renal biopsy; once the biopsy results showed GIN the patient's treatment was tailored towards the diagnosis with significant improvement in overall condition. Thus, a renal biopsy should be performed when the suspicion for renal sarcoidosis is high without any other organ involvement in order to make a definitive diagnosis and guide management.

In conclusion, sarcoidosis is a disease involving multiple different organs including the kidney. Acute kidney injury as the initial presentation of sarcoidosis as was seen in our case is a rare entity. It is necessary to combine clinical presentation, laboratory results, and renal pathology to make a correct diagnosis which often responds well to treatment with steroids.

Conflict of Interests

The authors declare that there is no conflict of interests regarding the publication of this paper.

References

[1] M. Mahévas, F. X. Lescure, J.-J. Boffa et al., "Renal sarcoidosis: clinical, laboratory, and histologic presentation and outcome in 47 patients," *Medicine*, vol. 88, no. 2, pp. 98–106, 2009.

[2] D. Valeyre, A. Prasse, H. Nunes, Y. Uzunhan, P.-Y. Brillet, and J. Müller-Quernheim, "Sarcoidosis," *The Lancet*, vol. 383, no. 9923, pp. 1155–1167, 2014.

[3] A. S. Morgenthau and M. C. Iannuzzi, "Recent advances in sarcoidosis," *Chest*, vol. 139, no. 1, pp. 174–182, 2011.

[4] N. Joss, S. Morris, B. Young, and C. Geddes, "Granulomatous interstitial nephritis," *Clinical Journal of the American Society of Nephrology*, vol. 2, no. 2, pp. 222–230, 2007.

[5] A. Ikeda, S. Nagai, M. Kitaichi et al., "Sarcoidosis with granulomatous interstitial nephritis: report of three cases," *Internal Medicine*, vol. 40, no. 3, pp. 241–245, 2001.

[6] T. Hannedouche, G. Grateau, L. H. Noel et al., "Renal granulomatous sarcoidosis: report of six cases," *Nephrology Dialysis Transplantation*, vol. 5, no. 1, pp. 18–24, 1990.

[7] P. Nagaraja and M. R. Davies, "Granulomatous interstitial nephritis causing acute renal failure: a rare presenting feature of sarcoidosis," *QJM*, vol. 107, no. 6, pp. 467–469, 2014.

[8] J. Rema, M. Carvalho, R. Vaz et al., "Acute renal failure as a form of presentation of sarcoidosis in a young adult: a case report," *Journal of Medical Case Reports*, vol. 8, no. 1, article 274, 2014.

[9] V. Manjunath, G. Moeckel, and N. K. Dahl, "Acute kidney injury in a patient with sarcoidosis: hypercalciuria and hypercalcemia leading to calcium phosphate deposition," *Clinical Nephrology*, vol. 80, no. 2, pp. 151–155, 2013.

[10] V. Bijol, G. P. Mendez, V. Nosé, and H. G. Rennke, "Granulomatous interstitial nephritis: a clinicopathologic study of 46 cases from a single institution," *International Journal of Surgical Pathology*, vol. 14, no. 1, pp. 57–63, 2006.

[11] P. D. Thomas and G. W. Hunninghake, "Current concepts of the pathogenesis of sarcoidosis," *American Review of Respiratory Disease*, vol. 135, no. 3, pp. 747–760, 1987.

[12] S. Kobak, "Sarcoidosis: a rheumatologist's perspective," *Therapeutic Advances in Musculoskeletal Disease*, vol. 7, no. 5, pp. 196–205, 2015.

[13] O. P. Sharma, "Vitamin D, calcium, and sarcoidosis," *Chest*, vol. 109, no. 2, pp. 535–539, 1996.

[14] D. G. Gardner, "Hypercalcemia and sarcoidosis—another piece of the puzzle falls into place," *American Journal of Medicine*, vol. 110, no. 9, pp. 736–737, 2001.

[15] H. Reichel, H. P. Koeffler, R. Barbers, and A. W. Norman, "Regulation of 1,25-dihydroxyvitamin D_3 production by cultured alveolar macrophages from normal human donors and from patients with pulmonary sarcoidosis," *The Journal of Clinical Endocrinology & Metabolism*, vol. 65, no. 6, pp. 1201–1209, 1987.

[16] R. S. Mason, T. Frankel, Y. L. Chan, D. Lissner, and S. Posen, "Vitamin D conversion by sarcoid lymph node homogenate," *Annals of Internal Medicine*, vol. 100, no. 1, pp. 59–61, 1984.

[17] J. S. Adams, O. P. Sharma, M. A. Gacad, and F. R. Singer, "Metabolism of 25-hydroxyvitamin D3 by cultured pulmonary alveolar macrophages in sarcoidosis," *The Journal of Clinical Investigation*, vol. 72, no. 5, pp. 1856–1860, 1983.

[18] O. P. Sharma, J. Trowell, N. Cohen et al., "Abnormal calcium metabolism in sarcoidosis," in *La Sarcoidose: Rapport, IV Conférence Internationale*, J. Turiaf and J. Chabot, Eds., pp. 627–632, Maison et Cie, 1967.

[19] E. Lebacq, H. Verhaegen, and V. Desmet, "Renal involvement in sarcoidosis," *Postgraduate Medical Journal*, vol. 46, no. 538, pp. 526–529, 1970.

[20] J. D. Reid and M. E. Andersen, "Calcium oxalate in sarcoid granulomas. With particular reference to the small ovoid body and a note on the finding of dolomite," *American Journal of Clinical Pathology*, vol. 90, no. 5, pp. 545–558, 1988.

[21] M. C. Iannuzzi, B. A. Rybicki, and A. S. Teirstein, "Sarcoidosis," *The New England Journal of Medicine*, vol. 357, no. 21, pp. 2153–2165, 2007.

[22] M. Brause, K. Magnusson, S. Degenhardt, U. Helmchen, and B. Grabensee, "Renal involvement in sarcoidosis—a report of 6 cases," *Clinical Nephrology*, vol. 57, no. 2, pp. 142–148, 2002.

[23] Z. Korzets, M. Schneider, R. Taragan, J. Bernheim, and J. Bernheim, "Acute renal failure due to sarcoid granulomatous infiltration of the renal parenchyma," *American Journal of Kidney Diseases*, vol. 6, no. 4, pp. 250–253, 1985.

[24] P. F. Williams, D. Thomson, and J. L. Anderton, "Reversible renal failure due to isolated renal sarcoidosis," *Nephron*, vol. 37, no. 4, pp. 246–249, 1984.

[25] S. Ikeda, T. Hoshino, and T. Nakamura, "A case of sarcoidosis with severe acute renal failure requiring dialysis," *Clinical Nephrology*, vol. 82, no. 4, pp. 273–277, 2014.

[26] M. G. Robson, D. Banerjee, D. Hopster, and H. S. Cairns, "Seven cases of granulomatous interstitial nephritis in the absence of extrarenal sarcoid," *Nephrology Dialysis Transplantation*, vol. 18, no. 2, pp. 280–284, 2003.

[27] I. Hilderson, S. Van Laecke, A. Wauters, and J. Donck, "Treatment of renal sarcoidosis: is there a guideline? Overview of the different treatment options," *Nephrology, Dialysis, Transplantation*, vol. 29, no. 10, pp. 1841–1847, 2014.

[28] J. Thumfart, D. Müller, B. Rudolph, M. Zimmering, U. Querfeld, and D. Haffner, "Isolated sarcoid granulomatous interstitial nephritis responding to infliximab therapy," *American Journal of Kidney Diseases*, vol. 45, no. 2, pp. 411–414, 2005.

45

Three-Dimensional Imaging of a Central Venous Dialysis Catheter Related Infected Thrombus

Diana Yuan Yng Chiu,[1,2] **Darren Green,**[1,2] **Philip A. Kalra,**[1,2] **and Nik Abidin**[3]

[1]*Vascular Research Group, Institute of Population Health, The University of Manchester, Manchester Academic Health Sciences Centre, Manchester M13 9PL, UK*
[2]*Department of Renal Medicine, Salford Royal NHS Foundation Trust, Stott Lane, Salford M6 8HD, UK*
[3]*Department of Cardiology, Salford Royal Hospital, Salford Royal NHS Foundation Trust, Stott Lane, Salford M6 8HD, UK*

Correspondence should be addressed to Nik Abidin; nik.abidin@srft.nhs.uk

Academic Editor: Kostas C. Siamopoulos

Three-dimensional (3D) echocardiography is becoming widely available and with novel applications. We report an interesting case of a 68-year-old lady with a central venous thrombosis coincident with both a dialysis catheter infection and a recent pacemaker insertion. Two-dimensional transesophageal echocardiography was unable to delineate whether the thrombosis was involved with the pacemaker wire or due to the tunneled catheter infection. The use of 3D echocardiography was able to produce distinct images aiding diagnosis. This circumvented the need for invasive investigations and inappropriate, high-risk removal of the pacing wire. This case highlights the emerging application of 3D echocardiography in routine nephrology practice.

1. Introduction

Central venous catheters are a crucial form of access for hemodialysis, especially when providing acute dialysis therapy or as a therapeutic bridge whilst waiting for an arteriovenous graft formation. But dialysis catheters are not without risks. Thrombosis is one well-recognized complication, second in prevalence to catheter related infection. Contrast venography is considered the gold standard for visualization of central venous thrombosis. However, this is invasive and associated with contrast and radiation exposure. We present the case of a lady who had a dialysis catheter related thrombus in which two-dimensional (2D) imaging could not delineate the extent of thrombus and the novel application of three-dimensional (3D) echocardiography aided diagnosis.

2. Case Presentation

2.1. Clinical History and Initial Laboratory Data. A 68-year-old lady with End Stage Kidney Disease (ESKD) secondary to IgA nephropathy had been established on maintenance hemodialysis for three years via a tunneled central venous dialysis catheter. She presented with fever after a routine dialysis session having had a change of tunneled dialysis catheter due to a split in the catheter 6 weeks before. She had no focal symptoms such as dysuria or productive cough to indicate an alternative source of infection. Other medical history included type 2 diabetes mellitus, hypothyroidism, and an aortic tissue valve replacement for severe aortic stenosis two months previously. This was complicated by complete heart block and a pacemaker inserted. She was a nonsmoker and did not drink alcohol. Medications were simvastatin and levothyroxine. On physical examination, the patient was febrile with temperature 38.2°C, blood pressure 112/72 mmHg, heart rate 105 beats/min, respiratory rate 20 breaths/min, and oxygen saturations 99% on air. Her chest was clear on auscultation, jugular venous pressure was not raised, and cardiac heart sounds were heard with a grade 2 apical pansystolic murmur. She had pitting sacral edema, but no splinter hemorrhages, Roth's spots, or Janeway lesions.

Laboratory tests showed albumin 3 g/dL, hemoglobin 8.4 g/dL, white blood cell count 3.7 × 10^3/μL, platelets 86 × 10^3/μL, and C-reactive protein 126 mg/L. Urine culture

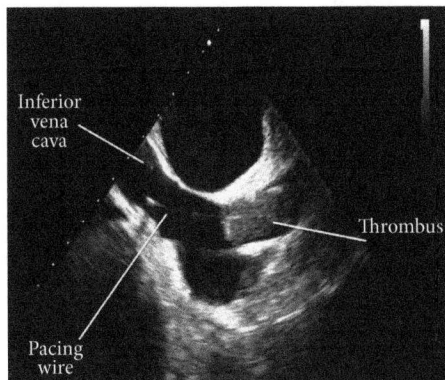

FIGURE 1: Transesophageal echocardiogram demonstrating a large thrombus in the superior vena cava. The pacing wire appears to overlay the thrombus. Because this is a 2D image, hence no spatial depth, it is unclear if there is a space between the thrombus and wire or whether it is independent of this.

displayed mixed growth without pyuria. An electrocardiogram showed sinus rhythm, and a plain chest radiograph confirmed a right tunnelled central venous dialysis catheter and left pacemaker wire *in situ*, but no other abnormalities. Central and peripheral blood cultures were positive with *Staphylococcus aureus* sensitive to vancomycin, gentamicin, and rifampicin.

2.2. Imaging Studies. Dialysis catheter associated infection with possible infective endocarditis was the presumed diagnosis and therefore the central venous dialysis catheter was removed under local anesthetic. The patient then underwent a 2D transesophageal echocardiogram that demonstrated normal heart valves but showed a large thrombus at the superior vena cava/right atrial junction with some protrusion into the right atrial cavity and in proximity to her pacing wire. It was not possible to delineate the spatial relationship of the thrombus to the pacemaker wire because the ultrasound image can only depict a sector, originating from the rotation axis of the transducer (Figure 1). It was therefore not clear whether the infection and/or thrombus was caused by or involved the pacing wire. This is a vital consideration as there would be increased technical difficulty and risk of thrombus dislodgement for pacemaker removal if the thrombus was entangled with the pacemaker wire. Therefore, using the same echocardiography machine and with selection of the 3D function (echocardiography machine, Philips IE 33 x MATRIX; Transducer: X5-1; 3D analysis software: QLAB 9), 3D images were acquired (Figure 2). These images clearly demonstrated the tracts of the pacemaker wires (2 pacing leads: right atrial and right ventricular leads) and showed that the venous thrombosis was separate from the wires.

2.3. Diagnosis. A diagnosis of infected venous thrombosis without involvement of pacemaker wire was therefore reliably made. This meant that there was no need for further invasive investigation and also that no inappropriate, high-risk attempts to remove and replace the pacing wire were undertaken.

2.4. Clinical Follow-Up. The patient received sensitivity-specific antibiotics for 4 weeks and was commenced on peritoneal dialysis. She was warfarinized to an international normalized ratio target of 2.5 intended for lifelong treatment. Her fever settled and she was discharged without the need for pacemaker removal.

3. Discussion

The reported incidence of central catheter venous thrombosis varies between 1.5 and 33% depending on the definition [1, 2]. Factors that predispose to thrombosis are described in Virchow's triad: hypercoagulability, hemodynamic disturbance (stasis or turbulence), and endothelial damage. The risk factors associated with tunneled dialysis catheters are multiple lumen [3], catheters *in situ* for >2 weeks, and multiple previous catheter insertions at the same site. Our patient had a recent pacemaker insertion, cardiac surgery, and exchange of tunneled dialysis catheter and therefore had repeated vascular trauma.

In this case, the thrombosis was further complicated by infection. The fibrin sheath formed around the catheter lumen and external portions provide an ideal surface for microorganisms such as *Staphylococcus aureus* and *Staphylococcus epidermidis* to adhere to [4]. In turn, the infection increases the incidence of thrombosis.

The novelty in this case rests on the use of 3D echocardiographic imaging to delineate the course of the thrombosis. Contrast venography is considered the gold standard for diagnosis of catheter related deep vein thrombosis. However, this investigation requires radiation exposure and intravenous contrast which may be problematic for dialysis patients who are sensitive to a fluid load or allergic to contrast agents. Furthermore, the image obtained with venography may only demonstrate a filling defect and it may be difficult to visualize the exact involvement of wires in relation to the thrombus.

For this patient the thrombosis was identified by transesophageal echocardiography performed to detect infective endocarditis. This was easy to perform and did not require intravenous contrast. However, 2D transesophageal echocardiography could not accurately delineate the course of the thrombosis (Figure 1). Due to inadequate spatial visualization it is unclear whether the pacemaker wire is entangled with the thrombus or independent of this, but with 3D echocardiography a clear diagnosis was obtained. Moreover, 3D echocardiography was carried out in the same sitting with the same machine.

Real time 3D echocardiography is an advanced technique that is becoming widely available in clinical practice. A 3D image is acquired in a manner similar to 2D echocardiography with a specialised transducer. A pyramidal volume of tissue is scanned with the apex at the probe. The images may then be manipulated in different ways by the echocardiographic software to allow visualization from different angles. Image may be rotated in three different axes (viewed from top to bottom, front to back, or left to right) or progressively sliced to the plane of interest. As a result, the depth of the image may be appreciated much better than 2D echocardiographic images and provides better visualization of adjacent cardiac

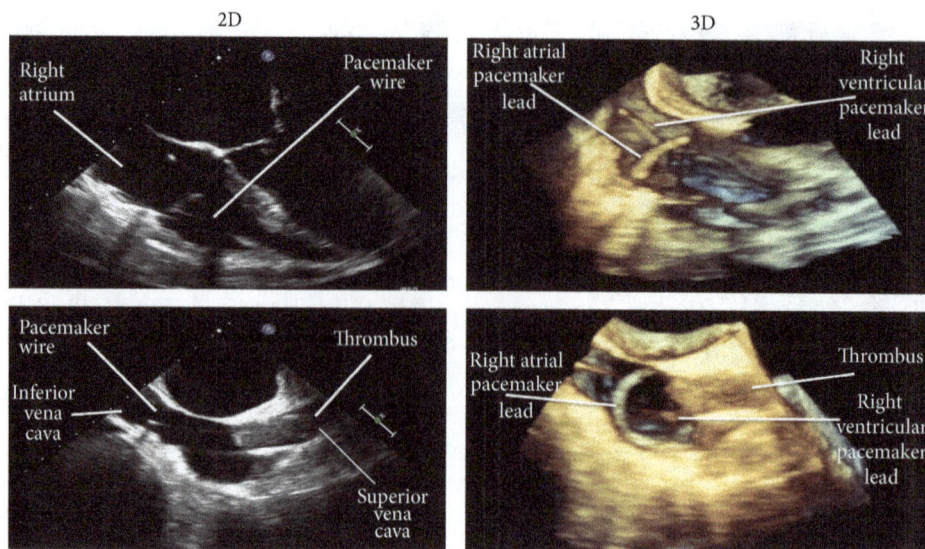

FIGURE 2: 3D echocardiogram demonstrated the tract of the pacemaker wires clearly and showed that the venous thrombosis was separate from the pacemaker wires. In comparison, 2D echocardiography is less distinct.

structures and masses (e.g., thrombus). For this patient, use of 3D imaging subverted the need for the invasive contrast venography.

The image produced by 3D is easy to interpret, even by a nonspecialist (Figure 2). A more common application for 3D echocardiography is in measurements of left ventricular mass and function. Limitations of 2D echocardiography in determining left ventricular ejection fraction and mass are that it involves calculations that assume the left ventricle to be elliptical in shape and frequently 2D echocardiography Forshortens the left ventricular apex; hence, there will be inaccuracies in the measurements. 3D echocardiography does not make any geometric assumptions and hence has been shown to produce calculations of left ventricular volume and ejection fraction comparable to the gold standard of cardiac magnetic resonance [5, 6]. Furthermore, there is reduced interobserver variability and high reproducibility compared with conventional 2D echocardiography [7]. As a result, this has been utilized in research studies in patients with chronic kidney disease and end stage renal failure for more accurate cardiac volume assessments [8, 9]. In this case, we demonstrate another useful application of 3D echocardiography in patients with ESKD undergoing hemodialysis via a tunneled venous catheter.

Treatment of tunneled dialysis catheter related thrombosis prevents later complications such as pulmonary embolism, vascular compromise of the limb, or death. There is no standardized method of treatment, although it may involve thrombolysis, systemic anticoagulants, and/or removal of catheter [10]. In this case, the lady responded well to treatment, dialysis catheter was removed safely, and the pacing wire was left *in situ* with no adverse events.

In conclusion, we present a case whereby the use of 3D echocardiography has provided an accurate diagnosis and aided management for an infected dialysis catheter related venous thrombosis. It is likely that further clinical applications may be further defined for this useful investigation.

Conflict of Interests

None of the authors have any relevant financial interests to declare.

References

[1] R. S. Boersma, K.-S. G. Jie, A. Verbon, E. C. M. van Pampus, and H. C. Schouten, "Thrombotic and infectious complications of central venous catheters in patients with hematological malignancies," *Annals of Oncology*, vol. 19, no. 3, pp. 433–442, 2008.

[2] R. Kujur, S. M. Rao, G. Badwaik, and R. Paraswani, "Thrombosis associated with right internal jugular central venous catheters: a prospective observational study," *Indian Journal of Critical Care Medicine*, vol. 16, no. 1, pp. 17–21, 2012.

[3] B. J. Eastridge and A. T. Lefor, "Complications of indwelling venous access devices in cancer patients," *Journal of Clinical Oncology*, vol. 13, no. 1, pp. 233–238, 1995.

[4] J. R. Mehall, D. A. Saltzman, R. J. Jackson, and S. D. Smith, "Fibrin sheath enhances central venous catheter infection," *Critical Care Medicine*, vol. 30, no. 4, pp. 908–912, 2002.

[5] V. Mor-Avi, L. Sugeng, L. Weinert et al., "Fast measurement of left ventricular mass with real-time three-dimensional echocardiography: comparison with magnetic resonance imaging," *Circulation*, vol. 110, no. 13, pp. 1814–1818, 2004.

[6] L. Macron, P. Lim, A. Bensaid et al., "Single-beat versus multibeat real-time 3D echocardiography for assessing left ventricular volumes and ejection fraction: a comparison study with cardiac magnetic resonance," *Circulation: Cardiovascular Imaging*, vol. 3, no. 4, pp. 450–455, 2010.

[7] C. Jenkins, K. Bricknell, L. Hanekom, and T. H. Marwick, "Reproducibility and accuracy of echocardiographic measurements of left ventricular parameters using real-time three-dimensional

echocardiography," *Journal of the American College of Cardiology*, vol. 44, no. 4, pp. 878–886, 2004.

[8] B. J. Krenning, M. M. Voormolen, M. L. Geleijnse et al., "Three-dimensional echocardiographic analysis of left ventricular function during hemodialysis," *Nephron. Clinical Practice*, vol. 107, no. 2, pp. c43–c49, 2007.

[9] R. J. Glassock, R. Pecoits-Filho, and S. H. Barberato, "Left ventricular mass in chronic kidney disease and ESRD," *Clinical Journal of the American Society of Nephrology*, vol. 4, supplement 1, pp. S79–S91, 2009.

[10] C. J. Van Rooden, M. E. T. Tesselaar, S. Osanto, F. R. Rosendaal, and M. V. Huisman, "Deep vein thrombosis associated with central venous catheters—a review," *Journal of Thrombosis and Haemostasis*, vol. 3, no. 11, pp. 2409–2419, 2005.

46

Nonsecretory Multiple Myeloma and AL Amyloidosis Presenting with Nephrotic Range Proteinuria

Ozlem Beyler Kilic,[1] Ali Kemal Oguz,[1] Ihsan Ergun,[2] Dilek Ertoy Baydar,[3] and Meltem Ayli[4]

[1]Department of Internal Medicine, Ufuk University School of Medicine, 06520 Ankara, Turkey
[2]Division of Nephrology, Department of Internal Medicine, Ufuk University School of Medicine, 06520 Ankara, Turkey
[3]Department of Pathology, Hacettepe University School of Medicine, 06100 Ankara, Turkey
[4]Division of Hematology, Department of Internal Medicine, Ufuk University School of Medicine, 06520 Ankara, Turkey

Correspondence should be addressed to Ihsan Ergun; ihsanerg@yahoo.com

Academic Editor: Raoul Bergner

Nonsecretory multiple myeloma (NSMM) is the absence of a detectable monoclonal protein in serum and urine of a multiple myeloma (MM) patient and immunoglobulin light chain (AL) amyloidosis is a significantly rare complication. A case of NSMM with AL amyloidosis and nephrotic range proteinuria is presented. Sharing clinical, therapeutic, and prognostic characteristics with MM, real challenge may be during initial diagnosis of NSMM and assessment of treatment response. In elderly patients with unexplained renal dysfunction, MM should be in the differential diagnosis and the absence of a monoclonal protein should not rule out MM but should remind us of the possibility of NSMM.

1. Introduction

Multiple myeloma (MM) is a hematological neoplasm of the bone marrow arising from monoclonal proliferation of plasma cells secreting a monoclonal paraprotein (M protein) which may be an immunoglobulin or one of its constituent chains [1]. Nonsecretory multiple myeloma (NSMM) is by definition the absence of a detectable M protein in the serum and the urine of an MM patient and constitutes approximately 1–5% of all patients newly diagnosed with MM [2–4].

Amyloidosis occurs with the extracellular deposition of one of a variety of abnormally folded fibrillar proteins which characteristically display a beta-pleated sheet structure. According to the Nomenclature Committee of the International Society of Amyloidosis, the clinical classification of the amyloidosis should be based on the amyloid fibril forming protein [5]. In AL amyloidosis, the deposited amyloid protein is derived from immunoglobulin light chains (i.e., lambda [λ] or kappa [κ]) originating from plasma cells [5]. One of the plasma cell dyscrasias such as MM, Waldenstrom macroglobulinemia (WM), and monoclonal gammopathy of undetermined significance (MGUS) or a B-cell non-Hodgkin's lymphoma is identified in approximately 5–15% of AL amyloidosis cases.

In the case of NSMM, the development of an AL amyloidosis is reported to be extremely rare. Herein, we present a case of NSMM complicated with AL amyloidosis resulting in nephrotic range proteinuria.

2. Case Presentation

A 74-year-old man was referred to our nephrology clinic on the occasion of his complaints of swollen legs and difficulty in walking. His past medical history revealed a well-controlled hypertension by valsartan/hydrochlorothiazide and doxazosin. On physical examination, he had truncal obesity, severe bilateral pretibial pitting edema, and varicose veins in his lower extremities. His routine admission laboratory tests (i.e., complete blood count, basic metabolic panel [glucose, blood urea nitrogen, creatinine, sodium, potassium, chloride, and calcium], liver panel, urinalysis, and TSH) were normal with the exceptions of low serum total protein

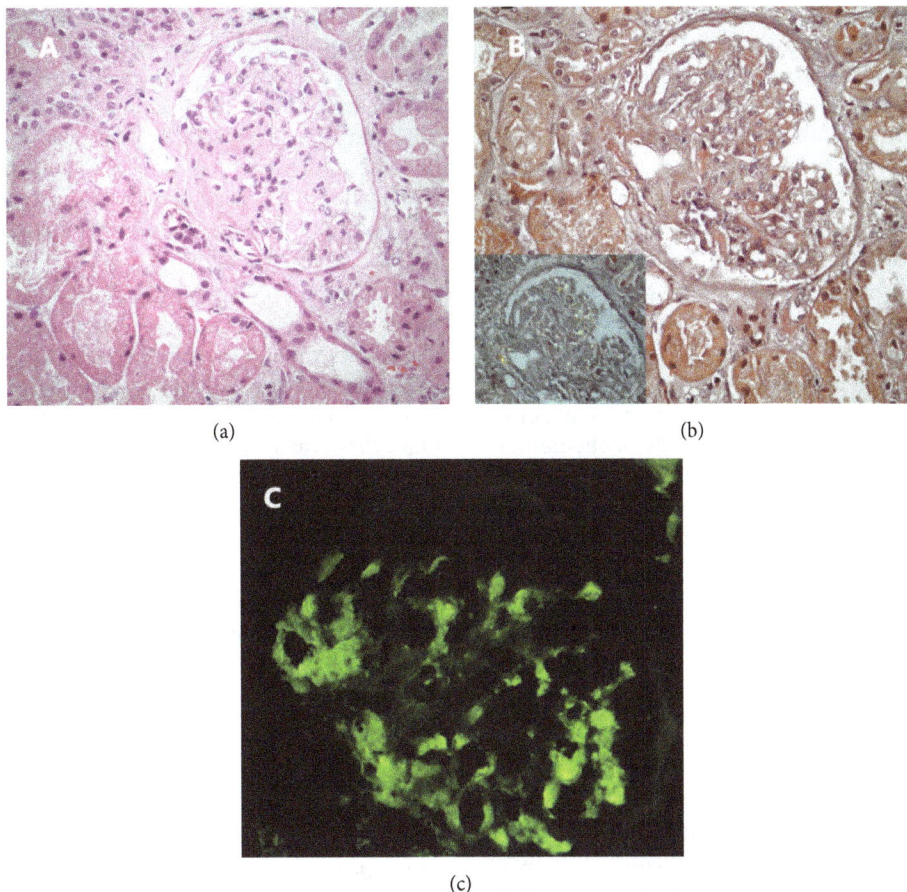

(a)

(b)

(c)

FIGURE 1: (a) Homogenous pale eosinophilic material accumulation in the glomerulus and in the hilar arteriole (H&E, ×400). (b) Positive Congo red staining in the areas of glomerular deposition (Congo red stain, ×400). Inset shows apple green birefringence given by deposits under polarized light (Congo red stain with polarized microscopy, ×200). (c) Amyloid was strongly reactive for lambda light chain on immunofluorescence microscopy (immunofluorescence, fluorescein isothiocyanate-conjugated anti-lambda antibody, ×400).

(5.00 g/dL [6.00–8.30 g/dL]) and albumin (2.50 g/dL [3.00–5.00 g/dL]) levels together with a 300 mg/dL proteinuria on dipstick testing. While the patient's serum creatinine and eGFR (by the MDRD equation) were 0.81 mg/dL and 99 mL/min/1.73 m^2, a 24-hour urine collection documented a proteinuria of 4.6 g/day. Simultaneously ordered serum and urine protein electrophoreses and immunofixation studies, serum-free light chain (FLC) measurements (lambda 93 mg/dL [90–210 mg/dL] and kappa 170 mg/dL [170–370 mg/dL], by nephelometry) and FLC ratio, and serum IgG, IgA, and IgM levels were all found to be normal. Antinuclear and anti-neutrophil cytoplasmic antibodies were negative and serum C3c and C4 levels were within the normal ranges.

Patient's abdominal ultrasonography documented bilaterally increased renal parenchymal echogenicities (grade 1) with renal dimensions and parenchymal thicknesses of 97 × 57 × 52/18 mm and 118 × 70 × 63/18 mm for the right and the left kidneys, respectively. A thoracic computerized tomography performed on the occasion of vague respiratory complaints revealed pleural thickening, loss of volume, and subpleural linear atelectases in the right hemithorax. As these findings were in accordance with a probable previous

tuberculosis infection, a rectal mucosa biopsy was performed to search for a secondary amyloidosis. Histopathologically, no deposition of amyloid was documented in the rectal biopsy.

The absence of direct and clear clues about the etiology of the nephrotic range proteinuria dictated a renal biopsy which was promptly performed. Microscopic examination of the renal biopsy showed homogenous eosinophilic deposits in the glomeruli and the vessel walls which proved to be amyloid depositions with Congo red staining (Figure 1, Panels (a) and (b)). Immunofluorescence examination for lambda and kappa light chains documented a strong and a weak staining, respectively (Figure 1, Panel (c)). Consequently, the patient was diagnosed with lambda-type AL amyloidosis.

Following the diagnosis of AL amyloidosis, a bone marrow aspiration and biopsy were performed to exclude an underlying plasma cell tumor or B-cell lymphoproliferative disease. The bone marrow examination documented a uniformly appearing monotonous infiltrate of plasma cells with a percentage of 25%, which was consistent with a diagnosis of MM, in the patient's case an NSMM. Both conventional and fluorescent in situ hybridization (t[9;22], t[4;14], t[11;14], and trisomies 7 and 8 were negative) cytogenetic analyses revealed a normal karyotype (46,XY). There were lytic bone lesions of cranial and pelvic bones on conventional skeletal survey. In search of systemic involvement of AL amyloidosis, a thorough cardiac evaluation and an electroneuromyography were performed. The patient's NT-proBNP and troponin I levels were 78 pg/mL (10–110 pg/mL) and 0.04 ng/mL (≤0.04 ng/mL), respectively. On echocardiography, an interventricular septum thickness of 13 mm consistent with a mild left ventricular hypertrophy was the only abnormal finding with an ejection fraction of 64% (55–70%). Clinically, the patient was in NYHA class I. The result of the electrophysiological examination was normal.

As for chemotherapy, a combination regimen with bortezomib and dexamethasone was instituted. The response evaluation performed following the second cycle of chemotherapy documented a complete remission with a bone marrow plasma cell percentage of 4%. At the time of writing the paper, the patient was doing well with a complete remission and was waiting for a scheduled autologous stem cell transplant.

3. Discussion

Multiple myeloma is a hematologic neoplasm significantly more prevalent in the elderly patients [3]. The International Myeloma Working Group updated (2014) criteria for the diagnosis of MM require presence of ≥10% clonal bone marrow plasma cells and any one or more of the CRAB features (hypercalcemia, renal failure, anemia, and bone lesions) [6]. At the age of 74, having 25% monoclonal plasma cells in the bone marrow, nephrotic range proteinuria, and lytic bone lesions, the case presented herein was a typical MM patient with a nonsecretory disease. Here, it is important to note and remember that the diagnosis of MM frequently results from the diagnostic workup of elderly patients with unexplained renal dysfunction [3]. The same was true for our patient in whom a clear etiological diagnosis of nephrotic range proteinuria was made by the renal biopsy and the bone marrow examinations following the initial workup.

Conventionally, NSMM is defined as the absence of a detectable amount of M protein in the serum and urine of an MM patient [2, 4]. The previous frequency figure of NSMM among newly diagnosed MM patients was around 5%. With the widespread use of sensitive immunoassays which precisely quantify serum-free light chains, this figure is now about 3% [2, 3]. Moreover, if examined at the cellular level, great majority of NSMM plasma cells demonstrate intracellular presence of immunoglobulins or their components [7–10]. Taking this into account, some researchers group NSMM patients into two, namely, the nonproducers (about 15%; no immunoglobulin or any of its components is present in the plasma cells) and the producers (about 85%; an immunoglobulin or a component is demonstrable in the plasma cells). Consequently, it can be stated that in NSMM patients true nonproduction is unusual [8]. Although not investigated at a cellular level, the neoplastic plasma cell clone of the presented patient was presumably of the producer type as the disease resulted in a lambda-type AL amyloidosis. In addition to the state of nonproduction, several mechanisms

are proposed to account for the absence of an M protein in NSMM cases. These are a decrease in M protein synthesis secondary to increased cytoplasmic immunoglobulins, accelerated degradation of abnormal intracellular immunoglobulins, impaired intracellular transport of immunoglobulins, intermittent excretion of M protein, altered secretion ability of plasma cell, reduced plasma cell membrane permeability, and rapid degradation of abnormal immunoglobulin following its secretion [8, 9].

Depending on the clinical definitions used and the diagnostic methods implemented, the incidence of renal disease in patients with MM varies between 15% and 40% [11]. The spectrum of renal diseases associating MM is considerably wide and includes many distinct clinicopathologic entities. Light chain cast nephropathy also known as myeloma kidney remains the most common form of MM related renal disease. Nonetheless, in NSMM the occurrence of light chain cast nephropathy is an unexpected situation owing to the absence of a detectable M protein, in this case a light chain in the serum and the urine of the patient [4]. The other two most common forms of M protein mediated renal disease are AL amyloidosis and monoclonal immunoglobulin deposition disease. When becoming manifest, significant proteinuria/nephrotic syndrome is present in approximately 70% of AL amyloidosis cases. The case presented had an AL amyloidosis which is documented to be very rare in patients with NSMM. Whether in series of NSMM patients or in presentations of single cases, NSMM patients with an AL amyloidosis had always been reported as individual cases and are scarce in the literature [7, 12–15]. As previously stated, the amyloid fibrils deposited in AL amyloidosis are made up of monoclonal immunoglobulin light chains secreted by the responsible plasma cell clone. Using electron microscopy, Azar et al. had also provided additional support for this fact [12].

Except for renal involvement due to light chain cast nephropathy, clinical manifestations of NSMM are consistent with MM. As such, bone marrow failure, lytic bone lesions, osteoporosis, and hypogammaglobulinemia have all been reported [4, 8, 9, 16]. In addition to a nephrotic range proteinuria, the presented case also demonstrated lytic bone lesions of cranial and pelvic bones. With respect to treatment approaches, treatment responses, and prognosis, NSMM and MM harbour shared characteristics [2, 4, 9]. A challenging point in patients with NSMM was the lack of a detectable M protein to be used during assessment of treatment responses. For this purpose, serum-free light chain measurements seem to offer a new opportunity in cases with NSMM [17].

To conclude, especially in elderly patients with unexplained renal dysfunction, MM should be included in the differential diagnosis and the absence of a detectable M protein should not rule out MM but should remind us of the possibility of an NSMM.

Consent

Written informed consent was obtained from the patient for publication of this case report and the accompanying images.

Conflict of Interests

The authors declare no potential conflict of interests with respect to the authorship and/or publication of this paper.

References

[1] J. Laubach, P. Richardson, and K. Anderson, "Multiple myeloma," *Annual Review of Medicine*, vol. 62, pp. 249–264, 2011.

[2] S. Lonial and J. L. Kaufman, "Non-secretory myeloma: a clinician's guide," *Oncology*, vol. 27, no. 9, pp. 924–930, 2013.

[3] S. M. Korbet and M. M. Schwartz, "Multiple myeloma," *Journal of the American Society of Nephrology*, vol. 17, no. 9, pp. 2533–2545, 2006.

[4] J. Bladé and R. A. Kyle, "Nonsecretory myeloma, immunoglobulin D myeloma, and plasma cell leukemia," *Hematology/Oncology Clinics of North America*, vol. 13, no. 6, pp. 1259–1272, 1999.

[5] J. D. Sipe, M. D. Benson, J. N. Buxbaum et al., "Nomenclature 2014: amyloid fibril proteins and clinical classification of the amyloidosis," *Amyloid*, vol. 21, no. 4, pp. 221–224, 2014.

[6] S. V. Rajkumar, M. A. Dimopoulos, A. Palumbo et al., "International Myeloma Working Group updated criteria for the diagnosis of multiple myeloma," *The Lancet Oncology*, vol. 15, no. 12, pp. e538–e548, 2014.

[7] J. L. Preud'Homme, D. Hurez, F. Danon, J. C. Brouet, and M. Seligmann, "Intracytoplasmic and surface bound immunoglobulins in 'nonsecretory' and Bence Jones myeloma," *Clinical and Experimental Immunology*, vol. 25, no. 3, pp. 428–436, 1976.

[8] D. B. Smith, M. Harris, E. Gowland, J. Chang, and J. H. Scarffe, "Non-secretory multiple myeloma: a report of 13 cases with a review of the literature," *Hematological Oncology*, vol. 4, no. 4, pp. 307–313, 1986.

[9] D. Rubio-Felix, M. Giralt, M. Pilar Giraldo et al., "Nonsecretory multiple myeloma," *Cancer*, vol. 59, no. 10, pp. 1847–1852, 1987.

[10] T. Ishida and H. D. Dorfman, "Plasma cell myeloma in unusually young patients: a report of two cases and review of the literature," *Skeletal Radiology*, vol. 24, no. 1, pp. 47–51, 1995.

[11] E. C. Heher, H. G. Rennke, J. P. Laubach, and P. G. Richardson, "Kidney disease and multiple myeloma," *Clinical Journal of the American Society of Nephrology*, vol. 8, no. 11, pp. 2007–2017, 2013.

[12] H. A. Azar, E. C. Zaino, T. D. Pham, and K. Yannopoulos, "'Nonsecretory' plasma cell myeloma: observations on seven cases with electron microscopic studies," *American Journal of Clinical Pathology*, vol. 58, no. 6, pp. 618–629, 1972.

[13] J. M. Nores, J. M. Remy, A. D. Nenna, and J. Dalayeun, "Twelve-year profile of a non-secretory myeloma with amyloidosis," *British Journal of Clinical Practice*, vol. 44, no. 11, pp. 529–530, 1990.

[14] G. Lugassy, A. Ducach, C. Yossefi, and J. Michal, "Unusual case of amyloidosis complicating nonsecretory multiple myeloma," *American Journal of Hematology*, vol. 43, no. 4, pp. 332–333, 1993.

[15] E. Laurat, C. Cazalets, M. Sébillot, M. Bernard, S. Caulet-Maugendre, and B. Grosbois, "Localized epidural and bone amyloidosis, rare cause of paraplegia in multiple myeloma," *Amyloid*, vol. 10, no. 1, pp. 47–50, 2003.

[16] J. Amir, W. B. Forman, A. Rassiga, and G. M. Bernier, "Nonsynthetizing multiple myeloma," *Haematologia*, vol. 11, no. 1-2, pp. 73–77, 1977.

[17] M. Drayson, L. X. Tang, R. Drew, G. P. Mead, H. Carr-Smith, and A. R. Bradwell, "Serum free light-chain measurements for identifying and monitoring patients with nonsecretory multiple myeloma," *Blood*, vol. 97, no. 9, pp. 2900–2902, 2001.

47

Donor-Derived Myeloid Sarcoma in Two Kidney Transplant Recipients from a Single Donor

Amudha Palanisamy,[1] Paul Persad,[2] Patrick P. Koty,[2] Laurie L. Douglas,[3] Robert J. Stratta,[4] Jeffrey Rogers,[4] Amber M. Reeves-Daniel,[1] Giuseppe Orlando,[4] Alan C. Farney,[4] Michael W. Beaty,[2] Mark J. Pettenati,[2] Samy S. Iskandar,[2] David D. Grier,[2] Scott A. Kaczmorski,[5] William H. Doares,[5] Michael D. Gautreaux,[4] Barry I. Freedman,[1] and Bayard L. Powell[3]

[1]Department of Internal Medicine, Section on Nephrology, Wake Forest School of Medicine, Winston-Salem, NC 27103, USA
[2]Department of Pathology, Wake Forest School of Medicine, Winston-Salem, NC 27103, USA
[3]Department of Internal Medicine, Section on Hematology and Oncology, Comprehensive Cancer Center of Wake Forest University, Winston-Salem, NC 27103, USA
[4]Department of General Surgery, Wake Forest School of Medicine, Winston-Salem, NC 27103, USA
[5]Department of Pharmacy, Wake Forest School of Medicine, Winston-Salem, NC 27103, USA

Correspondence should be addressed to Amudha Palanisamy; apalanis@wakehealth.edu

Academic Editor: Gianna Mastroianni Kirsztajn

We report the rare occurrence of donor-derived myeloid sarcoma in two kidney transplant patients who received organs from a single deceased donor. There was no evidence of preexisting hematologic malignancy in the donor at the time of organ recovery. Both recipients developed leukemic involvement that appeared to be limited to the transplanted organ. Fluorescence *in situ* hybridization (FISH) and molecular genotyping analyses confirmed that the malignant cells were of donor origin in each patient. Allograft nephrectomy and immediate withdrawal of immunosuppression were performed in both cases; systemic chemotherapy was subsequently administered to one patient. Both recipients were in remission at least one year following the diagnosis of donor-derived myeloid sarcoma. These cases suggest that restoration of the immune system after withdrawal of immunosuppressive therapy and allograft nephrectomy may be sufficient to control HLA-mismatched donor-derived myeloid sarcoma without systemic involvement.

1. Introduction

Donor-derived malignancies occur in less than 0.1% of kidney transplant recipients [1]. However, increased utilization of older donors in the last decade has the potential to increase recipient risk for the development of donor-derived malignancy [2]. Although the most common donor-derived cancers after kidney transplantation are renal cell carcinomas, various types of donor-derived malignancies have been reported [3]. We report the rare occurrence of two cases of myeloid sarcoma that developed following kidney transplantation from a single deceased donor, in which the donor origin of the neoplastic clone was verified by molecular genotyping in each case.

2. Case Report: Donor

A 38-year-old female nursing home resident with a body mass index (BMI) of 44 kg/m² and bilateral sequential lower extremity amputations was found unresponsive and pulseless for an unknown period of time and was immediately intubated at the scene. Cardiopulmonary resuscitation was initiated with restoration of circulation. Following transfer to a nearby acute care hospital, neurological examination revealed apnea and a computerized tomographic (CT) scan of the head revealed diffuse cerebral edema. She was pronounced dead by brain death criteria and the family consented to organ donation.

Past medical history provided by the family and skilled nursing facility revealed that the patient had been hypertensive for 3 years and had a history of diabetes mellitus for 20 years. She also smoked tobacco and had resultant chronic obstructive pulmonary disease. However, she did not have any history of cancer or chronic weight loss. On the day of admission, the white blood cell count was 4800 cells/microL (differential 83% neutrophils, 4% monocytes, and 13% lymphocytes), hemoglobin was 10.3 grams/dL, and platelet count was 125,000/microL. Peripheral blasts were not detected on a blood smear. Both kidneys were recovered for transplantation. No other organs were used (the liver was not recovered because of steatosis). Although an autopsy was not performed, a preimplantation kidney biopsy revealed changes that were consistent with long-standing diabetes mellitus.

3. Recipient 1

The first kidney transplant recipient was a 72-year-old European American male with a history of type 2 diabetes mellitus and hypertension culminating in end-stage renal disease (ESRD) who had been on hemodialysis for 2 years. He had previously undergone thyroidectomy for papillary adenocarcinoma of the thyroid and radical prostatectomy with pelvic lymphadenectomy for prostate cancer. He also had a remote history of tobacco use. The recipient and donor were a two-human leukocyte antigen (HLA) mismatch. During the transplant procedure, he received intravenous induction therapy with a single intraoperative dose of alemtuzumab (30 mg) and dexamethasone (100 mg). Cold ischemia time was 13.5 hours; the kidney reperfused well and appeared anatomically normal. A reperfusion biopsy of the renal cortex showed mild to moderate donor transmitted chronic changes and acute tubular injury. Following transplantation, maintenance immunosuppression was initiated and included tacrolimus and mycophenolic acid. The patient experienced slow graft function but did not receive any hemodialysis treatments postoperatively. A one-month surveillance biopsy of the renal allograft revealed residual acute tubular injury and donor transmitted diffuse and nodular diabetic glomerulosclerosis. Serum creatinine levels subsequently stabilized in the 2.5–3.0 mg/dL range.

Two months following transplantation, he was readmitted for dyspnea attributed to bilateral pneumonia and pulmonary edema thought to be cardiac in nature. He improved with diuresis and antibiotic therapy. Recurrent dyspnea and pulmonary edema developed four months following transplantation at which time he was readmitted and found to have acute kidney injury (serum creatinine level 4.5 mg/dL) and volume overload. An ultrasound examination of the renal allograft demonstrated a significant increase in volume of the transplanted kidney and elevated resistance

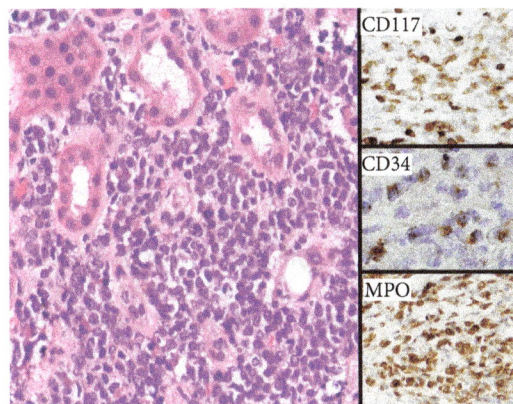

FIGURE 1: Recipient 1, kidney biopsy: A diffuse proliferation of immature myeloid cells is seen dissecting between renal tubules. Immunohistochemical analysis for blasts (CD117 and CD34) and myeloid lineage (MPO, myeloperoxidase) were strongly positive.

indices. A subsequent renal allograft biopsy revealed diffuse parenchymal infiltration with immature mononuclear cells. Immunohistochemical studies revealed CD34, CD117, and myeloperoxidase (MPO) positive blasts consistent with a diagnosis of myeloid sarcoma (Figure 1). Fluorescence in situ hybridization (FISH) studies showed normal chromosomes and confirmed that 93% of the cells in the biopsy were of donor (female, XX) origin, suggesting a donor-derived myeloid sarcoma transmitted with the transplanted kidney. At the time of kidney biopsy, the white blood cell count was 2800 cells/microL, hemoglobin was 11 grams/dL, and platelet count was 95,000/microL. There were no peripheral blasts detected and a bone marrow biopsy was negative for leukemic involvement. Positron Emission Tomography/CT (PET/CT) did not reveal any other foci of involvement beyond the renal allograft. Conventional metaphase cytogenetic analysis of the bone marrow biopsy revealed a normal male karyotype with no apparent leukemic involvement.

Initial treatment included planned embolization of the transplant renal artery to induce allograft infarction followed by uneventful nephrectomy performed on the following day. Immunosuppression was immediately discontinued. Direct tissue sample following nephrectomy showed 5.5% XY and 94.5% XX chromosomes. He subsequently completed induction therapy with one cycle of cytarabine and daunorubicin (7 + 3). A repeat bone marrow biopsy performed 5 months following the initial diagnosis did not reveal any evidence of disease. He remained in remission and on dialysis for another 8 months before sustaining a cardiovascular death 13 months following nephrectomy.

4. Recipient 2

The second kidney transplant recipient was a 77-year-old European American woman with ESRD secondary to interstitial nephritis who had been on hemodialysis for 2 years. She had a history of a prior failed renal transplant at another center secondary to early renal artery thrombosis that resulted in allograft nephrectomy. The recipient and donor were a three-HLA mismatch. Cold ischemia time was 28 hours; the kidney reperfused well and appeared normal anatomically. A reperfusion biopsy of the renal cortex showed mild to moderate donor transmitted chronic changes and acute tubular injury. Induction therapy consisted of alemtuzumab and dexamethasone with tacrolimus and mycophenolic acid maintenance immunosuppression. She experienced immediate graft function and serum creatinine levels eventually stabilized in the 1.4–1.7 mg/dL range. She was admitted with fever two weeks following kidney transplantation and was successfully treated for a urinary tract infection. Three weeks following transplantation, she underwent a surveillance allograft biopsy that revealed recovering acute tubular injury, donor transmitted nodular diabetic glomerulosclerosis, and hyalinosis.

The patient was readmitted 4 months following transplantation to another facility for acute kidney injury (serum creatinine level > 4.0 mg/dL) and recurrent urinary tract infections. A kidney biopsy showed acute and chronic thrombotic microangiopathy and immunosuppression was changed from tacrolimus to a cyclosporine-based regimen. However, upon further review, atypical cells were noted in the biopsy and renal function did not improve with conversion to cyclosporine. By this time, the diagnosis of myeloid sarcoma had been confirmed in Recipient 1 (above), who received the mate kidney from the same donor. Recipient 2 was notified of these findings and she opted for allograft nephrectomy. Laboratory analysis at the time of readmission to our facility revealed allograft dysfunction with a serum creatinine level of 4.3 mg/dL. Her white blood cell count was 2700 cells/microL, hemoglobin was 8.3 grams/dL, and platelet count was 109,000/microL. There were no peripheral blasts and PET/CT scan did not reveal any fluorodeoxyglucose (FDG) avid lesions other than the renal allograft. The patient refused a bone marrow biopsy.

Allograft nephrectomy was performed following planned preoperative embolization. Pathologic examination of the explant demonstrated a monotonous population of myeloid blasts morphologically identical to the first transplant recipient (Figure 2). Molecular genotyping analysis performed on renal tissue from each recipient yielded identical haplotypes and confirmed that both myeloid sarcomas were of donor origin (Figure 3). Immunosuppression was immediately withdrawn. The patient chose not to receive systemic chemotherapy and she remained in remission and on dialysis for another 18 months following nephrectomy before sustaining a cardiovascular death.

5. Discussion

This report describes the rare development of donor-derived myeloid sarcoma in two kidney transplant recipients from a single donor. Donor-derived leukemia has been reported after solid organ transplantation in liver transplant recipients and in a renal transplant recipient [4–6]. In these cases, the authors hypothesized that the most likely mechanism of disease was transformation of normal hematopoietic stem cells residing in the allograft into a malignant clone

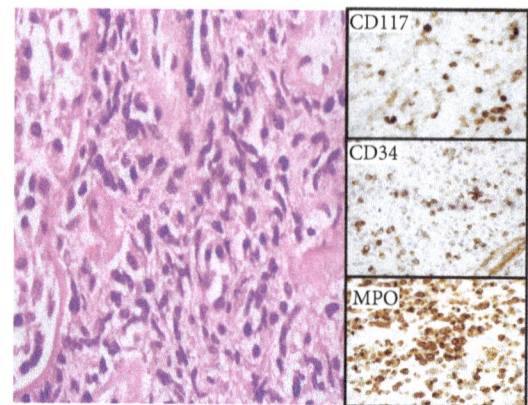

FIGURE 2: Recipient 2, kidney biopsy: A diffuse proliferation of immature myeloid cells is seen dissecting between renal tubules. Immunohistochemical analysis for blasts (CD117 and CD34) and myeloid lineage (MPO, myeloperoxidase) were strongly positive.

following transplantation. The authors favored this hypothesis given the absence of clinically evident disease in the donor prior to donation, a greater than two-year interval between transplantation and leukemic presentation, and the lack of involvement in recipients who received other organs from the same donor [4–6]. In the present report, although there was no evidence of preexisting hematologic malignancy in the donor, it appears most likely that a leukemic clone was transplanted through kidney tissue as both kidney transplant recipients were affected, disease was renal-limited, and both FISH and molecular genotyping analyses confirmed that the malignant cells were of donor origin.

It is remarkable that, despite partial HLA mismatch, the leukemic clone proliferated in both recipients. It has been reported that leukemic cells with normal karyotypes can display genomic instability in the form of uniparental disomy in myeloid cancers [7–9]. Vago et al. demonstrated that leukemic cells are able to elude antitumor donor T cells after haploidentical hematopoietic stem cell transplantation with infusion of donor T cells, by failing to express the mismatched HLA haplotype [10]. This effect leads to relapse of leukemia. It is plausible that a similar phenomenon occurred in these two recipients, whereby genomic instability of the transplanted leukemic clones resulted in decreased expression of mismatched HLA allowing leukemic cells to escape from alloreactive recipient T cells and proliferate. We also hypothesize that immunosenescence associated with the advanced age of the recipients and need for immunosuppressive drugs following transplantation impaired the recipient's immune response to a partially HLA-mismatched leukemic clonal proliferation.

As opposed to previous reports of leukemia after solid organ transplantation, this report demonstrates leukemic involvement of only the transplanted organs [4–6]. We believe that these cases may be the first reported cases of donor transmitted renal-limited myeloid sarcoma to two recipients from the same deceased organ donor. Both recipients lacked peripheral blasts and had negative PET/CT scans looking for systemic involvement, so a high index of

(a)

(b)

(c)

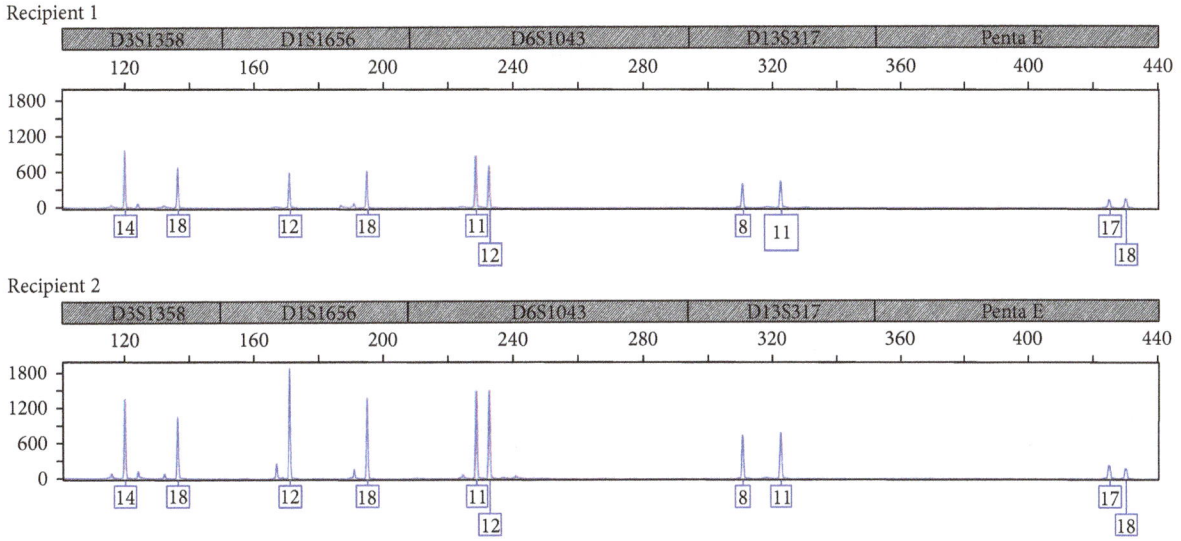

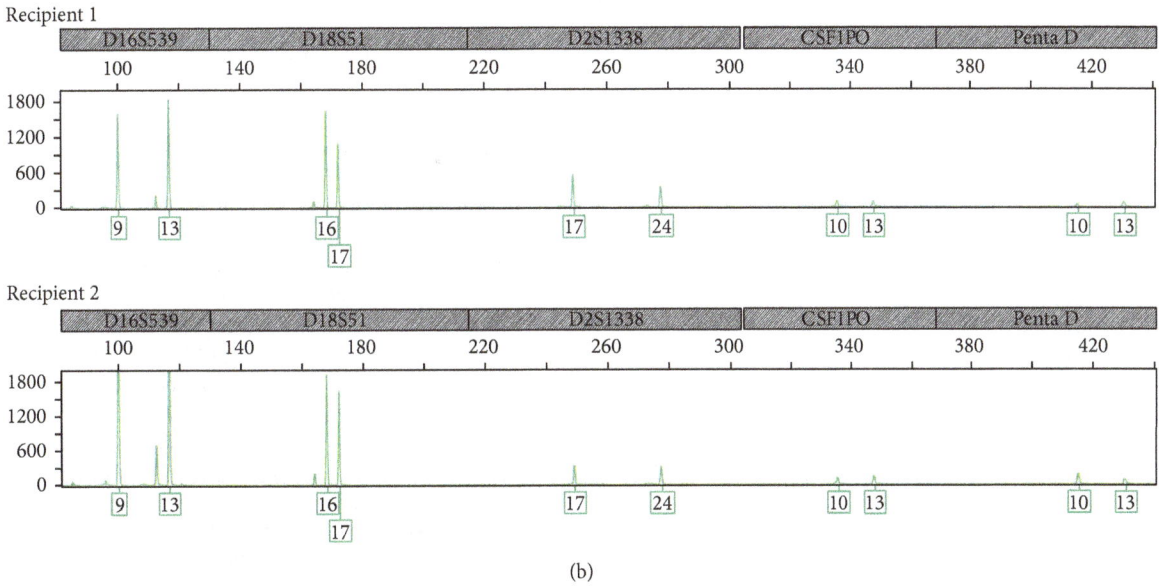

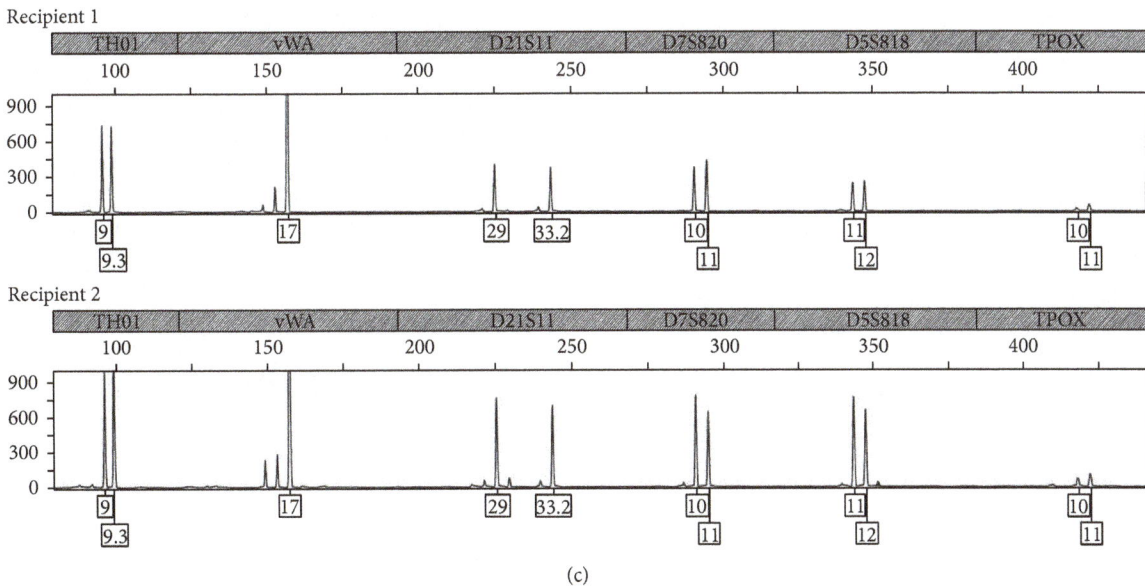

FIGURE 3: Continued.

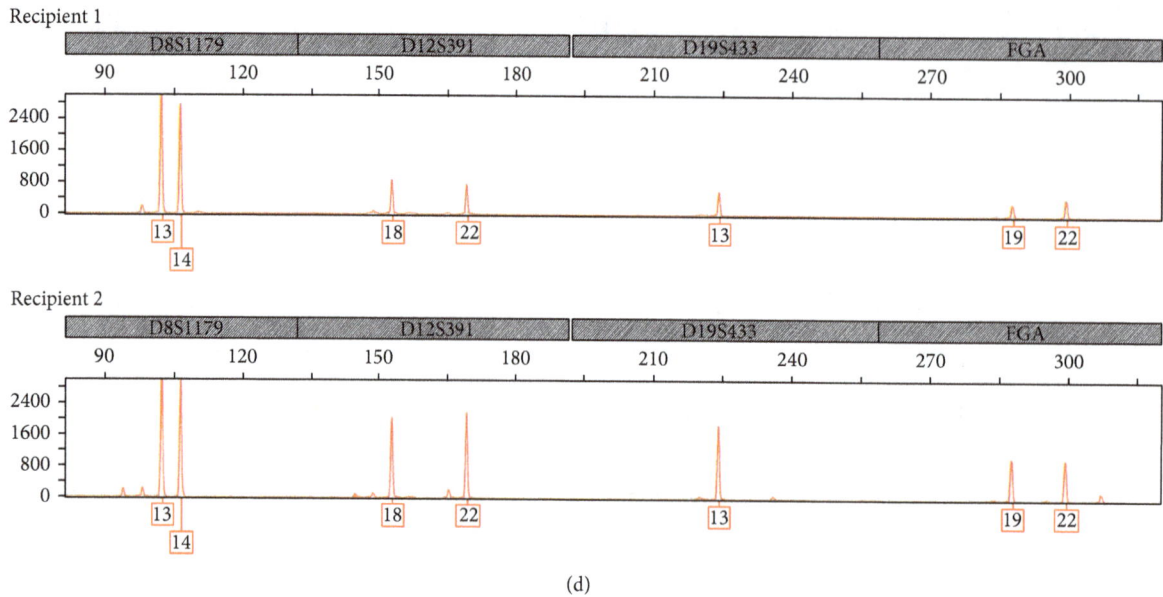

FIGURE 3: Molecular genotyping of Recipients 1 and 2 tumors for 21 informative markers (PowerPlex 21, Promega Corp).

suspicion is required to make this diagnosis. Bone marrow biopsy was also negative in the first recipient. The treatment regimens differed in each recipient based upon patient preference. Allograft nephrectomy and immediate withdrawal of immunosuppression were performed in both patients, while systemic chemotherapy was only administered to one. Both recipients remained in remission for at least one year following transplantation. These unusual cases suggest that restoration of the immune system after withdrawal of immunosuppressive therapy and allograft nephrectomy may be sufficient to control HLA-mismatched donor-derived myeloid sarcoma without systemic involvement.

Conflict of Interests

The authors declare that there is no conflict of interests regarding the publication of this paper.

References

[1] H. M. Kauffman, M. A. McBride, W. S. Cherikh, P. C. Spain, and F. L. Delmonico, "Transplant tumor registry: donors with central nervous system tumors," *Transplantation*, vol. 73, no. 4, pp. 579–582, 2002.

[2] A. J. Collins, R. N. Foley, B. Chavers et al., "US renal data system 2013 annual data report," *American Journal of Kidney Diseases*, vol. 63, no. 1, p. A7, 2014.

[3] D. Xiao, J. C. Craig, J. R. Chapman, B. Dominguez-Gil, A. Tong, and G. Wong, "Donor cancer transmission in kidney transplantation: a systematic review," *The American Journal of Transplantation*, vol. 13, no. 10, pp. 2645–2652, 2013.

[4] M. Subklewe, M. Nagy, C. Schoch et al., "Extramedullary manifestation of a donor-derived acute myeloid leukemia in a liver transplant patient," *Leukemia*, vol. 18, no. 12, pp. 2050–2053, 2004.

[5] I. Bodó, M. Peters, J. P. Radich et al., "Donor-derived acute promyelocytic leukemia in a liver-transplant recipient," *The New England Journal of Medicine*, vol. 341, no. 11, pp. 807–813, 1999.

[6] S. Girsberger, C. Wehmeier, P. Amico et al., "Donor-derived acute myeloid leukemia in a kidney transplant recipient." *Blood*, vol. 122, no. 2, pp. 298–300, 2013.

[7] M. Raghavan, D. M. Lillington, S. Skoulakis et al., "Genome-wide single nucleotide polymorphism analysis reveals frequent partial uniparental disomy due to somatic recombination in acute myeloid leukemias," *Cancer Research*, vol. 65, no. 2, pp. 375–378, 2005.

[8] T. A. Gorletta, P. Gasparini, M. M. D'Elios, M. Trubia, P. G. Pelicci, and P. P. Di Fiore, "Frequent loss of heterozygosity without loss of genetic material in acute myeloid leukemia with a normal karyotype," *Genes Chromosomes and Cancer*, vol. 44, no. 3, pp. 334–337, 2005.

[9] A. J. Dunbar, L. P. Gondek, C. L. O'Keefe et al., "250K single nucleotide polymorphism array karyotyping identifies acquired uniparental disomy and homozygous mutations, including novel missense substitutions of c-Cbl, in myeloid malignancies," *Cancer Research*, vol. 68, no. 24, pp. 10349–10357, 2008.

[10] L. Vago, S. K. Perna, M. Zanussi et al., "Loss of mismatched HLA in leukemia after stem-cell transplantation," *The New England Journal of Medicine*, vol. 361, no. 5, pp. 478–488, 2009.

48

Crossed Renal Ectopia without Fusion: An Uncommon Cause of Abdominal Mass

Ana Ratola,[1] **Maria Miguel Almiro,**[1] **Rita Lacerda Vidal,**[1]
Nuno Neves,[2] **Adelaide Bicho,**[1] **and Sofia Figueiredo**[1]

[1]*Pediatrics Department, Baixo Vouga Hospital Center, Avenida Artur Ravara, 3814-501 Aveiro, Portugal*
[2]*Radiology Department, Baixo Vouga Hospital Center, Avenida Artur Ravara, 3814-501 Aveiro, Portugal*

Correspondence should be addressed to Ana Ratola; anaratola@hotmail.com

Academic Editor: John A. Sayer

Crossed renal ectopia is a rare congenital anomaly usually associated with fused kidneys (90%). Most cases are asymptomatic and remain undiagnosed. We report an unusual case of nonfused crossed renal ectopia. The 11-year-old adolescent female patient was admitted with abdominal pain, anorexia, weight loss, and periumbilical mass. Although the initial clinical suspicion was a tumoral lesion, abdominal ultrasound and magnetic resonance examination revealed crossed renal ectopia without fusion. The renal ectopy was incidentally diagnosed, as described in 20 to 30% of cases. In this case, the associated nonspecific symptoms were a coincidence.

1. Introduction

Crossed renal ectopia (CRE) is a rare congenital anomaly consisting of the transposition of a kidney to the opposite side. Nevertheless, the ectopic kidney's ureter crosses the midline to insert in its normal position in the bladder [1]. Ninety percent of the crossed ectopic kidneys are fused [2–4].

The majority of pediatric patients are asymptomatic, but they often have nonspecific or unrelated symptoms such as abdominal or flank pain, palpable mass, hematuria, or dysuria. In some reported cases, the patient develops additional symptoms arising from complications such as infection, renal calculi, or urinary obstruction [5]. Accordingly, most cases remain unnoticed whereas 20 to 30% of the cases are only incidentally detected [1–4].

Here, we report the case of crossed nonfused renal ectopia incidentally diagnosed.

Given that the adolescent had an abdominal mass and pain, it was therefore necessary to discard other diagnoses first.

2. Case Report

An 11-year-old adolescent female was admitted to the emergency department with lower abdominal pain for 2 months associated with anorexia and weight loss of about 2 kg in the last month (approximately 4.3% of body weight loss). This was the first time these complaints required medical assistance. The patient had a healthy appearance, but the physical examination revealed a periumbilical, well-defined, and painless mass (9 × 6 cm) and a stool-filled dilated descending colon. The weight, height, and body mass index were, respectively, at the 81st, 83rd, and 78th percentiles on the CDC pediatric growth charts (see Supplementary Material available online at http://dx.doi.org/10.1155/2015/679342) [6]. Breast and pubic hair development were Tanner stage 4 [7]. Blood pressure (BP) measures were below the 50th percentile on BP tables for children and adolescents, by height, sex, and age [8].

Constipation was the only condition reported in the personal medical history. The prenatal ultrasounds scans did not detect any structural abnormalities and were described as normal and no urinary tract infections were diagnosed in the past. No relevant family background was found.

Based on the clinical data (abdominal mass, anorexia, and weight loss), an abdominal tumoral lesion was initially suspected; namely, the most common in this age was lymphoproliferative disease (lymphoma), germ cell tumor (teratoma, germinoma), or sarcoma. However, an abdominal ultrasound was performed and revealed crossed ectopic left kidney not fused to the right kidney. Both kidneys showed normal renal parenchymal thickness, echogenicity, and parenchyma-sinus differentiation. The left ectopic kidney was located in the right hemiabdomen with the hilum anteriorly faced.

The discharge planning took into account the good health appearance and the fact that the adolescent's growth had not crossed the percentile lines (see Supplementary Material). It was recommended to increase fluid and dietary fiber intake and a laxative treatment was prescribed. The patient was reevaluated 3 weeks later in pediatric nephrology consultation. At this time, she already had recovered the previous weight (see Supplementary Material) and the symptoms of constipation had improved.

To complete the renal ectopia investigation, a magnetic resonance imaging and DMSA renal scintigraphy were performed. The magnetic resonance imaging showed the left kidney on the right side, slightly below and anterior to the other kidney (Figures 1 and 2). It also revealed a malrotation of the ectopic kidney with the renal pelvis anteriorly oriented and an apparent left ureteropelvic duplication without dilatation of the excretory system. DMSA renal scintigraphy revealed left renal crossed ectopy, with preserved differential function (46.2% in the left kidney) and without renal scarring. One year follow-up of the patient revealed no further symptoms or no additional complications.

3. Discussion

Renal ectopy and fusion are common congenital anomalies of the kidney and urinary tract, and they result from the disruption of the normal embryologic migration of the kidneys [5]. Renal ectopy occurs when the kidney does not ascend normally to the retroperitoneal renal fossa (level of the second lumbar vertebra) [4, 5, 9]. Simple congenital ectopy refers to a kidney that lies on the correct side of the body but in an abnormal position. When kidneys cross the midline the condition is known as CRE. This can occur with or without fusion to the contralateral kidney [5].

CRE can be anatomically differentiated into four groups: (1) CRE with fusion (the majority of cases, 90%); (2) CRE without fusion (uncommon); (3) solitary CRE (very rare); and (4) unfused bilateral CRE (also very rare) [1–3]. In the first two groups, the ectopic kidney is usually located below the orthotopic kidney. Malrotation of the crossed ectopic kidney is the predominant form. CRE is more frequent in males (M/F = 1.4/1) and is two to three times more common on the right than on the left side [1].

Our patient had the uncommon CRE without fusion identified after investigation of nonspecific symptoms (abdominal pain and palpable mass). The pain was probably associated with constipation. Although weight loss and anorexia were unrelated to the anomaly, these features made the ectopic kidney palpable, facilitating the diagnosis. The renal ectopy was therefore incidentally diagnosed as it occurs in 20 to 30% of the cases [2].

A high incidence of other urological abnormalities has been associated with renal ectopy [1–5]. Vesicoureteral reflux

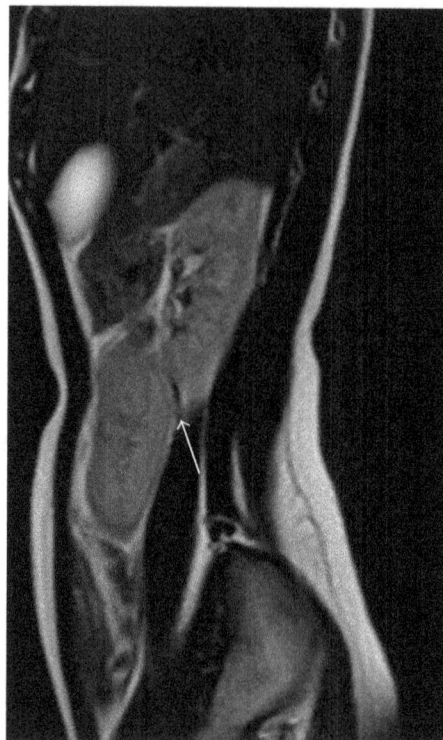

FIGURE 1: 11-year-old adolescent female with left-to-right crossed renal ectopia. Sagittal RM scan, showing a clear plane of separation between the two kidneys (white arrow) and each kidney, having its own Gerota's fascia.

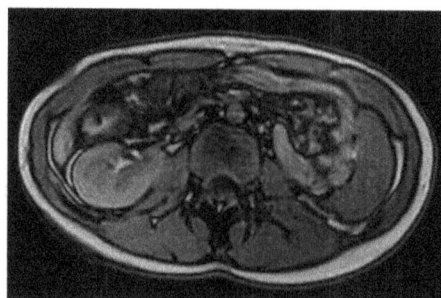

FIGURE 2: 11-year-old adolescent female with left-to-right crossed renal ectopia. Axial RM scan demonstrates two normal enhancing kidneys on the right.

is the most common and occurs in 20% of the CRE cases [5, 9]. Other genitourinary abnormalities include megaureter, hypospadias, cryptorchism, urethral valve and cystic dysplasia, and unilateral agenesis of fallopian tubes and ovaries [1, 5, 10]. Our patient had an apparent left ureteropelvic duplication without dilatation of the bilateral excretory system. No other anomalies were found.

Ectopic kidney can also be associated with other nonrenal anomalies (adrenal, cardiopulmonary, gastrointestinal, and skeletal abnormalities) and genetic syndromes [1, 4, 5, 10].

Moreover, ectopic kidneys are likely to be associated with urological complications, such as urinary infections, renal calculi, and ureteropelvic junction obstruction, due to their frequent abnormal shape, malrotation, and aberrant vasculature [1, 5]. When an ectopic kidney is detected, associated renal and urinary anomalies and structural extrarenal malformations should be evaluated [10].

4. Conclusion

CRE without fusion is a rare condition that can be diagnosed when other diseases are being investigated, as in this case. Treatment is only indicated for the complications.

Patients may need a follow-up and should be examined to check for potential complications.

Conflict of Interests

The authors declare that there is no conflict of interests regarding the publication of this paper.

References

[1] G. N. Nursal and G. Büyükdereli, "Unfused renal ectopia: a rare form of congenital renal anomaly," *Annals of Nuclear Medicine*, vol. 19, no. 6, pp. 507–510, 2005.

[2] B. J. Birmole, S. S. Borwankar, A. S. Vaidya, and B. K. Kulkarni, "Crossed renal ectopia," *Journal of Postgraduate Medicine*, vol. 39, no. 3, pp. 149–151, 1993.

[3] D. P. Ramaema, W. Moloantoa, and Y. Parag, "Crossed renal ectopia without fusion—an unusual cause of acute abdominal pain: a case report," *Case Reports in Urology*, vol. 2012, Article ID 728531, 4 pages, 2012.

[4] C. Oliveira, D. Santos, D. Gomes, G. Choukroun, and M. Kubrusly, "Ectopia renal cruzada com fusão: Relato de dois casos e revisão da literatura," *Jornal Brasileiro de Nefrologia*, vol. 34, no. 3, pp. 283–287, 2012.

[5] A. Waters and N. Rosenblum, *Renal Ectopic and Fusion Anomalies*, UpToDate, 2014, http://www.uptodate.com.

[6] R. J. Kuczmarski, C. L. Ogden, S. S. Guo et al., "2000 CDC Growth Charts for the United States: methods and development," *Vital and Health Statistics*, vol. 11, no. 246, pp. 1–190, 2002.

[7] W. A. Marshall and J. M. Tanner, "Variations in pattern of pubertal changes in girls," *Archives of Disease in Childhood*, vol. 44, no. 235, pp. 291–303, 1969.

[8] National High Blood Pressure Education Program Working Group on High Blood Pressure in Children and Adolescents, "The fourth report on the diagnosis, evaluation and treatment of high blood pressure in children and adolescents," *Pediatrics*, vol. 114, supplement 2, pp. 555–576, 2004.

[9] F. Macedo, "Radiological case," *Nascer e Crescer*, vol. 17, no. 3, pp. 152–153, 2008.

[10] M. Arrieta, R. Trapote, and D. Lizarraga, "Anomalías renales de posición y de fusión," *Anales de Pediatria (Barcelona)*, vol. 75, no. 5, pp. 329–333, 2011.

49

Necrotizing ANCA-Positive Glomerulonephritis Secondary to Culture-Negative Endocarditis

Sophie Van Haare Heijmeijer,[1] **Dunja Wilmes,**[2] **Selda Aydin,**[3]
Caroline Clerckx,[1] **and Laura Labriola**[4]

[1]*Department of Nephrology, Clinique Saint-Pierre, Ottignies, Belgium*
[2]*Department of Internal Medicine, Cliniques universitaires Saint-Luc, Université catholique de Louvain, Brussels, Belgium*
[3]*Department of Pathology, Cliniques universitaires Saint-Luc, Université catholique de Louvain, Brussels, Belgium*
[4]*Department of Nephrology, Cliniques universitaires Saint-Luc, Université catholique de Louvain, Brussels, Belgium*

Correspondence should be addressed to Laura Labriola; laura.labriola@uclouvain.be

Academic Editor: Sofia Lionaki

Infective endocarditis (IE) and small-vessel vasculitis may have similar clinical features, including glomerulonephritis. Furthermore the association between IE and ANCA positivity is well documented, making differential diagnosis between IE- and ANCA-associated vasculitis particularly difficult, especially in case of culture-negative IE. We report on one patient with glomerulonephritis secondary to culture-negative IE caused by *Bartonella henselae* which illustrates this diagnostic difficulty.

1. Introduction

Infective endocarditis (IE) and small-vessel vasculitis may have a similar clinical presentation. Cardiac involvement has been documented in patients with Wegener granulomatosis [1]. Conversely, patients with IE often have renal complications, including glomerulonephritis. Moreover the association between IE and ANCA positivity is well documented, making differential diagnosis between IE- and ANCA-associated vasculitis particularly difficult, especially in case of culture-negative IE. We report on one patient with glomerulonephritis secondary to culture-negative IE caused by *Bartonella henselae* which highlights this diagnostic difficulty.

2. Case

A 67-year-old man presented with asthenia and weight loss (12 kg over 5 months). His medical history included hypertension, bicuspid aortic valve, and thoracic aortic aneurysm repair. He owned four pet dogs and one cat. Medications included amlodipine and acetylsalicylic acid. There was no history of recent dental procedure or use of intravenous drugs. He did not report fever, chills, night sweats, hematuria, or oliguria. On admission he was afebrile and normotensive. Physical examination revealed palpable purpura on his legs without edema.

Three months prior to admission, serum creatinine and CRP levels were 1.6 mg/dL [eGFR 43 mL/min/1.73 m^2 by the 4-variable MDRD (Modification of Diet in Renal Disease Study equation)] and 2.1 mg/dL, respectively. On admission laboratory data revealed serum creatinine 3.5 mg/dL (eGFR 18 mL/min/1.73 m^2), serum urea 88 mg/dL, hemoglobin 8.8 g/dL, normal platelet count, and moderate inflammatory syndrome (CRP 2.3 mg/dL) with polyclonal hypergammaglobulinemia. Urinalysis showed hematuria (1370 red blood cells/μL) with red blood cell casts and moderate proteinuria (protein/creatinine ratio 0.72 g/g; 830 mg/24 h). Further laboratory investigations revealed both positive myeloperoxidase antineutrophil cytoplasmic (MPO-ANCA) (89 RU/mL, normal <20) and proteinase 3 antibodies (PR3-ANCA) (41 RU/mL, normal <20); low complement levels of C3 (80 mg/dL; normal 90–180 mg/dL); normal C4 levels; and increased rheumatoid factor (189 IU/mL; normal <40). Anti-nuclear

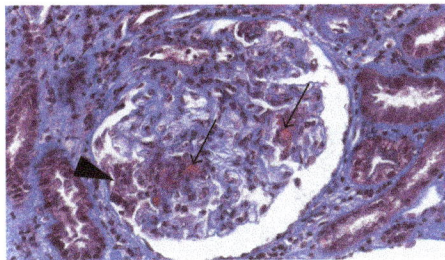

FIGURE 1: Kidney biopsy findings (Masson's trichrome, 46x): glomeruli showing foci of necrosis (arrows) with a recent cellular crescent (arrowhead).

and anti-cardiolipin antibodies were negative. There was no cryoglobulinemia. Serologic tests for hepatitis B, C and HIV were negative. Multiple blood cultures were negative.

Renal biopsy showed segmental necrosis involving 1 out of 16 nonsclerotic glomeruli, as well as one cellular crescent and one fibrous crescent (Figure 1). Two glomeruli were globally sclerosed. Foci of acute interstitial infiltrate and acute tubular necrosis were associated. Mild significant interstitial fibrosis was observed. Immunofluorescence showed moderate granular parietal staining for IgM, C3, and C1q (Figure 2), which suggested infection-related glomerulonephritis. However transesophageal echocardiography did not show any signs of endocarditis. Imaging by positron-emission tomography only showed mild splenomegaly.

Because of this rapidly progressive renal failure secondary to necrotizing and crescentic glomerulonephritis without any evidence of infective endocarditis, treatment with cyclophosphamide (500 mg) and intravenous pulses of methylprednisolone was started, followed by oral corticotherapy (1 mg/kg/day). The patient felt rapidly better and renal function improved.

However, ten days later, creatinine level acutely peaked at 9.2 mg/dL and hemodialysis was started. Two weeks later the patient presented with thoracic pain. Coronary angiography showed a double coronary vessel disease. Repeated transesophageal echocardiography showed severe aortic and moderate mitral insufficiency with possible perforation. Broad-spectrum antibiotics were started and the patient underwent mitral valve repair, aortic valve replacement, and triple coronary artery bypass. He had an uneventful postoperative course. Hemodialysis therapy was discontinued 13 days later. Histopathological examination of the excised valve was consistent with bacterial endocarditis, but cultures of the valve remained negative. Serological test results for atypical pathogens turned negative except for Bartonella henselae (IgM: 1/100; IgG: 1/1280). Bartonella henselae DNA was detected by polymerase chain reaction (PCR) on the resected valve. The patient was administered doxycycline and gentamycin for two weeks. He was discharged home and continued treatment by doxycycline and rifampicin for four more weeks. Methylprednisolone doses were slowly tapered. Three months later, creatinine level was 1.5 mg/dL, and ANCA were negative.

3. Discussion

Renal disease in the setting of IE is a well-known extracardiac complication of IE, affecting as many as 40–50% of patients with IE [2]. Kidney lesions include abscess from septic emboli, immune complex-mediated glomerulonephritis, ANCA-associated glomerulonephritis, and renal toxicity secondary to antibiotics.

Among the causes of infection-related glomerulonephritis in adults, 6–20% are related to endocarditis [3] and glomerulonephritis is considered as a minor Duke criterion for the diagnosis of IE [4]. In a recent large biopsy-based clinicopathologic series on IE-related glomerulonephritis ($n = 49$), acute kidney injury was the most common presenting condition (79%) with hematuria present in almost all cases. However, typical nephritic and nephrotic syndromes were relatively uncommon (9 and 6%, resp.) [5]. Hypocomplementemia (low C3 and/or C4 levels) was found in 56% of patients tested and ANCA antibodies in as many as 28%, with mostly anti-PR3 specificity, although anti-MPO and dual-positive anti-PR3 and anti-MPO were also seen. As in previous reports (summarized in [3]), the most frequent infectious organism identified on blood cultures was Staphylococcus aureus (53%), followed by Streptococcus species (23%) [5]. Importantly, culture-negative endocarditis accounts for almost 10% of the patients with IE-related glomerulonephritis [5, 6].

The spectrum of glomerular histopathologic lesions of IE-related glomerulonephritis is variable. Diffuse necrotizing crescentic GN is the most common pattern (53%), followed by diffuse proliferative glomerulonephritis (37%) and mild mesangial hypercellularity without endocapillary proliferation or crescents (10%) [5]. The immunofluorescence patterns include classic postinfectious type (with prominent IgG and C3 deposition and subepithelial humps on electron microscopy), although IgM- or IgA-dominant staining (particularly with Staphylococcus aureus) has also been reported with variable frequency [3, 5, 7]. Interestingly, the association between IE and pauci-immune glomerulonephritis has been documented in as many as 44% of cases [5].

Our patient has experienced blood culture negative endocarditis, which represents 2.5–31% of all cases of IE [8]. The most often, previous antibiotic therapy is the reason for negative blood cultures. The namely "true" blood culture-negative IE is caused by intracellular bacteria that cannot be routinely cultured in blood with currently available techniques. In a large reference laboratory series, Bartonella sp. was the second most common aetiology in Europe (28%), after Coxiella burnetii [8]. B. quintana has been associated with body-louse infested alcoholic homeless persons, whereas B. henselae has been associated with patients with exposure to cats or their fleas, and previous structural valvulopathy, with most cases occurring in native aortic valves [8].

Diagnostic tests for Bartonella IE include cultures and serologic and DNA amplification techniques. PCR from valvular tissue has been demonstrated to have a higher sensitivity than blood and valvular culture (92% versus 20 and 31%, resp.), even in patients receiving antibiotics [8]. In a recent large series of Bartonella IE, serum Western

TABLE 1: Characteristics of published cases of *Bartonella* endocarditis-associated glomerulonephritis.

Case	Serum complement level		ANCA	Light microscopy	IF microscopy	Diagnostic	Therapy
	C3	C4					
van Tooren et al. [9]	ND	ND	Negative	Diffuse proliferative GN / Focal crescents	ND	Serology	Antibiotics / Valvular surgery
Bookman et al. [10] Case 1	↓	↓	Negative	Segmental necrosis / Crescents	IgM-dominant staining C3 deposits	Serology	Prednisolone / Antibiotics
Bookman et al. [10] Case 2	N	↓	Negative	Segmental necrosis / Crescents	IgM-dominant staining C3 deposits	Serology	Prednisolone / Antibiotics / Valvular surgery
Bookman et al. [10] Case 3	↓	↓	Negative	Segmental necrosis / Crescents	IgM-dominant staining C3 deposits	Serology	Antibiotics / Valvular surgery
Turner et al. [11]	ND	ND	Anti-PR3	Focal crescents	IgA-dominant staining	PCR on valvular tissue	Prednisolone / Cyclophosphamide / Antibiotics / Valvular surgery
Vikram et al. [12]	ND	ND	Anti-PR3	Segmental necrosis / Focal crescents	Pauci-immune	Serology / PCR on valvular tissue	Prednisolone / Cyclophosphamide / Antibiotics / Valvular surgery
Forbes et al. [13]	↓	↓	Anti-PR3	Diffuse proliferative GN	IgG/C3/C1q	Serology	Antibiotics
Salvado et al. [14]	↓	N	Anti-PR3	Diffuse proliferative GN / Diffuse crescents	IgM/C3/C1q	Serology	Antibiotics
Khalighi et al. [15]	↓	↓	Anti-PR3	Diffuse proliferative GN / Focal crescents	IgM-dominant staining C3/C1q deposits	Serology / PCR on blood	Antibiotics / Prednisolone
Shah et al. [16]	ND	ND	Anti-PR3	Necrotizing GN	Pauci-immune	Serology / Culture of valvular tissue	Prednisolone / Cyclophosphamide / Antibiotics / Valvular surgery
Present report	↓	N	Anti-PR3 and anti-MPO	Focal/segmental necrosis/crescents	IgM/C3/C1q	Serology / PCR on valvular tissue	Prednisolone / Cyclophosphamide / Antibiotics / Valvular surgery

Ref IF: immunofluorescence; GN: glomerulonephritis; N: normal; and ND: not determined.

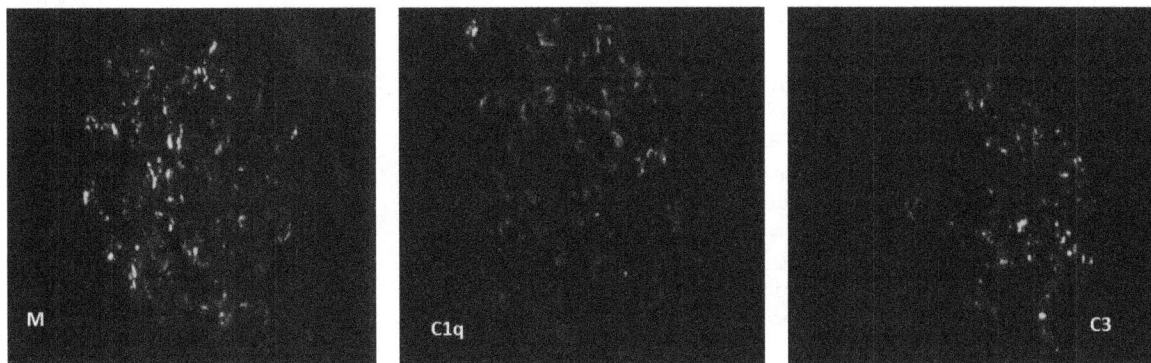

FIGURE 2: Immunofluorescence shows subepithelial granular staining for IgM and C3 and parietal granular staining for C1q.

blotting (WB), PCR, and 16S rRNA gene amplification in valvular tissue exhibited sensitivities of 100%, 92%, and 60%, respectively [17]. Although PCR on total blood and serum may enable the diagnosis before cardiac surgery, its sensitivity is low (33% and 36%, resp.) [17]. *Bartonella* species IgG titer >1 : 800 using an immunofluorescence assay has a predictive value of 95% to detect *Bartonella* IE, but a titer <800 does not exclude the diagnosis [17, 18]. Therefore, any patient with IgG titer <800 and a medical history evocative of IE should be tested by WB and PCR following cardiac valve removal. Currently, it is considered that a positive PCR from a cardiac valve or blood specimen, an IgG titer of >800, and a positive WB assay should be major criteria for *Bartonella* IE [17].

Glomerular disease in the setting of *Bartonella* IE seems to be a rare complication, but its true incidence is unknown. To the best of our knowledge, there have been only 10 cases published to date (Table 1); all of them are caused by *B. henselae*. Hypocomplementemia was documented in the 6 patients in whom complement levels were tested. ANCA were positive in 7/11 cases, with anti-PR3 specificity in 6. Of note, dual anti-PR3 and anti-MPO specificity was documented in only one case (this present case). The predominant light microscopy pattern of injury was segmental necrotizing crescentic glomerulonephritis. On immunofluorescence, the predominant immunoglobulin was IgM, with strong C3 deposits, although in two cases there was a dominant staining for IgA [11] and IgG [14]. Only two cases showed a pauci-immune pattern. Most cases required valvular surgery. Interestingly, in 7/11 cases, immunosuppressive agents were first administered for a suspected vasculitis and withdrawn when the diagnosis of endocarditis was made.

This case highlights the difficulty to make the differential diagnosis between occult infection with secondary glomerular involvement and ANCA-associated vasculitis. Distinguishing these two conditions is crucial, particularly when immunosuppressive treatment is considered. Although delayed, the diagnosis of culture-negative IE was finally suggested by a proliferative immune complex-mediated glomerulonephritis in a patient with a structural cardiac valve anomaly. The association of rapidly progressive renal failure secondary to necrotizing and crescentic glomerulonephritis and palpable purpura on the legs without any evidence of IE has initially supported the diagnosis of ANCA-associated vasculitis. However, even in case of negative blood cultures, the concomitant presence of hypocomplementemia and positive ANCA antibodies is strongly suggestive of immune complex-mediated disease. Moreover the dual-positive ANCA specificity anti-PR3 and anti-MPO is very unusual and should always trigger the screening for secondary causes of ANCA positivity, that is, occult infection, including IE due to atypical pathogens [5], or levamisole-contaminated cocaine use [19].

Conflict of Interests

The authors declare that there is no conflict of interests regarding the publication of this paper.

Authors' Contribution

Sophie Van Haare Heijmeijer and Dunja Wilmes have contributed equally to this paper.

References

[1] G. S. Hoffman, G. S. Kerr, R. Y. Leavitt et al., "Wegener granulomatosis: an analysis of 158 patients," *Annals of Internal Medicine*, vol. 116, no. 6, pp. 488–498, 1992.

[2] D. J. Sexton and D. Spelman, "Current best practices and guidelines. Assessment and management of complications in infective endocarditis," *Cardiology Clinics*, vol. 21, no. 2, pp. 273–282, 2003.

[3] S. H. Nasr, J. Radhakrishnan, and V. D. D'Agati, "Bacterial infection-related glomerulonephritis in adults," *Kidney International*, vol. 83, no. 5, pp. 792–803, 2013.

[4] J. S. Li, D. J. Sexton, N. Mick et al., "Proposed modifications to the Duke criteria for the diagnosis of infective endocarditis," *Clinical Infectious Diseases*, vol. 30, no. 4, pp. 633–638, 2000.

[5] C. L. Boils, S. H. Nasr, P. D. Walker, W. G. Couser, and C. P. Larsen, "Update on endocarditis-associated glomerulonephritis," *Kidney International*, vol. 87, no. 6, pp. 1241–1249, 2015.

[6] P.-E. Fournier, F. Thuny, H. Richet et al., "Comprehensive diagnostic strategy for blood culture-negative endocarditis: a

prospective study of 819 new cases," *Clinical Infectious Diseases*, vol. 51, no. 2, pp. 131–140, 2010.

[7] A. Majumdar, S. Chowdhary, M. A. S. Ferreira et al., "Renal pathological findings in infective endocarditis," *Nephrology Dialysis Transplantation*, vol. 15, no. 11, pp. 1782–1787, 2000.

[8] P. Houpikian and D. Raoult, "Blood culture-negative endocarditis in a reference center: etiologic diagnosis of 348 cases," *Medicine*, vol. 84, no. 3, pp. 162–173, 2005.

[9] R. M. van Tooren, R. van Leusen, and F. H. Bosch, "Culture negative endocarditis combined with glomerulonephritis caused by *Bartonella* species in two immunocompetent adults," *Netherlands Journal of Medicine*, vol. 59, no. 5, pp. 218–224, 2001.

[10] I. Bookman, J. W. Scholey, S. V. Jassal, G. Lajoie, and A. M. Herzenberg, "Necrotizing glomerulonephritis caused by *Bartonella henselae* endocarditis," *American Journal of Kidney Diseases*, vol. 43, no. 2, pp. e25–e30, 2004.

[11] J. W. Turner, B. C. Pien, S. A. Ardoin et al., "A man with chest pain and glomerulonephritis," *The Lancet*, vol. 365, no. 9476, article 2062, 2005.

[12] H. R. Vikram, A. K. Bacani, P. A. DeValeria, S. A. Cunningham, and F. R. Cockerill III, "Bivalvular *Bartonella henselae* prosthetic valve endocarditis," *Journal of Clinical Microbiology*, vol. 45, no. 12, pp. 4081–4084, 2007.

[13] S. H. Forbes, S. C. Robert, J. E. Martin, and R. Rajakariar, "Acute kidney injury with hematuria, a positive ANCA test, and low levels of complement," *American Journal of Kidney Diseases*, vol. 59, no. 1, pp. A28–A31, 2012.

[14] C. Salvado, A. Mekinian, P. Rouvier, P. Poignard, I. Pham, and O. Fain, "Rapidly progressive crescentic glomerulonephritis and aneurism with antineutrophil cytoplasmic antibody: *Bartonella henselae* endocarditis," *Presse Medicale*, vol. 42, no. 6, pp. 1060–1061, 2013.

[15] M. A. Khalighi, S. Nguyen, J. A. Wiedeman, and M. F. Palma Diaz, "*Bartonella endocarditis*-associated glomerulonephritis: a case report and review of the literature," *American Journal of Kidney Diseases*, vol. 63, no. 6, pp. 1060–1065, 2014.

[16] S. H. Shah, C. Grahame-Clarke, and C. N. Ross, "Touch not the cat bot a glove: ANCA-positive pauci-immune necrotizing glomerulonephritis secondary to *Bartonella henselae*," *Clinical Kidney Journal*, vol. 7, no. 2, pp. 179–181, 2014.

[17] S. Edouard, C. Nabet, H. Lepidi, P. E. Fournier, and D. Raoult, "*Bartonella*, a common cause of endocarditis: a report on 106 cases and review," *Journal of Clinical Microbiology*, vol. 53, no. 3, pp. 824–829, 2015.

[18] P.-E. Fournier, J.-L. Mainardi, and D. Raoult, "Value of microimmunofluorescence for diagnosis and follow-up of *Bartonella* endocarditis," *Clinical and Diagnostic Laboratory Immunology*, vol. 9, no. 4, pp. 795–801, 2002.

[19] A. Q. Carlson, D. S. Tuot, K.-Y. Jen et al., "Pauci-immune glomerulonephritis in individuals with disease associated with levamisole-adulterated cocaine: a series of 4 cases," *Medicine*, vol. 93, no. 17, pp. 290–297, 2014.

50

Homozygosity for the E526V Mutation in Fibrinogen A Alpha-Chain Amyloidosis: The First Report

Isabel Tavares,[1,2] **Luísa Lobato,**[3,4] **Carlos Matos,**[3] **Josefina Santos,**[3,4] **Paul Moreira,**[5] **Maria João Saraiva,**[5] **and António Castro Henriques**[3,4]

[1] *Department of Nephrology, Centro Hospitalar de São João, 4200-319 Porto, Portugal*
[2] *Nephrology and Infectious Diseases Research and Development Group, INEB (I3S), University of Porto, 4150-180 Porto, Portugal*
[3] *Department of Nephrology, Centro Hospitalar do Porto, Hospital de Santo António, 4099-001 Porto, Portugal*
[4] *Unit for Multidisciplinary Research in Biomedicine, Instituto de Ciências Biomédicas Abel Salazar, University of Porto, 4050-313 Porto, Portugal*
[5] *Molecular Neurobiology, Institute of Molecular and Cellular Biology, University of Porto, 4150-180 Porto, Portugal*

Correspondence should be addressed to Isabel Tavares; isabel.salome@hsjoao.min-saude.pt

Academic Editor: Raoul Bergner

Systemic hereditary amyloidoses are autosomal dominant diseases associated with mutations in genes encoding ten different proteins. The clinical phenotype has implications on therapeutic approach, but it is commonly variable and largely dependent on the type of mutation. Except for rare cases involving gelsolin or transthyretin, patients are heterozygous for the amyloidogenic variants. Here we describe the first patient identified worldwide as homozygous for a nephropathic amyloidosis, involving the fibrinogen variant associated with the fibrinogen alpha-chain E526V (p.Glu545Val) mutation. In 1989, a 44-year-old woman presented with hypertension, hepatosplenomegaly, nephrotic syndrome, and renal failure. She started hemodialysis in 1990 and 6 years later underwent isolated kidney transplantation from a deceased donor. Graft function and clinical status were unremarkable for 16 years, despite progressively increased left ventricular mass on echocardiography. In 2012, 4 months before death, she deteriorated rapidly with severe heart failure, precipitated by *Clostridium difficile* colitis and urosepsis. Affected family members developed nephropathy, on average, nearly three decades later, which may be explained by the gene dosage effects on the phenotype of E526V (p.Glu545Val) fibrinogen A alpha-chain amyloidosis.

1. Introduction

Hereditary fibrinogen A alpha-chain (AFib) amyloidosis is a systemic amyloid disease first characterized in 1993 in a Peruvian kindred [1–4]. It presents with proteinuria and features a progressive decline in kidney function to end stage renal failure (ESRF) within 5 years of diagnosis [3]. Nonetheless, there is a wide variability in disease onset, systemic involvement, and penetrance. Renal replacement therapy and transplantation are currently the mainstay of therapy. However, because the liver is the source of the amyloidogenic variant fibrinogen and there is no evidence that WT fibrinogen can be amyloidogenic, the only curative treatment is liver transplantation [5].

AFib amyloidosis appears to be more common worldwide than previously recognized [6]. The R554L (p.Arg573Leu) mutation was the first fibrinogen amyloidogenic variant identified [1]. To date, thirteen amyloidogenic mutations have been reported in the fibrinogen alpha-chain gene (*FGA*) (http://amyloidosismutations.com/mut-afib.php), accounting for 8% of hereditary amyloidosis cases [7]. The most common mutant variant, E526V (p.Glu545Val), was identified heterozygously in kindred members of Irish, British, Polish, Portuguese, French, German, and Brazilian origin [2, 3, 8–11]. Homozygosity has only been reported for hereditary gelsolin and transthyretin amyloidosis (Table 1). In gelsolin (AGel) amyloidosis, homozygotes have been reported to show earlier onset and more severe clinical manifestations

TABLE 1: Homozygous amyloidogenic variants reported in the literature.

Gene	Protein variant	Sequence variant (mRNA)	Patients (n)	Geographic origin/ethnicity	Reported phenotype	Clinical course	References
GSN	Asp187Asn (p.Asp214Asn)	c.640G>A	2	Finland	CN, CLD, SC, CRF	Severe nephropathy	[12, 13]
TTR	Val30Met (p.Val50Met)	c.148G>A	19	Japan Spain Sweden Turkey	PN, AN, VO, GI, H, CN	Wide variability, from asymptomatic carriers to slightly more severe phenotypes with higher incidence rate and earlier onset than heterozygotes within the same family	[14–19]
	Leu58His (p.Leu78His)	c.233T>G	1	American/German	PN, CMP	More rapid course of disease	[20]
	Phe64Leu (p.Phe84Leu)	c.250T>C	1	Italy	PN, AN, CMP	More severe phenotype	[21]
	Val122Ile (p.Val142Ile)	c.424G>A	24	African/American	CMP	Earlier age at onset and uncertain penetrance, particularly with respect to gender	[22, 23]

AN: autonomic neuropathy; CLD: corneal lattice dystrophy; CMP: cardiomyopathy; CN: cranial neuropathy; CRF: chronic renal failure; GI: gastrointestinal symptoms; H: heart conduction disturbance; PN: peripheral polyneuropathy; SC: skin changes; VO: vitreous opacities.

than heterozygotes, explained by the lethal effects of the mutant genes [12, 13]. However, in transthyretin (ATTR) amyloidosis, the underlying molecular mechanisms are largely unknown [14–23].

Here, we report the first homozygous patient with AFibE526V (p.Glu545Val) amyloidosis, identified in 1989 and followed up for 23 years. In this reported kindred, the comparison of the clinical pictures of homozygote and heterozygotes provides important information about the gene dosage effects on the phenotype of AFib amyloidosis.

2. Case Report

2.1. Proband. A 44-year-old Caucasian northern Portuguese woman who had suffered a single previous episode of upper gastrointestinal hemorrhage presented with hypertension, nephrotic syndrome, and renal failure in April 1989. Renal biopsy 1 year later revealed abundant glomerular amyloid deposition (Figure 1(a)); her serum creatinine was 4.0 mg/dL and proteinuria of 7.5 g/day was detected. In the absence of any underlying inflammatory disease and unawareness of family history, she was presumed to have immunoglobulin light chain (AL) amyloidosis. However, there was no evidence of cardiac amyloidosis, and neither a monoclonal immunoglobulin nor a plasma cell disorder was identified. She was treated with melphalan and corticosteroids but progressed rapidly to ESRF and started hemodialysis in December 1990. During hemodialysis, her functional status remained good.

Successful isolated renal transplantation (RTx) was performed in August 1996. At the time, she had no other health problems. Physical examination revealed an enlarged liver and spleen. There was no anemia or thrombocytopenia and liver function tests were normal. Blood coagulation tests revealed low fibrinogen levels. Echocardiography showed mild left ventricular hypertrophy without the typical speckle appearance. Abdominal ultrasonography showed hepatomegaly (17.5 cm), splenomegaly (14.5 cm), and bilateral kidney atrophy. A neurophysiologic study of the lower limbs found mild sensory peripheral neuropathy. Induction and maintenance immunosuppression for transplantation involved corticosteroids, cyclosporine, and azathioprine.

2.2. Histology and Immunohistochemistry. In 2001, we began an extensive investigation to determine the patient's amyloid type. Congo red staining of 6 μm formalin fixed, paraffin embedded section of the native kidney biopsy confirmed abundant glomerular amyloid deposition and absence of vascular and interstitial involvement. Immunohistochemical staining was performed on 2 μm sections of amyloid-containing tissue using standard methods and a rabbit/mouse, peroxidase/diaminobenzidine detection system (REAL EnVision: Dako, Glostrup, Denmark). mAbs were directed against serum amyloid A (Dako), apolipoprotein A-II (Abcam, Cambridge, UK), and transthyretin [24]; polyclonal antibodies were used for kappa light chain, lambda light chain, fibrinogen A alpha-chain (FGA), transthyretin, apolipoprotein A-I, and lysozyme (Dako). For light chains and FGA, sections were treated with 10 μg/mL proteinase K for 10 min at 37°C and 10 min at room temperature. Blocking was performed with 5% bovine serum albumin/phosphate buffered saline (BSA/PBS). Sections were incubated with the antibodies for 2 h at room temperature and diluted in 1% BSA/PBS as follows: monoclonal anti-transthyretin, used directly; polyclonal anti-transthyretin, 1 : 500; anti-serum amyloid A, 1 : 100; anti-kappa light chain, 1 : 1000; anti-lambda light chain, 1 : 2000; anti-FGA, 1 : 800; anti-lysozyme, 1 : 300; anti-apolipoprotein A-I, 1 : 400; and anti-apolipoprotein A-II, 1 : 600. Positive control tissues containing these amyloid proteins were also stained during each run. The glomerular amyloid deposits in the patient's kidney biopsy reacted with the anti-serum to FGA (Figure 1(a)).

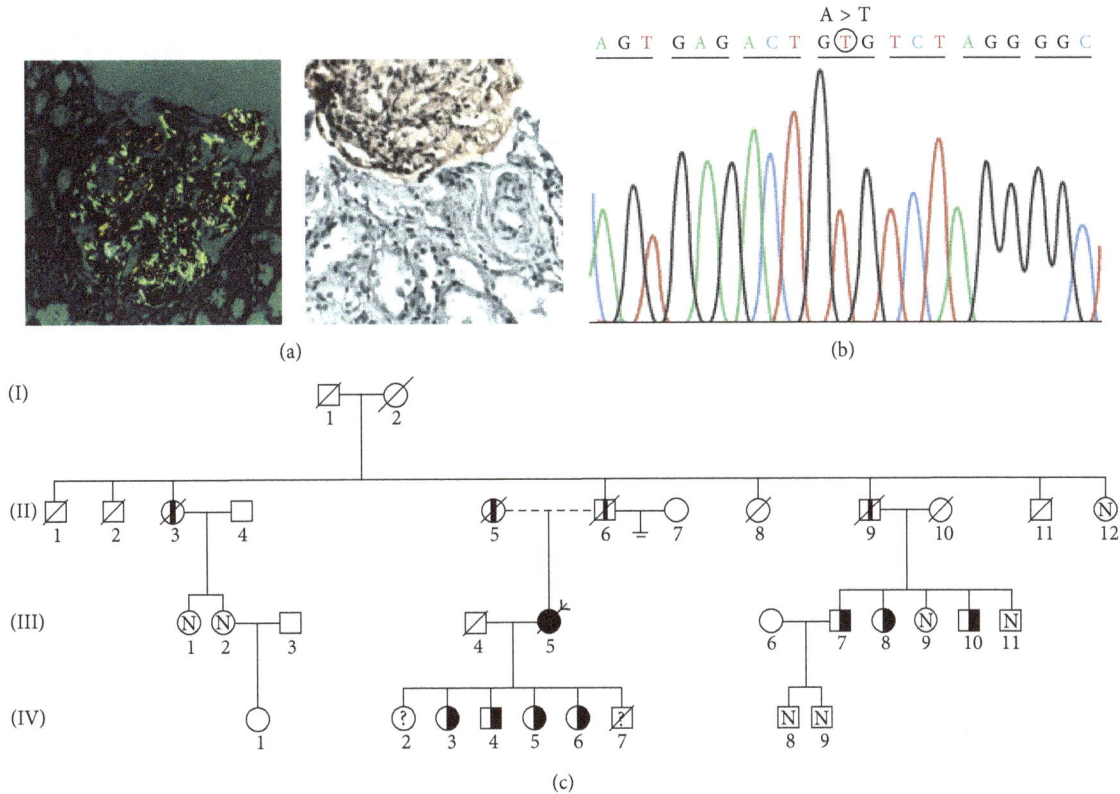

FIGURE 1: Homozygous E526V (p.Glu545Val) mutation in the fibrinogen alpha-chain gene (*FGA*) associated with fibrinogen A alpha-chain amyloidosis in a Portuguese patient. (a) shows abundant glomerular amyloid deposition with typical apple-green birefringence (Congo red staining under polarized light, ×200, left). Immunohistochemical staining was positive with polyclonal anti-fibrinogen antibodies, (×200, right). (b) shows a partial sequence chromatogram of *FGA*. The mutation identified in the proband, which alters codon 545 (position 526 of the mature protein) from GAG (glutamic acid) to GTG (valine), is depicted in a circle. (c) shows the pedigree of the affected kindred. The homozygous patient (proband) is indicated by the arrow. The *FGA* p.Glu545Val mutation was identified heterozygously in family members III7, III8, III10, IV3, IV4, IV5, and IV6 (indicated by half-solid symbols). Obligatory heterozygotes IV2 and IV7 (indicated by question marks) did not perform genotyping because the former was abroad and the latter died at young age. Those with chronic renal failure who have not undergone histologic or genetic testing are indicated by a black column inside the symbol. Familiars whose genetic tests were negative are indicated by an N inside the symbol. Blank symbols indicate that tests have not been conducted and/or information is unavailable for these individuals. Slashes denote deceased members.

2.3. Genetic Evaluation. DNA was extracted from peripheral white blood cells obtained from whole blood. Exon 5 of the *FGA* gene was amplified by the polymerase chain reaction (PCR) with primers flanking the coding region (forward 5′-CCT TCT TCG ACA CTG CCT CAA CTG-3′ and reverse 5′-TCC TCT GTT GTA ACT CGT GCT-3′), which amplified a fragment of 224 base pairs encompassing nucleotide 4827 to 5051. PCR products were analyzed by agarose gel electrophoresis, purified, and sequenced with Big Dye Terminator Cycle Sequencing Kit (Applied Biosystems, Foster City, CA, USA) in an Applied Biosystems 3700 sequencer. Sequences were analysed using ChromasPro. A homozygous A to T transversion at nucleotide 4909 in *FGA* was detected; this changes codon 526 of the mature protein (corresponding to position 545 of the unprocessed gene product), from GAG, encoding glutamic acid, to GTG, encoding valine (Figure 1(b)). Codons are numbered according to reference sequence NM_000508.3.

2.4. Proband Outcome. During 16 years of follow-up after RTx, there were no episodes of rejection and she was normotensive. Maximal proteinuria of 0.9 g/day was detected in 2009 and renal graft function remained good until 4 months before her death; thus, no renal allograft biopsy was performed. Peptic ulcer due to *Helicobacter pylori* infection was diagnosed after an episode of upper gastrointestinal hemorrhage. Apparent progression of extrarenal amyloid disease was mainly cardiovascular and hepatic. Repeated electrocardiography found sinus rhythm, normal intervals, and no criteria for hypertrophy. Serial echocardiography showed left atrial enlargement (53 mm), severely abnormal left ventricular hypertrophy (left ventricular mass index increased from $154 \, \text{g/m}^2$ in 2006 to $170 \, \text{g/m}^2$ in 2012, with a reference range of 43–$95 \, \text{g/m}^2$), mild degenerative valvular disease, preserved systolic ventricular function, and moderate pulmonary hypertension. These findings were consistent with cardiac amyloidosis. Hepatic involvement was characterized by mild elevations of gamma-glutamyl transferase

TABLE 2: Laboratory data.

Parameter/date	02.14.2006	04.07.2009	08.17.2010	08.14.2012	11.26.2012	12.05.2012
Urea (mg/dL)	69	41	89	136	135	188
Creatinine (mg/dL)	0.80	0.75	1.03	1.22	1.44	4.62
Creatinine clearance (mL/min/1.73 m^2)	67.9	84.7	68.3	45.9	37.6	9.2
Albumin (g/L)	43.0		45.7			
HbA1c (%)			5.9			
Uric acid (mg/dL)		6.7	8.9	7.0		
Total bilirubin (mg/dL)	0.79	0.60	0.60	0.72	1.13	0.96
AST (U/L)	21	23	23	19	14	22
ALT(U/L)	19	14	20	15	2	12
ALP (U/L)	102	106	134	139	160	170
GGT (U/L)	90	86	88	81	106	65
Sodium (mmol/L)	144		134	136	132	122
Potassium (mmol/L)	4.73		4.17	4.50	4.87	5.73
Chloride (mmol/L)	106		96	101	96	98
Calcium (mmol/L)	2.52		2.56			2.02
Phosphorus (mmol/L)	1.03		1.18			2.09
iPTH (pg/mL)	75	80	103			
Total cholesterol (mg/dL)	203	207	196	155		
Triglycerides (mg/dL)	127	78	105	111		
NT-proBNP (pg/mL)					14 056	
CRP (mg/dL)						85.62
Cyclosporine (ng/mL)		80.5	94.7			130.2
Proteinuria (g/24 h)	0.15	0.90	0.51			

HbA1c: glycated hemoglobin; AST: aspartate aminotransferase; ALT: alanine aminotransferase; ALP: alkaline phosphatase; GGT: gamma-glutamyl transferase; iPTH: intact parathyroid hormone; NT-proBNP: N-terminal pro-B-type natriuretic peptide; CRP: C-reactive protein.

and alkaline phosphatase with increasing hepatomegaly; the liver's ultrasound diameter reached 22.7 cm in September 2012. At that time, the spleen diameter was 9.4 cm and there were several calcifications. There was no sign of portal hypertension. Relevant laboratory data are listed in Table 2.

In August 2012, 4 months before her death, the patient was hospitalized for *Clostridium difficile* colitis, which was successfully treated with metronidazole. One month later, she was admitted for congestive heart failure with an N-terminal pro-B-type natriuretic peptide (NT-proBNP) level of 31 937 pg/mL; this was controlled with diuretic therapy. In November 2012, she was hospitalized for hyponatremia associated with effective circulating volume depletion. She died in December 2012 after admission for *Klebsiella pneumoniae* urosepsis, congestive heart failure with NT-proBNP 14 056 pg/mL unresponsive to diuretic therapy, and acute kidney allograft injury. Autopsy was not performed.

2.5. Kindred. After some years of research, a family tree was obtained (Figure 1(c)). The research protocol was approved by the Health Ethics Commission of Centro Hospitalar de São João. The mother of the proband (II5) presented with hypertension aged 67 years. She had a stroke at 76 years and died from chronic renal failure (CRF) 1 year later. The father (II6) had hypertension from the age of 55 years, significant cardiovascular disease (peripheral artery disease, ischemic cardiopathy), and CRF from 77 years, dying from

pneumonia at 82 years. One paternal aunt (II3) died at 84 years due to hemorrhagic cerebrovascular accident. She had hypertension from the age of 59 years and CRF from 69 years and had started hemodialysis at 79 years. One paternal uncle (II9) had hypertension from the age of 61 years, significant cardiovascular disease (peripheral artery disease, ischemic cardiopathy), and CRF from 72 years, dying from uremia at 78 years. Three first cousins (III7, III8, and III10) had hypertension (from 57, 55, and 53 years, resp.) and carried the same amyloidogenic fibrinogen mutation. As patient III5 was homozygous for the *FGA* p.Glu545Val mutation, all her offspring are obligatory heterozygotes. This condition was confirmed by genotyping in all, except IV2, who was abroad, and IV7, who died at young age. Members IV3 and IV4 had hypertension from the age of 45 and 43 years, respectively.

3. Discussion

Here, we describe the first AFib amyloidosis patient homozygous for the E526V (p.Glu545Val) mutation and her long term outcome after isolated RTx. The unexpected etiology and outcome of this case highlight important aspects of the clinical management of systemic amyloidosis in general. Our patient's prolonged survival without treatment and the absence of an identifiable monoclonal plasma cell disorder led us to question the diagnosis of AL amyloidosis. Retrospective finding that the amyloid deposits in her kidney biopsy were derived from FGA and the complete concordance between the presence of the E526V (p.Glu545Val) and the development of amyloidosis indicated that this mutation was the cause of the disease in the proband's family. This approach ensured family screening.

Immunohistochemical classification of 102 northern Portuguese patients with amyloidosis diagnosed in native kidney biopsies disclosed 4 (3.9%) cases of AFib, including our proband. They were all from the same rural geographical area and belonged to apparently unrelated families [25]. In the case of our homozygous patient, both parents had CRF and consanguinity was not possible to prove, but they may share a common ancestor given the possibility of an endemic focus of the disease in their region. In this context, homozygosity proposal was based on DNA sequencing (Figure 1(b)).

Previously reported AFib amyloidosis phenotypes result from the heterozygous genotype. The effect of homozygosity on phenotype has been reported for patients with hereditary transthyretin [14–23] or gelsolin [12, 13] amyloidosis (Table 1), but this is the first report for AFib amyloidosis. Our patient presented at a relatively early age and during long term follow-up apparently developed a heavy disease burden with multisystem involvement. After RTx, serial echocardiography demonstrated increased wall thickness, despite normotension and normal graft function, consistent with cardiac amyloidosis. The main forms of amyloidosis that affect the heart are light chain and ATTR amyloidosis. Cardiac involvement of AFib amyloidosis was described in a cohort of 22 AFib patients [4], 52% had abnormal echocardiographic findings suggestive of amyloid cardiomyopathy, and 55% had parasympathetic dysfunction and risk of bradycardia. Coronary atherosclerosis was identified in 68%. In the present case, cardiac involvement in the setting of established AFib amyloidosis, with left ventricular hypertrophy on echocardiography and a relative low-voltage electrocardiogram, complicated by congestive heart failure refractory to standard medical therapy, was considered cardiac amyloidosis. Two of the family members developed atherosclerotic cardiovascular disease with no echocardiographic evidence of cardiac amyloidosis. Affected family members developed nephropathy almost three decades later and five heterozygous carriers developed hypertension in their forties and fifties. Thus, the clinical phenotype of our homozygous patient was more severe (earlier onset of nephropathy, cardiac and hepatic involvement) than those of heterozygotes in the same family, consistent with gene dosage effects on the phenotype of AFib amyloidosis. The follow-up of hypertensive heterozygous carriers will be helpful in the study of the pathogenesis of hypertension in AFib amyloidosis.

In systemic amyloidosis, solid organ transplantation has been used to replace failing organ function [26–29]. Isolated RTx alone has been performed for ESRF in several patients with AFib and probably remains appropriate when there is good evidence that amyloid deposition does not threaten the function of other vital organs. Gillmore et al. reported that RTx in AFib is associated with recurrence of amyloid in the graft with resultant loss of transplanted kidneys after a median of 6.7 years [3]. CLKT in a patient with amyloidotic renal failure caused by the *FGA* p.Glu545Val

mutation was first performed in 1995 [28]. Despite liver transplantation being the only currently available curative treatment for AFib, it seems reasonable to propose it for younger and fitter patients, weighing the high risk of early perioperative death following CLKT against the elimination of the risk of recurrent amyloid disease in the allograft [3, 29]. Transplantation in our patient aimed to replace her failing organ function, because in 1996 her amyloid type was unknown; it was 5 years later that we made a retrospective diagnosis of hereditary fibrinogen amyloidosis. Despite isolated RTx, our patient's outcome was not unfavourable compared to the results with CLKT [3, 4]. Her apparent cardiac and hepatic AFib involvement progressed despite clinical absence of disease recurrence in the allograft. Mild proteinuria appeared 13 years after transplantation, but allograft function remained good until 4 months before the patient's death. At that time, cardiovascular symptoms were her principal problem, due to cardiac amyloidosis suggested by echocardiography. In patients with cardiac AFib involvement, combined heart-liver, heart-kidney, or heart-liver-kidney transplantation could be discussed [30, 31], but, given the high risk in our 67-year-old patient, she received recommended drug treatment only. She died 16 years after renal transplantation due to severe heart failure in the context of sepsis.

4. Conclusions

In conclusion, correct identification of amyloidogenic protein should always be pursued, even retrospectively, because it enables the choice of the most appropriate therapy, avoids unnecessary and potentially harmful treatments, and ensures family screening. This first report of a homozygous AFibE526V (p.Glu545Val) amyloidosis expands our knowledge about the phenotype and the outcome of isolated renal transplantation and may be relevant for understanding the molecular mechanisms of dominance in hereditary amyloidosis.

Conflict of Interests

The authors declare that there is no conflict of interests regarding the publication of this paper.

Authors' Contribution

Isabel Tavares and Luísa Lobato, the first and second authors, contributed equally to this paper.

Acknowledgments

The authors thank posthumously Dr. Elísio Carvalho of the Department of Nephrology and Renal Pathology of Centro Hospitalar de São João, Porto, Portugal, for his contribution to this work. They thank Professor João Paulo Oliveira for his critical revision of the paper. This work was supported by the National Funds through the FCT, Fundação para a Ciência e Tecnologia (Portuguese National Funding Agency for Science, Research and Technology) in the frameworks of the PEst-OE/SAU/UI0215/2014 project, Unit for Multidisciplinary Research in Biomedicine, UMIB/ICBAS/UP.

References

[1] M. D. Benson, J. Liepnieks, T. Uemichi, G. Wheeler, and R. Correa, "Hereditary renal amyloidosis associated with a mutant fibrinogen α-chain," *Nature Genetics*, vol. 3, no. 3, pp. 252–255, 1993.

[2] M. De Carvalho, R. P. Linke, F. Domingos et al., "Mutant fibrinogen A-α-chain associated with hereditary renal amyloidosis and peripheral neuropathy," *Amyloid*, vol. 11, no. 3, pp. 200–207, 2004.

[3] J. D. Gillmore, H. J. Lachmann, D. Rowczenio et al., "Diagnosis, pathogenesis, treatment, and prognosis of hereditary fibrinogen Aalpha-chain amyloidosis," *Journal of the American Society of Nephrology*, vol. 20, no. 2, pp. 444–451, 2009.

[4] A. J. Stangou, N. R. Banner, B. M. Hendry et al., "Hereditary fibrinogen a α-chain amyloidosis: phenotypic characterization of a systemic disease and the role of liver transplantation," *Blood*, vol. 115, no. 15, pp. 2998–3007, 2010.

[5] G. A. Tennent, S. O. Brennan, A. J. Stangou, J. O'Grady, P. N. Hawkins, and M. B. Pepys, "Human plasma fibrinogen is synthesized in the liver," *Blood*, vol. 109, no. 5, pp. 1971–1974, 2007.

[6] M. M. Picken, "Fibrinogen amyloidosis: the clot thickens!," *Blood*, vol. 115, no. 15, pp. 2985–2986, 2010.

[7] D. M. Rowczenio, I. Noor, J. D. Gillmore et al., "Online registry for mutations in hereditary amyloidosis including nomenclature recommendations," *Human Mutation*, vol. 35, pp. E2403–E2412, 2014.

[8] T. Uemichi, J. J. Liepnieks, and M. D. Benson, "Hereditary renal amyloidosis with a novel variant fibrinogen," *The Journal of Clinical Investigation*, vol. 93, no. 2, pp. 731–736, 1994.

[9] T. Uemichi, J. J. Liepnieks, F. Alexander, and M. D. Benson, "The molecular basis of renal amyloidosis in Irish-American and Polish-Canadian kindreds," *QJM*, vol. 89, no. 10, pp. 745–750, 1996.

[10] M. Eriksson, S. Schönland, R. Bergner et al., "Three German fibrinogen Aα-chain amyloidosis patients with the p.Glu526Val mutation," *Virchows Archiv*, vol. 453, no. 1, pp. 25–31, 2008.

[11] J. R. Machado, M. V. D. Silva, P. D. M. D. M. Neves et al., "Fibrinogen A alpha-chain amyloidosis: report of the first case in Latin America," *Amyloid*, vol. 20, no. 1, pp. 52–55, 2013.

[12] C. P. J. Maury, J. Kere, R. Tolvanen, and A. de la Chapelle, "Homozygosity for the Asn187 gelsolin mutation in Finnish-type familial amyloidosis is associated with severe renal disease," *Genomics*, vol. 13, no. 3, pp. 902–903, 1992.

[13] C. P. J. Maury, "Homozygous familial amyloidosis, finnish type: demonstration of glomerular gelsolin-derived amyloid and non-amyloid tubular gelsolin," *Clinical Nephrology*, vol. 40, no. 1, pp. 53–56, 1993.

[14] J. Skare, H. Yazici, E. Erken et al., "Homozygosity for the met30 transthyretin gene in a Turkish kindred with familial amyloidotic polyneuropathy," *Human Genetics*, vol. 86, no. 1, pp. 89–90, 1990.

[15] T. Yoshinaga, M. Nakazato, S.-I. Ikeda, and A. Ohnishi, "Homozygosity for the transthyretin-Met30 gene in three Japanese siblings with type I familial amyloidotic polyneuropathy," *Neurology*, vol. 42, no. 10, pp. 2045–2047, 1992.

[16] M. Munar-Qués, J. M. L. Domínguez, C. Viader-Farré, P. Moreira, and M. J. M. Saraiva, "Two Spanish sibs with familial amyloidotic polyneuropathy homozygous for the V30M-TTR gene," *Amyloid*, vol. 8, no. 2, pp. 121–123, 2001.

[17] A. Yoshioka, Y. Yamaya, S. Saiki et al., "A case of familial amyloid polyneuropathy homozygous for the transthyretin Val30Met gene with motor-dominant sensorimotor polyneuropathy and unusual sural nerve pathological findings," *Archives of Neurology*, vol. 58, no. 11, pp. 1914–1918, 2001.

[18] G. Holmgren, U. Hellman, H. E. Lundgren, O. Sandgren, and O. B. Suhr, "Impact of homozygosity for an amyloidogenic transthyretin mutation on phenotype and long term outcome," *Journal of Medical Genetics*, vol. 42, no. 12, pp. 953–956, 2005.

[19] K. Tojo, Y. Sekijima, K. Machida, A. Tsuchiya, M. Yazaki, and S.-I. Ikeda, "Amyloidogenic transthyretin Val30Met homozygote showing unusually early-onset familial amyloid polyneuropathy," *Muscle and Nerve*, vol. 37, no. 6, pp. 796–803, 2008.

[20] D. R. Jacobson, P. D. Gorevic, G. H. Sack, and R. L. Malamet, "Homozygous transthyretin His 58 associated with unusually aggressive familial amyloidotic polyneuropathy," *The Journal of Rheumatology*, vol. 20, p. 178, 1993.

[21] A. Ferlini, F. Salvi, A. Uncini et al., "Homozygosity and heterozygosity for the transthyretin Leu64 mutation: clinical, biochemical and molecular findings," *Clinical Genetics*, vol. 49, no. 1, pp. 10–14, 1996.

[22] I. M. Hamour, H. J. Lachmann, H. J. B. Goodman et al., "Heart transplantation for homozygous familial transthyretin (TTR) V122I cardiac amyloidosis," *The American Journal of Transplantation*, vol. 8, no. 5, pp. 1056–1059, 2008.

[23] H. V. Reddi, S. Jenkins, J. Theis et al., "Homozygosity for the V122I mutation in transthyretin is associated with earlier onset of cardiac amyloidosis in the african american population in the seventh decade of life," *Journal of Molecular Diagnostics*, vol. 16, no. 1, pp. 68–74, 2014.

[24] P. M. P. Costa, *Amiloidoses transtirretínicas, da biopatologia à terapêutica [Ph.D. dissertation]*, Porto University, 1993.

[25] I. Tavares, R. Vaz, L. Moreira et al., "Renal amyloidosis: classification of 102 consecutive cases," *Portuguese Journal of Nephrology and Hypertension*, vol. 28, no. 3, pp. 201–209, 2014.

[26] C. Mousson, B. Heyd, E. Justrabo et al., "Successful hepatorenal transplantation in hereditary amyloidosis caused by a frameshift mutation in fibrinogen Aα-chain gene," *American Journal of Transplantation*, vol. 6, no. 3, pp. 632–635, 2006.

[27] S. Y. Tan, M. B. Pepys, and P. N. Hawkins, "Treatment of amyloidosis," *American Journal of Kidney Diseases*, vol. 26, no. 2, pp. 267–285, 1995.

[28] J. D. Gillmore, D. R. Booth, M. Rela et al., "Curative hepatorenal transplantation in systemic amyloidosis caused by the Glu526Val fibrinogen α-chain variant in an English family," *QJM*, vol. 93, no. 5, pp. 269–275, 2000.

[29] J. H. Pinney, H. J. Lachmann, P. T. Sattianayagam et al., "Renal transplantation in systemic amyloidosis—importance of amyloid fibril type and precursor protein abundance," *The American Journal of Transplantation*, vol. 13, no. 2, pp. 433–441, 2013.

[30] E. Raichlin, R. C. Daly, C. B. Rosen et al., "Combined heart and liver transplantation: a single-center experience," *Transplantation*, vol. 88, no. 2, pp. 219–225, 2009.

[31] T. Legris, L. Daniel, and V. Moal, "Delayed diagnosis of fibrinogen Aα-chain amyloidosis after dual heart-kidney transplantation," *Transplant International*, vol. 26, no. 1, pp. e1–e3, 2013.

51

The Rarest of the Rare: Crossed Fused Renal Ectopia of the Superior Ectopia Type

Leyla Akdogan,[1,2] **Ali Kemal Oguz,**[1,2] **Tarkan Ergun,**[3,4] **and Ihsan Ergun**[5]

[1]*Department of Internal Medicine, Ufuk University School of Medicine, Ankara, Turkey*
[2]*Dr. Rıdvan Ege Hospital, Konya Bulvarı No. 86-88, Balgat, Çankaya, 06520 Ankara, Turkey*
[3]*Department of Radiology, Baskent University School of Medicine, Alanya, Antalya, Turkey*
[4]*Baskent University School of Medicine, Alanya Research and Education Hospital, Alanya, 07400 Antalya, Turkey*
[5]*Division of Nephrology, Department of Internal Medicine, Ufuk University School of Medicine, Ankara, Turkey*

Correspondence should be addressed to Ihsan Ergun; ihsanerg@yahoo.com

Academic Editor: John A. Sayer

Crossed fused renal ectopia is a rare congenital anomaly of the urinary system where one kidney crosses over to opposite side and the parenchyma of the two kidneys fuse. Herein, we present an atypical CFRE case whose renal anatomy does not exactly match any of the already defined CFRE types. Both of the kidneys are ectopic with the crossed ectopic right kidney lying superiorly and fused to the upper pole of the left kidney. Renal arteries were originating from the common iliac arteries. A focal 90% stenosis was observed on the right main renal artery. The patient is borderline hypertensive.

1. Introduction

Crossed fused renal ectopia (CFRE) is a markedly rare congenital malformation of the urinary system where one of the kidneys crosses the midline to become located on the opposite side of its ureter entrance to the bladder and the parenchymas of the two kidneys fuse. CFRE has a reported autopsy incidence of around 1 : 2000 and is the second most frequently observed fusion anomaly of the kidneys following the horseshoe kidney. Resulting from aberrant migration and crossing of the midline of the metanephric blastema and the ureteral bud, CFRE is thought to develop during the fourth to eighth weeks of gestation. Mostly remaining asymptomatic and detected as an incidental finding during imaging studies, six well-defined anatomical variations of CFRE have been reported [1, 2]. Herein, we present an atypical CFRE case whose renal anatomy does not exactly match any of the already defined CFRE types.

2. Case Presentation

A 25-year-old man with no current complaints was referred to our nephrology outpatient clinic on the occasion of an incidental finding of renal ectopia. His initial abdominal ultrasonography had reported renal ectopia with both kidneys located in the left iliac fossa. Except a blood pressure reading of 135/85 mmHg, a complete physical examination was nonrevealing. His body mass index was within the normal range. Routine laboratory studies did not document any abnormalities (i.e., blood urea nitrogen: 9 mg/dL, creatinine: 0.95 mg/dL, normal serum electrolyte concentrations, normal urinalysis). A repeated renal ultrasound documented two ectopic kidneys located superiorly and inferiorly in the same anatomic location. Renal dimensions and parenchymal thicknesses of the superiorly and the inferiorly situated kidneys were 115 × 36 × 33/11 mm and 116 × 59 × 53/21 mm, respectively. The superiorly located kidney also displayed irregular contours and a thinner parenchyma, especially prominent in its superior pole. No renal calculi or dilatation of the collecting systems was observed.

In order to exclude "white coat" hypertension, an ambulatory 24 hour blood pressure monitoring was performed which documented a mean blood pressure of 129/78 mmHg compatible with a borderline hypertension (the 24 hour average was higher than the expected limit of 115/75 mmHg, close to the upper limit of 130/80 mmHg). Accordingly, in search of a renovascular etiology of hypertension, renal Doppler

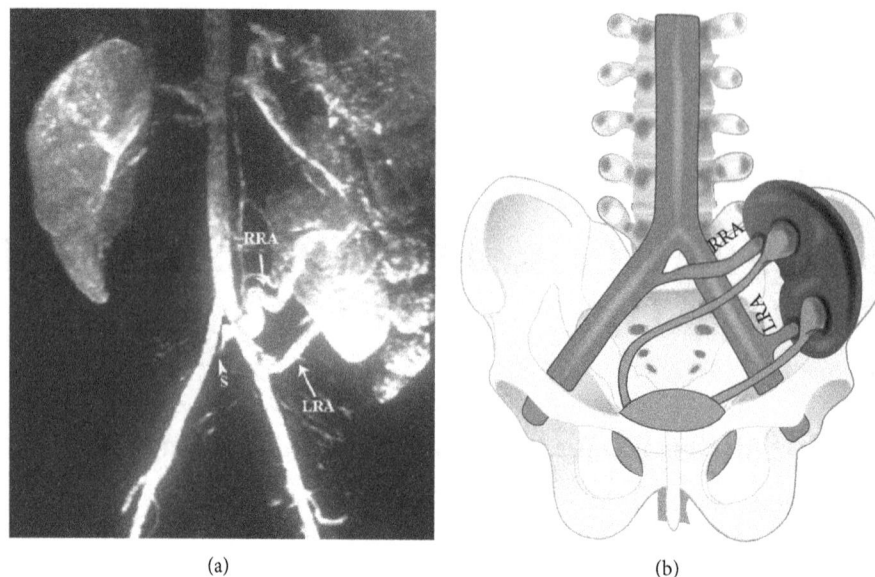

FIGURE 1: (a) The arterial phase of the 3D gadolinium-enhanced aortoiliac and renal magnetic resonance angiography of the patient. RRA and LRA (arrows) are pointing to the right and left main renal arteries, respectively, whereas S (arrow head) is marking the stenotic lesion closely located to the origin of the right main renal artery. (b) Schematic drawing of the renal and renal artery anatomy of the patient. Again, RRA and LRA are the right and left main renal arteries, respectively.

ultrasonography was performed. Excluding elevated renal resistive index values in both renal arteries, the Doppler study was not informative. A 3D gadolinium enhanced aortoiliac and renal magnetic resonance angiography was planned and it revealed the exact renal and renal vascular anatomy of the patient. According to the findings of the angiography, the left ectopic kidney was located in the left iliac fossa with the crossed ectopic right kidney lying superiorly and fused to the upper pole of the left kidney. Also, both main renal arteries were originating from the corresponding ipsilateral common iliac arteries and there was a focal 90% stenosis situated 5 mm distal to the origin of the right main renal artery (Figure 1).

With the aim of documenting the potential contribution of the stenotic lesion to the borderline hypertension, plasma renin activity (24.5 pg/mL (normal values, 5.41–34.53 pg/mL)) and aldosterone level (149 pg/mL (normal values, 30–160 pg/mL)) were measured. Additionally, a captopril Tc99m-MAG3 radioisotope renography was performed, revealing a right : left differential renal function of 38 : 62 and no depression or alteration of renal functions following the test dose of captopril. Consequently, no immediate intervention for the stenotic lesion was planned, whereas a close followup, the DASH diet, and therapeutic lifestyle modification were strongly advised. Any plans of renal artery intervention were reserved for future use in cases of increasing blood pressure or the emergence of overt hypertension. The patient's blood pressure is still under control without the need of any drug therapy.

3. Discussion

Crossed renal ectopia is classified into 4 main categories: crossed renal ectopia with or without fusion, unilateral crossed renal ectopia (with unilateral renal agenesis), and bilateral crossed renal ectopia (without fusion) [3]. In 85–90% of the crossed renal ectopia cases, the kidneys are partially or completely fused, hence given the name CFRE. CFRE is reported to be two times more prevalent in men than women [4]. Consistently, the patient we presented was also a young man. With respect to CFRE, six anatomical variations have been described [1], namely, inferior CFRE, sigmoid kidney, lump kidney, disc kidney, L-shaped kidney, and superior CFRE (Figure 2). While the inferior CFRE is the most frequent type observed, the superior CFRE is reported to be the least common. In the inferior CFRE type, the upper pole of the inferiorly situated crossed ectopic kidney is fused to the lower pole of the superiorly, normally positioned kidney. Another characteristic feature of CFRE is the three times more common occurrence of left-to-right ectopy [2]. Noteworthily, in our case both kidneys were ectopic and the crossed ectopic right kidney was positioned superiorly with its lower pole fused to the upper pole of the left kidney. To our best knowledge, in the current literature, there is only one case reported with superior CFRE of the right kidney [5].

As previously mentioned, most CFRE cases remain asymptomatic and are detected incidentally. This was also the case for our patient. When present, hydronephrosis, recurrent urinary tract infections, and renal calculi are the main reported complications of CFRE. Also, there may be associating congenital malformations affecting the urogenital, gastrointestinal, and musculoskeletal systems and vesicoureteral reflux is the most common accompanying urogenital abnormality [6, 7]. The only case with superior CFRE of the right kidney previously reported by Yin et al. had also associating retroiliac megaureter and thoracic scoliosis anomalies [5]. In our case, CFRE was present as an isolated congenital malformation.

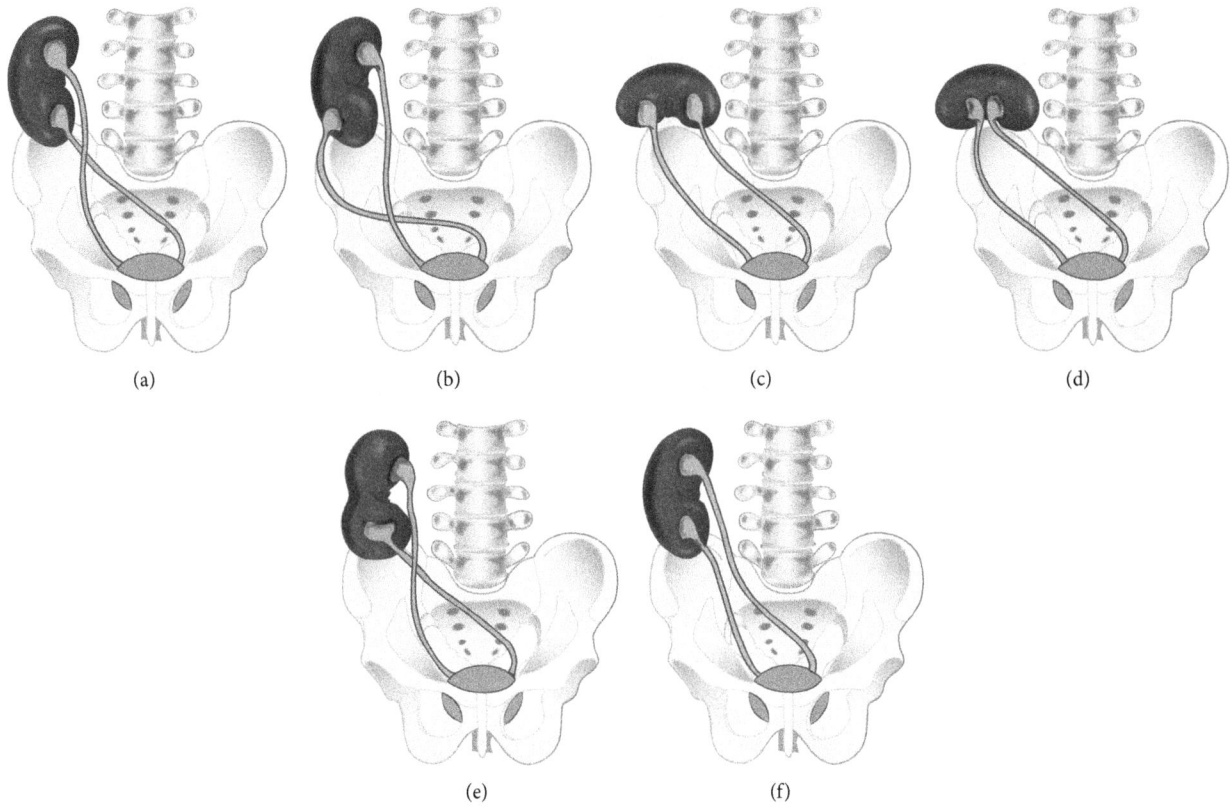

FIGURE 2: Six anatomical variations (types) of crossed fused renal ectopia: (a) inferior crossed fused renal ectopia; (b) sigmoid or S-shaped kidney; (c) lump kidney; (d) disc kidney; (e) L-shaped kidney; (f) superior crossed fused renal ectopia.

Hypertension is very rare in CFRE and there is no given single pathophysiologic mechanism for this entity in the literature [8]. Our patient had a borderline hypertension and a stenosis was documented in the proximal segment of the main renal artery of the crossed fused right kidney. The laboratory tests pertinent to a renovascular hypertension and the findings of the captopril radioisotope renography were not conclusive in his case. Although currently the stenotic lesion does not seem to contribute to the elevated blood pressure, it may prove to be so during the followup. So, a close followup was scheduled for our patient.

In crossed fused ectopic kidneys, the vascular anatomy is grossly aberrant and the crossed ectopic kidney generally demonstrates a decreased function. In accordance with the literature, the crossed ectopic right kidney of our patient also had a decreased renal function. In approximately 25% of the CFRE cases, the arteries originate from the superior abdominal aorta, whereas in the remainder the origin is from the inferior abdominal aorta or the iliac arteries [1, 4, 6, 7]. In our case, the origin of the main renal arteries was from the ipsilateral common iliac arteries, respectively.

In the absence of complications and associating additional abnormalities, the prognosis for a patient with CFRE is very good. There are no specific primary treatment approaches for the management of CFRE. Treatment of the associated pathologies is indicated which are most frequently nephrolithiasis and vesicoureteral reflux [6]. It is important to remember that a thorough understanding of the aberrant anatomy is vital before planning of any surgical intervention in the renal region. An angiography is certainly recommended before the surgical intervention. Finally, despite a significantly rare congenital renal abnormality, CFRE should be remembered in cases of renal ectopia with both kidneys located in close proximity.

Consent

Written informed consent was obtained from the patient for publication of this case report and accompanying images.

Conflict of Interests

The authors declare no potential conflict of interests with respect to the authorship and/or publication of this paper.

Acknowledgment

The authors would like to express their sincere thanks to Mrs. Yasemin Bilgin Karadağ (Freelance Illustrator) for her contribution to the figures of the paper.

References

[1] S. B. Bauer, "Anomalies of the upper urinary tract," in *Campbell's Urology*, P. C. Walsh, A. B. Retik, E. D. Vaughan, and A. J. Wein, Eds., pp. 1898–1906, WB Saunders, Philadelphia, Pa, USA, 8th edition, 2002.

[2] T. V. Patel and A. K. Singh, "Crossed fused ectopia of the kidneys," *Kidney International*, vol. 73, no. 5, p. 662, 2008.

[3] J. H. McDonald and D. S. McClellan, "Crossed renal ectopia," *The American Journal of Surgery*, vol. 93, no. 6, pp. 995–999, 1957.

[4] V. Sharma, C. S. R. Babu, and O. P. Gupta, "Crossed fused renal ectopia multidetector computed tomography study," *International Journal of Anatomy and Research*, vol. 2, no. 2, pp. 305–309, 2014.

[5] Z. Yin, J. R. Yang, Y. B. Wei, K. Q. Zhou, and B. Yan, "A new subtype of crossed fused ectopia of the kidneys," *Urology*, vol. 84, no. 6, article e27, 2014.

[6] N. Guarino, B. Tadini, P. Camardi et al., "The incidence of associated urological abnormalities in children with renal ectopia," *Journal of Urology*, vol. 172, no. 4, pp. 1757–1759, 2004.

[7] A. Türkvatan, T. Ölcer, and T. Cumhur, "Multidetector CT urography of renal fusion anomalies," *Diagnostic and Interventional Radiology*, vol. 15, no. 2, pp. 127–134, 2009.

[8] D. T. Mininberg, S. Roze, and M. Pearl, "Hypertension associated with crossed renal ectopia in an infant," *Pediatrics*, vol. 48, no. 3, pp. 454–457, 1971.

52

Sildenafil Induced Acute Interstitial Nephritis

Ryan Burkhart,[1] Nina Shah,[1] and Matthew Lewin[2]

[1]*William Beaumont Army Medical Center, 5005 N. Piedras Street, El Paso, TX 79920, USA*
[2]*ProPath Services, LLP, 1355 River Bend Drive, Dallas, TX 75247, USA*

Correspondence should be addressed to Ryan Burkhart; ryan.v.burkhart.mil@mail.mil

Academic Editor: Ichiei Narita

Acute interstitial nephritis (AIN) is characterized by inflammation of the renal interstitium and usually occurs in a temporal relationship with the medication. We present a case of an Asian male who had nephrotic range proteinuria and presented with acute kidney injury. The patient reported an acute change in physical appearance and symptomatology after the ingestion of a single dose of sildenafil. Renal biopsy was notable for minimal change disease (MCD) with acute and chronic interstitial nephritis. Renal replacement and glucocorticoid therapy were initiated. Renal recovery within six weeks permitted discontinuation of dialysis. AIN superimposed on MCD is a known association of NSAID induced nephropathy. The temporal association and the absence of any new drugs suggest that the AIN was most likely due to the sildenafil. NSAIDs are less likely to have caused the AIN given their remote use. The ease of steroid responsiveness would also suggest another cause as NSAID induced AIN is often steroid resistant. The MCD was most likely idiopathic given the lack of temporal association with a secondary cause. As the number of sildenafil prescriptions increases, more cases of AIN may be identified and physician awareness for this potential drug disease association is necessary.

1. Introduction

Acute interstitial nephritis (AIN) is a known cause of intrinsic acute kidney injury and is characterized by inflammation of the renal interstitium. AIN has been reported to occur in approximately 1–3% of all renal biopsies, and up to 15–27% when biopsy indication is due to renal failure [1]. Drug induced AIN notably occurs in approximately 70% of cases, with the majority of cases being due to antibiotics, proton pump inhibitors, or NSAIDs [2]. Drug induced AIN usually occurs in a temporal relationship with a medication. While its diagnosis may be apparent based on presentation and ruling out more common causes of acute kidney injury, definitive diagnosis is made by renal biopsy. Given that almost any drug can potentially cause AIN and frequent coinciding polypharmacy, the offending agent can often be difficult to identify.

To the best of our knowledge, there have been no published reports of AIN due to sildenafil. We present a case of biopsy proven AIN likely attributable to sildenafil in an individual who also had minimal change disease (MCD).

2. Case Report

This is an 81-year-old Asian male with a known past medical history of erectile dysfunction, chronic kidney disease stage 3a, hypertension, hyperlipidemia, coronary artery disease, gout with chronic allopurinol use for years, and osteoarthritis with remote NSAID use. The patient was admitted with generalized edema, rapid weight gain of 9.1 kg over the previous month, hyperkalemia 5.9 mmol/L (5.9 mEq/L), BUN 17.14 mmol/L (48 mg/dL), and serum creatinine of 327.08 μmol/L (3.7 mg/dL). His baseline serum creatinine was 123.76 μmol/L (1.4 mg/dL) and eGFR was 47 mL/min/1.73 m^2 by CKD-EPI. He was noted to have 1661.1 mg/mmol proteinuria (14.7 mg/mg), serum BUN 13.57 mmol/L (38 mg/dL), and serum creatinine of 167.96 μmol/L (1.9 mg/dL) two weeks before. The patient specifically noted an acute increase in peripheral and facial edema after ingesting a single dose of sildenafil four days prior to his admission.

His admission medications included lisinopril, diltiazem, atorvastatin, aspirin, allopurinol, tramadol, docusate, and sildenafil. The patient specifically denied any recent NSAID usage or over-the-counter medications. He was previously on sulindac as needed with the last dose thirteen months prior to his presentation. Sildenafil was the only new medication.

On admission, the patient had unremarkable cardiac and pulmonary exams and diffuse bilateral lower extremity edema. Blood pressure was 144/70 mmHg. Chest X-ray noted small bilateral pleural effusions. Renal ultrasound revealed normal parenchyma bilaterally, without evidence of hydronephrosis. Cardiac echo revealed an ejection fraction of 68% with structurally normal valves and chambers.

Additional labs on admission noted a WBC of 5.4×10^9/L with 5.6% eosinophils (normal, 0–7%). Albumin was 26 g/L (2.6 g/dL). Urinalysis was notable for specific gravity of 1.020, blood 4+, and protein 4+. Urine sediment noted 0–2 granular casts/lpf, no cellular casts/lpf, 0–5 nondysmorphic RBCs/hpf, and 0-1 WBC/hpf on microscopy.

Renal biopsy was performed. Twenty-three glomeruli were obtained. Six out of twenty-three glomeruli were obsolescent with capillary tuft collapse and collagen accumulation within Bowmen's space consistent with hypertensive nephrosclerosis. The viable glomeruli were without significant evidence of increased mesangial matrix or mesangial cellularity. There was hyperplasia of the visceral epithelial cells and occasional protein reabsorption granules noted on the PAS stain. The glomerular basement membranes were slightly thickened but without discrete subepithelial spikes, pinholes, deposits, or double contours noted. No definitive segmental sclerotic lesions were identified.

The tubulointerstitium had patchy moderate interstitial inflammation with numerous eosinophils observed consistent with acute interstitial nephritis. There was mild interstitial fibrosis consistent with chronic interstitial nephritis.

Immunofluorescence showed segmental protein reabsorption granular staining for IgM (2+), C3 (2+), albumin (2+), kappa light chain (2+), and lambda light chain (2+). There was nonspecific linear tubal basement membrane staining for albumin (1+). Staining for IgA, IgG, C1q, or fibrinogen was negative. Electron microscopy showed normal cell elements and mesangial matrix. The glomerular basement membranes were normal without subendothelial or subepithelial densities. There was diffuse global foot process effacement with associated microvillus hypertrophy consistent with minimal change disease.

Dialysis was initiated in the setting of progressive decline in renal function. The patient was treated with 1 gram of methylprednisolone for 3 days followed by a prednisone taper over 18 weeks. Renal recovery within six weeks permitted discontinuation of dialysis. Proteinuria decreased to 57.9 mg/mmol (0.512 mg/mg), and serum creatinine returned to its prior baseline of 123.76 μmol/L (1.4 mg/dL).

3. Discussion

Initial differential diagnosis included membranous nephropathy, minimal change disease, IgA nephropathy, focal segmental glomerulosclerosis, fibrillary glomerulonephritis, immunotactoid glomerulopathy, amyloidosis, light chain deposition disease, and myeloma kidney. AIN was also on the differential diagnosis for his AKI; however, it would not account for the nephrotic range proteinuria. The renal biopsy was performed in the setting of nephrotic syndrome and AKI of unclear etiology.

Our patient had a very complicated presentation of acute kidney injury and nephrotic syndrome in the setting of multiple medications, two of which have a very well-known association with AIN. His renal biopsy noted MCD, with acute and early chronic interstitial nephritis, which would notably be characteristic of an NSAID induced etiology [3, 4]. We have not been able to find any reports of sildenafil induced AIN. There are multiple factors that would argue against NSAID, or allopurinol induced AIN, and would argue for sildenafil as the culprit agent.

There was a temporal association with sildenafil ingestion and the patient's symptom onset. First exposure to a medication may take weeks for the development of AIN. Medication reexposure may allow for AIN to develop more quickly and usually occurs in 3–5 days [5] but may occur as early as one day [6]. The majority of NSAID induced AIN have been on the medication for approximately 6 months [7]. Our patient's symptoms developed rapidly following the ingestion of sildenafil. AKI was noted 4 days later. Review of his records noted that he was prescribed sildenafil for the first time 15 months before. We suspect that this prior exposure likely primed his immune system to allow for the rapidity of the AIN to develop.

The patient adamantly denied recent consumption of NSAIDs (aside from aspirin) including both over-the-counter or prescription based medications. The patient had previously been on sulindac 150 mg twice a day for his osteoarthritis, with his last consumption thirteen months prior to his presentation. He had been on sulindac for more than two years prior to its cessation. The patient had been on allopurinol for decades and was without evidence of AIN despite continuous allopurinol use. He was also without the characteristic rash and abnormal liver associated tests that often accompany allopurinol induced AIN. The patient was on aspirin 325 mg daily as well which has been described in the literature to be associated with AIN [7]. However, there was no temporal association with the initiation of these medications. The patient remained on aspirin during and after treatment. Despite remaining on aspirin, his renal function returned to baseline and the degree of proteinuria significantly improved. The lack of temporal association here strongly goes against an NSAID or allopurinol induced etiology.

NSAID induced AIN is classically known to be less responsive to corticosteroids [7, 8] and portends a worse prognosis [9]. The patient had MCD as well as AIN and had an excellent clinical response that allowed him to become dialysis independent at 6 weeks. In this case, the corticosteroids were treating his MCD as well as the AIN. His renal function continued to improve back to his baseline. The ease of steroid responsiveness would suggest another etiology as NSAID induced AIN is often steroid resistant.

The patient had evidence of acute and "early" chronic interstitial nephritis on the renal biopsy which refers to the degree of fibrosis. The chronic portion could potentially be attributed to his chronic hypertension, prior NSAID use, or the allopurinol. This may also be secondary to the sildenafil. The renal biopsy was performed approximately 10 days after the ingestion of sildenafil, and 9 days after the onset of the patient's symptoms. Fibrosis has been shown to develop in as little as a week with AIN [5, 10] as part of an inflammatory continuum resulting in fibrogenesis [5]. The interstitial nephritis may have been undergoing its natural progression following the sildenafil exposure, resulting in those chronic changes.

MCD in the elderly is not uncommon and has been reported in roughly 10–15% of cases of nephrotic syndrome in adults [11] and with increased incidence among Asians [12]. While NSAIDS are a common cause of secondary MCD, the most common etiology of MCD is idiopathic. The patient was noted to have nephrotic range proteinuria of 1661.1 mg/mmol (14.7 mg/mg) proteinuria and serum creatinine of 167.96 μmol/L (1.9 mg/dL) two weeks prior to presentation. The lack of temporal association with a secondary cause would argue for idiopathic MCD.

The patient's baseline serum creatinine was 123.76 μmol/L (1.4 mg/dL) and notably the serum creatinine was 167.96 μmol/L (1.9 mg/dL) seven days prior to his ingestion of the sildenafil. This may have been due to a variable change in volume status, or secondary to the underlying MCD which often has modest changes in serum creatinine on presentation.

Our patient was initially treated with 1 g of methylprednisolone for 3 days followed by steroid taper for his MCD. There is no standard treatment protocol for AIN. The treatment course for this disease process is usually shorter. In this case, the corticosteroids were treating an AIN as well as MCD.

4. Conclusion

We present a case of AIN suspected due to sildenafil in an 81-year-old Asian male who also had idiopathic MCD. In the United States, generic formulations of sildenafil are currently available for the treatment of pulmonary hypertension but not erectile dysfunction. The true incidence of renal issues with sildenafil is unknown as there is minimal published or postmarketing data. More cases of AIN may be identified as the number of sildenafil prescriptions increases. Physician awareness for this potential drug-disease association is necessary.

Consent

Verbal and written consent were obtained from the patient for the publication of this paper.

Disclosure

The views expressed in this document are those of the authors and do not reflect the official policy of William Beaumont Army Medical Center, the Department of the Army, or the United States Government. This case report was presented as poster presentation at the 2015 National ACP Conference.

Conflict of Interests

No conflict of interests.

References

[1] M. Praga and E. González, "Acute interstitial nephritis," *Kidney International*, vol. 77, no. 11, pp. 956–961, 2010.

[2] A. K. Muriithi, N. Leung, A. M. Valeri et al., "Biopsy-proven acute interstitial nephritis, 1993-2011: a case series," *American Journal of Kidney Diseases*, vol. 64, no. 4, pp. 558–566, 2014.

[3] G. V. Warren, S. M. Korbet, M. M. Schwartz, and E. J. Lewis, "Minimal change glomerulopathy associated with nonsteroidal antiinflammatory drugs," *American Journal of Kidney Diseases*, vol. 13, no. 2, pp. 127–130, 1989.

[4] P. J. Champion de Crespigny, G. J. Becker, B. U. Ihle, N. M. A. Walter, C. A. Wright, and P. Kincaid-Smith, "Renal failure and nephrotic syndrome associated with sulindac," *Clinical Nephrology*, vol. 30, no. 1, pp. 52–55, 1988.

[5] E. G. Neilson, "Pathogenesis and therapy of interstitial nephritis," *Kidney International*, vol. 35, no. 5, pp. 1257–1270, 1989.

[6] R. M. Ten, V. E. Torres, D. S. Milliner, T. R. Schwab, K. E. Holley, and G. J. Gleich, "Acute interstitial nephritis: immunologic and clinical aspects," *Mayo Clinic Proceedings*, vol. 63, no. 9, pp. 921–930, 1988.

[7] J. Rossert, "Drug-induced acute interstitial nephritis," *Kidney International*, vol. 60, no. 2, pp. 804–817, 2001.

[8] J. L. Porile, G. L. Bakris, and S. Garrella, "Acute interstitial nephritis with glomerulopathy due to nonsteroidal antiinflammatory agents: a review of its clinical spectrum and effects of steriod therapy," *Journal of Clinical Pharmacology*, vol. 30, no. 5, pp. 468–475, 1990.

[9] A. Schwarz, P. H. Krause, U. Kunzendorf, F. Keller, and A. Distler, "The outcome of acute interstitial nephritis: risk factors for the transition from acute to chronic interstitial nephritis," *Clinical Nephrology*, vol. 54, no. 3, pp. 179–190, 2000.

[10] E. G. Neilson, "Mechanisms of disease: fibroblasts—a new look at an old problem," *Nature Clinical Practice Nephrology*, vol. 2, no. 2, pp. 101–108, 2006.

[11] J. S. Cameron, "The nephrotic syndrome and its complications," *American Journal of Kidney Diseases*, vol. 10, no. 3, pp. 157–171, 1987.

[12] J. Feehally, N. P. Kendell, P. G. F. Swift, and J. Walls, "High incidence of minimal change nephrotic syndrome in Asians," *Archives of Disease in Childhood*, vol. 60, no. 11, pp. 1018–1020, 1985.

53

A Case of Methanol Poisoning in a Child

Reyner Loza[1,2] and Dimas Rodriguez[3]

[1] Unit of Pediatric Nephrology, Department of Pediatrics, Cayetano Heredia National Hospital,
  Avenida Honorio Delgado 265, SMP, Lima 31, Peru
[2] Cayetano Heredia University, Avenida Honorio Delgado 430, SMP, Lima 31, Peru
[3] Unit of Pediatric Nephrology, Sergio Bernales National Hospital, Avenida Tupac Amaru 8000, Comas, Lima 7, Peru

Correspondence should be addressed to Reyner Loza; reyner.loza@upch.pe

Academic Editors: R. Enríquez and J. Maesaka

We report the case of a girl admitted to the emergency room with a history of four hours' acute illness, characterized by nausea, vomiting, salivation, headache, blurred vision, and acidotic "Kussmaul" breathing. Arterial blood gases showed severe mixed acidosis, metabolic and respiratory with high anion gap. She had ingested the contents of a scent bottle containing methanol, which she thought was a soft drink bottle. The girl was managed with hemodialysis and strong intravenous hydration. She improved well and made a full recovery.

1. Introduction

Methanol poisoning in children is rarely described in the literature; some cases are reported as accidental ingestion. For this reason, we report here a case of accidental methanol poisoning, discussing clinical and laboratory manifestations, management, and evolution.

1.1. Case Report. A six-year-old female patient was admitted to the emergency room with her mother after four hours of disease characterized by nausea and vomiting of food content, abdominal pain, difficulty in breathing, salivation, headache, blurred vision, and psychomotor agitation. A physical examination found the following: weight 22 kg, blood pressure 80/60 mmHg, respiratory rate 32 breaths per minute, and heart rate 148 beats per minute.

Her skin was pale, and her eyes were sunken, underactive, clouded, and irritable to stimulus.

The patient was initially treated for severe dehydration resulting from food poisoning. However, with the development of wheezing and unresponsiveness to stimuli, she was transferred to the shock trauma unit for worsening respiratory distress, deep breathing with panting (Kussmaul) breathing, unresponsiveness to stimuli, Glasgow 10, to receive ventilator support.

The laboratory findings were as follows: yellow urine, specific gravity 1.025, pH 7.0, trace glucose, leukocytes 8–10x field, erythrocytes 2-3x field, the leukocyte blood count 8,180x mm^3, segmented 69%, eosinophils 5%, lymphocytes 26%, Hb 12 g/dL, sodium 133 mEq/L, potassium 6 mEq/L, chloride 107 mEq/L, aspartate aminotransferase 4490 IU/L, alanine aminotransferase 8030 IU/L, and lactate dehydrogenase 2609 UI/L.

Arterial blood gases showed severe mixed acidosis, metabolic and respiratory with high anion gap (pH 6.9, PaO$_2$: 108 mmHg, PaCO$_2$: 26 mmHg, and HCO$_3$: 3 mEq/L). We therefore assumed the possibility of diabetic ketoacidosis, salicylate poisoning, or methanol poisoning. Evaluation of renal function showed urea 33 mg/dL and creatinine 0.6 mg/dL; glucose was normal. Therapy was initiated with vigorous hydration with sodium chloride 9/1000 and supplemental intravenous sodium bicarbonate. The toxicology results showed a serum methanol of 1.47 mg/dL. Emergency

TABLE 1: Evolution of acid base status.

	PO$_2$ mmHg	PCO$_2$ mmHg	HCO$_3$ mEq/L	Sodium mEq/L	Potassium mEq/L	Chloride mEq/L	Anion gap
pH blood							
6.9	108	26	3	133	6	107	23
6.8	85	21	6.7	131	5.6	108	16.3
Hemodialysis							
7.1	85	22	6.4	131	5.9	108	16
7.4	95	45	23	140	4	103	14

TABLE 2: Evolution of laboratory tests.

Days	1	3	4	5
Urea mg/dL	33	18	—	—
Creatinine mg/dL	0.6	0.5	—	—
Albumin g/L	—	3.7	4.1	4.4
Glucose mg/dL		94		
AST UI/L[**]	4490	2942	1225	21
SGPT UI/L[**]	8030	924	248	37
Lactate dehydrogenase UI/L	2609	5600	2800	800
Blood pH	6.9	7.34	7.38	7.4
HCO$_3$ mmol/L	3	24	23	24
Methanol mg/dL[*]	1.47	—	0	0

[*]Toxicological examination: spectrophotometer method.
[**]Aspartate aminotransferase.
[**]Glutamic pyruvic transaminase.

hemodialysis therapy was initiated; the patient was dialyzed for an hour for two sessions.

The family gave us new information that the girl regularly took a drink called Kola Ingles. They stated that the patient had found a 250 mL pink perfume bottle and that she had ingested 200 mL of its contents, thinking it was the cola drink.

The patient improved progressively after hemodialysis with correction of her metabolic acidosis, liver function tests, and lactic dehydrogenase (Tables 1 and 2).

The child was discharged from the hospital in five days recovering full health.

2. Discussion

Methanol (CH$_3$OH), also known as methyl alcohol, wood burning alcohol, or carbinol, is highly toxic. It is the simplest of the alcohols used in paints, varnishes, solvents, perfumes, plastic manufacture, photographic materials, antifreeze, and household cleaning products.

The pathways for poisoning are inhalation, cutaneous, and digestive tract, in most cases by swallowing. Methanol poisoning in children is rare and there are only isolated reports of homicidal poisoning and seizures [1, 2].

In some European countries, it is reported that the main cause of hospitalization among teens is alcohol poisoning. Reasons range from recreational use to poisoning and self-harm [3].

Sometimes symptoms may mask an underlying condition, which may delay diagnosis [4].

Individual or collective poisoning is usually voluntary or accidental ingestion in the case of adulterated liquor.

The stages of intoxication are described as follows. In the first phase, there is minimal decrease in central nervous system activity, weakness, dizziness, and nausea. The second phase is marked by the development of metabolic acidosis characterized by vomiting, abdominal pain, confusion, visual disturbances, photophobia, blurred vision, bilateral mydriasis, unresponsiveness to light, and occasional blindness. In the third phase, in direct relation to the degree of metabolic acidosis, neuronal injury occurs with retinal necrosis and hemorrhage in the basal ganglia of the brain. At this stage there is hypotension, coma, and Kussmaul breathing. Our patient was considered to be in the second phase of methanol toxicity.

Diagnosis of methanol poisoning is based on the suspicion of ingestion, the presence of visual disturbances, the onset of metabolic acidosis with elevated anion and osmolar gaps, and markedly increased liver enzymes.

Confirmation is by determining the plasma levels of methanol. The toxic methanol dose is 10–30 mL (100 mg/kg), although lower intakes have caused blindness. It is lethal above 60–240 mL (340 mg/kg). A dose of 30 mL of 100% methanol can be considered fatal.

Concentrations above 0.2 g/L are toxic, values higher than 0.5 g/L indicate severe poisoning, and concentrations above 0.9 g/L are potentially deadly.

Methanol is rapidly absorbed from the gastrointestinal tract, giving peak plasma levels after 30–90 minutes. The serum half-life ranges from 14 to 30 hours and is distributed freely. The kidney, in untreated patients, removes less than 5%.

In the liver, methanol is removed by biotransformation via alcohol dehydrogenase (ADH), forming formaldehyde, and subsequently through conversion of the aldehyde dehydrogenase to formic acid.

That methanol by itself is not toxic. It is the degradation of methanol by alcohol dehydrogenase that releases the toxic metabolites, formaldehyde, and formic acid.

The rational for treatment is reducing the formation of the toxic metabolites, by cleaning in hemodialysis or administering ethanol, Fomepizole.

Hemodialysis treatment removes the methanol and his metabolites from the circulation, reducing the shelf life. This is preferable to peritoneal dialysis as it results in more rapid clearance. Further, ethanol is a treatment form that competitively inhibits the metabolism of methanol by alcohol dehydrogenase. The affinity of the enzyme for ethanol is 10 to 20 times higher than that of methanol, thus avoiding the formation of toxic metabolites. In the ethanol administration schedule, the goal is to maintain serum levels between 1 and 1.5 g/L. It should be administered as a bolus loading dose of 0.6 g/kg followed by a maintenance dose of 66–154 mg/kg/h. IV administration of ethanol is safer than oral administration, although it can produce irritation and thrombophlebitis [5, 6].

There is also the 4-methylpyrazole (4-MP) (fomepizole) antidote, which acts similarly to ethanol by competitively inhibiting ADH. The advantages with respect to ethanol are various, and its affinity for the enzyme is higher. It has a long half-life (meaning a long duration of action and dosing convenience), and it does not require continuous monitoring of plasma levels. It has fewer side effects. Its use in children has been described in [6, 7].

The purpose of this paper was to report the possibility of poisoning of children with accidental ingestion of methanol in perfumes and other household products that may contain this substance.

Conflict of Interests

The authors declare that there is no conflict of interests regarding the publication of the paper.

Authors' Contribution

Dimas Rodriguez drafted the initial paper and approved the final version of the paper as submitted. Reyner Loza carried out the initial analyses, reviewed and revised the paper, and approved the final version of the paper as submitted. Reyner Loza, M.D., is the author; Dimas Rodriguez, M.D., is the coauthor.

References

[1] J. M. Beno, R. Hartman, C. Wallace, D. Nemeth, and S. LaPoint, "Homicidal methanol poisoning in a child," *Journal of Analytical Toxicology*, vol. 35, no. 7, pp. 524–528, 2011.

[2] J. C. van Gaal, R. Petru, and L. T. J. Sie, "An infant with unexplained epilepsy," *Nederlands Tijdschrift voor Geneeskunde*, vol. 154, Article ID A2420, 2010.

[3] J. H. Liisanantti, T. I. Ala-Kokko, T. S. Dunder, and H. E. Ebeling, "Contributing factors in self-poisoning leading to hospital admission in adolescents in Northern Finland," *Substance Use and Misuse*, vol. 45, no. 9, pp. 1340–1350, 2010.

[4] U. Celik, T. Celik, A. Avci et al., "Metabolic acidosis in a patient with type 1 diabetes mellitus complicated by methanol and amitriptyline intoxication," *European Journal of Emergency Medicine*, vol. 16, no. 1, pp. 45–48, 2009.

[5] A. H. B. Wu, T. Kelly, C. McKay, D. Ostheimer, E. Forte, and D. Hill, "Definitive identification of an exceptionally high methanol concentration in an intoxication of a surviving infant: methanol metabolism by first-order elimination kinetics," *Journal of Forensic Sciences*, vol. 40, no. 2, pp. 315–320, 1995.

[6] N. de Brabander, M. Wojciechowski, K. de Decker, A. de Weerdt, and P. G. Jorens, "Fomepizole as a therapeutic strategy in paediatric methanol poisoning. A case report and review of the literature," *European Journal of Pediatrics*, vol. 164, no. 3, pp. 158–161, 2005.

[7] P. E. Wallemacq, R. Vanbinst, V. Haufroid et al., "Plasma and tissue determination of 4-methylpyrazole for pharmacokinetic analysis in acute adult and pediatric methanol/ethylene glycol poisoning," *Therapeutic Drug Monitoring*, vol. 26, no. 3, pp. 258–262, 2004.

54

A Rare Case of Central Pontine Myelinolysis in Overcorrection of Hyponatremia with Total Parenteral Nutrition in Pregnancy

Kalyana C. Janga, Tazleem Khan, Ciril Khorolsky,
Sheldon Greenberg, and Priscilla Persaud

Maimonides Medical Center, 4802 10th Avenue, Brooklyn, NY 11219, USA

Correspondence should be addressed to Kalyana C. Janga; kjanga@maimonidesmed.org

Academic Editor: Yoshihide Fujigaki

A 42-year-old high risk pregnant female presented with hyponatremia from multiple causes and was treated with total parenteral nutrition. She developed acute hypernatremia due to the stage of pregnancy and other comorbidities. All the mechanisms of hyponatremia and hypernatremia were summarized here in our case report. This case has picture (graph) representation of parameters that led to changes in serum sodium and radiological findings of central pontine myelinolysis on MRI. In conclusion we present a complicated case serum sodium changes during pregnancy and pathophysiological effects on serum sodium changes during pregnancy.

1. Introduction

Hyponatremia is defined as a sodium concentration less than 135 mEq/L. If hyponatremia is not corrected appropriately, it can lead to significant clinical symptoms. During pregnancy, hyponatremia can be caused by various mechanisms. A reset osmostat phenomenon is one of the physiologic changes that occur during pregnancy. The osmotic threshold is decreased to a lower steady state value due to excess ADH release and a heightened thirst stimulus. This results in a decrease in the average plasma-osmolality by 5–10 mmol and the sodium concentration by up to 5 mmol/L [1].

Another cause of hyponatremia that is related to pregnancy is HG. HG is a complication of pregnancy that is associated with assisted reproduction techniques and multiple gestations [2, 3]. It is characterized by intractable vomiting often requiring parenteral nutrition and can have a profound effect on the patient's fluid and electrolyte status. It can result in malnutrition, hyponatremia, and low serum urea levels [4, 5]. Hyponatremia in HG is due to both hypovolemic stimulus of AVP and also low osmoles intake that impairs free water excretion. TPN is a form of nutritional support that contains lipid emulsions, amino acids, utilizable nitrogen, and nonprotein calorie sources such as glucose, electrolytes,

and minerals. It is indicated when enteral nutrition is not possible [6]. It may be used in pregnancy complicated by severe HG when conservative treatment has failed [2]. Use of TPN can reverse weight loss and meet the specific requirements necessary for maternal anabolism and fetal embryologic growth [7]. Sodium may be increased in the TPN prescription. However, parenteral sodium should be administered carefully so as to avoid rapid and/or excessive correction to minimize the risk of CPM [8].

On the other end of the spectrum, dysregulation of the vasopressin system can lead to hypernatremia, defined as a sodium concentration above 145 mEq/L. Sepsis has been associated with decreased levels of vasopressin [9]. Proposed mechanisms include reduced production of vasopressin, depletion of vasopressin stores, inhibition of vasopressin release (in a septic state, the inhibition of vasopressin overcomes the excess vasopressin release in pregnancy), impaired baroreflex mediated vasopressin secretion, and increased vasopressin degradation [9]. Significant clinical consequences can occur due to a rapid increase in sodium levels. CPM is a rare syndrome that typically occurs as a consequence of rapid correction of hyponatremia. In a hyponatremic state of greater than 2-3-day duration, there is loss of osmotically active substances (sodium, potassium, chloride, and organic osmolytes such as myoinositol, glutamate, and glutamine), which normally protect against cerebral edema. If there is a rapid correction of hyponatremia, these substances (with the exception of sodium) are not replaced efficiently, leading to cerebral edema and CPM [10]. Hypertonic saline was not used to correct the sodium as it is only indicated if neurological symptoms prevail with the severe hyponatremia [6]. Although vasopressin receptor 2 antagonists such as tolvaptan and hypertonic saline are treatments for hyponatremia, they could not be used in this case. Tolvaptan is category C in pregnancy and can be used with caution but was contraindicated in this patient due to hypovolemia and excessive vomiting.

2. Case Description

A 42-year-old woman, G2P0 at 14 weeks of gestation with diamniotic-dichorionic twins from an in vitro fertilization, presented to the hospital with refractory hyperemesis gravidarum (HG). She had protein calorie malnutrition with a 25% decreased PO intake and 7% weight loss. The serum sodium concentration on admission was 125 mEq/L. During the hospital course, she was treated with normal saline and increased protein intake. Urine electrolytes and urine osmolality were measured showing urine sodium of 90 mmol/L, urine potassium of 11.5 mmol/L, and urine osmolality of 440 mOsm/kg. The patient's symptoms failed to improve and she had a peripherally inserted central catheter (PICC) placed and TPN was initiated. The patient experienced improvement in symptoms and normalization of the sodium in pregnancy, where the sodium corrected 0.3 mEq/hr during the first 24 hours. The sodium corrected by day 2 of this admission and persisted to be normal by day 5. The discharge was delayed due to home care issues.

Two weeks later, the patient was readmitted for persistent HG, psychomotor retardation, intention tremor, fluctuating altered mental status, and incontinence of 2-day duration. On physical exam, the patient was tachycardic with stable blood pressure. Neurological exam demonstrated ankle clonus, hyperreflexia, saccadic breakdown of smooth pursuit, facial diparesis, and dysarthria. Laboratory data revealed leucocytosis of 16.8 and sodium of 163 mEq/L. She was found to have an infected PICC line with bacteremia and fungemia and met criteria for sepsis. An MRI of the brain was performed which revealed changes consistent with CPM (Figure 1). The patient's neurological symptoms persisted for 6 days into this admission and improved slowly as the sodium corrected from 163 mEq/L to 141 mEq/L. During this time, the patient also had hypokalemia to normokalemia ranging from 2.9 to 3.9 mmol/L. The potassium was supplemented with oral replacements as well as TPN which was constituted with 2.8–3.8 mEq/dL of potassium and other electrolytes such as calcium, magnesium, and phosphorus. During the hospitalization, urine osmolality was measured showing a level of 104 mOsm/kg. Urine output however could not be measured due to strict intensive care policies on minimizing Foley catheter placements. Subsequently, the patient underwent termination of pregnancy with improvement of CPM signs on MRI done 2 months later (Figure 2).

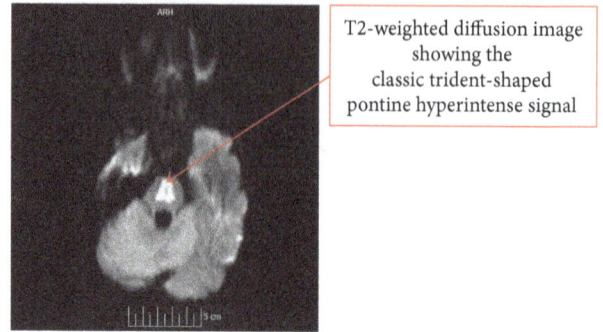

T2-weighted diffusion image showing the classic trident-shaped pontine hyperintense signal

FIGURE 1: Initial MRI of brain.

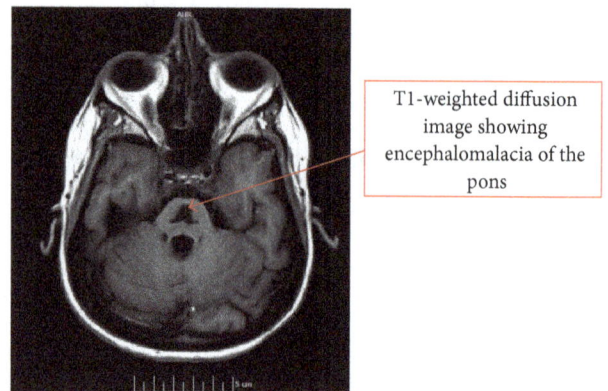

T1-weighted diffusion image showing encephalomalacia of the pons

FIGURE 2: Repeat MRI of brain after recovery.

3. Discussion

In this case, hyponatremia that was caused by hypovolemia and low osmotic intake (e.g., proteins) in the setting of HG was treated with hydration, protein supplementation, and nausea control. Concentrated TPN, consisting of high salt and protein supplements, via PICC line was the treatment of choice. As the patient's serum sodium increased, the TPN prescription was recalculated with lower volume and a decreased salt load.

Although not in septic shock this patient had tachycardia, leucocytosis, and bacteremia with Enterococcus faecalis and fungemia with Candida albicans meeting the criteria for sepsis. Sepsis has been established as a cause of diabetes insipidus and could have led to the overcorrection of sodium leading to CPM (Figure 1). The proposed mechanisms are increased metabolic clearance rate via increased vasopressinase activity [11], decreased production, or decreased release of vasopressin from the pituitary gland.

In our patient, despite having several risk factors for developing CPM including protein denutrition and potassium depletion, the primary cause favors the rapid correction of hypovolemia. In addition, the contribution of high vasopressinase activity (and thus high vasopressin clearance) due to diamniotic-dichorionic gestation can also explain the acute hyponatremia [12]. This is supported by the decrease in urine osmolality from 440 mOsm/kg on the first admission to 104 mOsm/kg on the second admission.

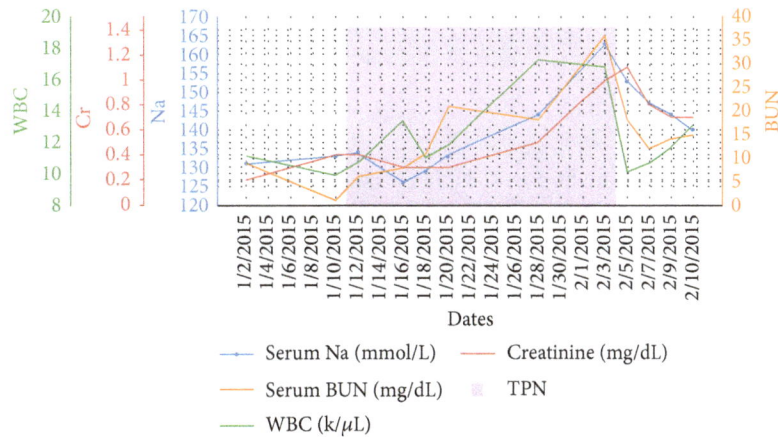

FIGURE 3: Correlation of serum Na, BUN, WBC, Cr, and TPN.

This patient's sodium was slowly corrected with hypotonic solution administration. Improvement in her neurological symptoms paralleled the correction of hypernatremia. A repeat MRI two months later showed resolution of CPM signs (Figure 2). Correlation of serum Na, BUN, WBC, Cr, and TPN is shown in Figure 3.

4. Conclusion

This case report describes the occurrence of rapid overcorrection of hyponatremia in pregnancy and sepsis. The outcome of treating hyponatremia in pregnancy associated with sepsis can be unpredictable. There is a high risk of overcorrection and developing hypernatremia given the complexities of the physiology of vasopressinase associated with pregnancy and sepsis. These risk factors should be taken into account when planning the rate of correction of sodium and volume in HG. In addition, serum sodium must be followed closely when correcting hyponatremia in this group of patients.

Conflict of Interests

The authors declare that there is no conflict of interests regarding the publication of this paper.

References

[1] J. Jellema, J. Balt, K. Broeze, F. Scheele, and M. Weijmer, "Hyponatraemia during pregnancy," *The Internet Journal of Gynecology and Obstetrics*, vol. 12, no. 1, pp. 1–6, 2009.

[2] T. M. Goodwin, "Hyperemesis gravidarum," *Clinical Obstetrics and Gynecology*, vol. 41, no. 3, pp. 597–605, 1998.

[3] T. J. Roseboom, A. C. J. Ravelli, J. A. van der Post, and R. C. Painter, "Maternal characteristics largely explain poor pregnancy outcome after hyperemesis gravidarum," *European Journal of Obstetrics Gynecology & Reproductive Biology*, vol. 156, no. 1, pp. 56–59, 2011.

[4] L. J. Wegrzyniak, J. T. Repke, and S. H. Ural, "Treatment of hyperemesis gravidarum," *Reviews in Obstetrics & Gynecology*, vol. 5, no. 2, pp. 78–84, 2012.

[5] N. K. Kuşcu and F. Koyuncu, "Hyperemesis gravidarum: current concepts and management," *Postgraduate Medical Journal*, vol. 78, no. 916, pp. 76–79, 2002.

[6] G. Zara, V. Codemo, A. Palmieri et al., "Neurological complications in hyperemesis gravidarum," *Neurological Sciences*, vol. 33, no. 1, pp. 133–135, 2012.

[7] M. G. Levine and D. Esser, "Total parenteral nutrition for the treatment of severe hyperemesis gravidarum: maternal nutritional effects and fetal outcome," *Obstetrics and Gynecology*, vol. 72, no. 1, pp. 102–107, 1988.

[8] G. Domínguez-Cherit, D. Borunda, and E. Rivero-Sigarroa, "Total parenteral nutrition," *Current Opinion in Critical Care*, vol. 8, no. 4, pp. 285–289, 2002.

[9] J.-L. Vincent and F. Su, "Physiology and pathophysiology of the vasopressinergic system," *Best Practice and Research: Clinical Anaesthesiology*, vol. 22, no. 2, pp. 243–252, 2008.

[10] UpToDate, *Osmotic Demyelination Syndrome and Overly Rapid Correction of Hyponatremia*, 2015, http://www.uptodate.com/contents/osmotic-demyelination-syndrome-and-overly-rapid-correction-of-hyponatremia?source=search_result&search=central+pontine+myelinolysis&selectedTitle=1~39.

[11] T. Sharshar, R. Carlier, A. Blanchard et al., "Depletion of neurohypophyseal content of vasopressin in septic shock," *Critical Care Medicine*, vol. 30, no. 3, pp. 497–500, 2002.

[12] J. A. Durr, J. G. Hoggard, J. M. Hunt, and R. W. Schrier, "Diabetes insipidus in pregnancy associated with abnormally high circulating vasopressinase activity," *The New England Journal of Medicine*, vol. 316, no. 17, pp. 1070–1074, 1987.

Permissions

List of Contributors

Sami Safadi, Michael Mao and John J. Dillon
Division of Nephrology and Hypertension, Mayo Clinic, 200 1st Street SW, Rochester, MN 55905, USA

Lohit Garg
Department of Internal Medicine, Oakland UniversityWilliam Beaumont School of Medicine, Royal Oak, MI 48073, USA

Sagar Gupta
Department of Nephrology, Washington University in St. Louis, St. Louis, MO 63130, USA

Abhishek Swami
Department of Nephrology, Oakland University William Beaumont School of Medicine, Royal Oak, MI 48073, USA

Ping Zhang
Department of Pathology, William Beaumont Hospital, Royal Oak, MI 48073, USA

Remi Goupil and Annie-Claire Nadeau-Fredette
Nephrology Division, Hôpital Maisonneuve-Rosemont, Montreal, QC, Canada H1T 2M4

Virginie Royal
Pathology Department, HôpitalMaisonneuve-Rosemont, Montreal,QC, Canada H1T 2M4

Alexandre Dugas
Radiology Division, Hôpital Maisonneuve-Rosemont, Montreal, QC, Canada H1T 2M4

Jean-Philippe Lafrance
Medicine Department, Universite de Montreal, Montreal, QC, Canada H3T 1J4
Centre de Recherche Hôpital Maisonneuve-Rosemont, Montreal, QC, Canada H1T 2M4
Nephrology Division, Hôpital Maisonneuve-Rosemont, Montreal, QC, Canada H1T 2M4

Maheswara S. Golla, Subasit Acharjee, Bertrand L. Jaber and Lawrence A. Garcia
Department of Medicine, St. Elizabeth's Medical Center, Department of Medicine, Tufts University School of Medicine, Boston, MA 02135, USA

David Callau Monje, Niko Braun, Joerg Latus, Kerstin Amann and Martin Kimmel
Department of Internal Medicine, Division of Nephrology, Robert-Bosch-Hospital, Auerbach Street 110, 70179 Stuttgart, Germany

Mark Dominik Alscher
Department of Pathology, Erlangen University Hospital, Krankenhaus Street 8-10, 91054 Erlangen, Germany

Stephanie M. Toth-Manikowski
Department of Medicine, Boston Medical Center, 72 East Concord Street, Evans 124, Boston, MA 02118, USA

Hanni Menn-Josephy and Jasvinder Bhatia
Renal Section, Boston University School of Medicine, 650 Albany Street, Rm 504, Boston, MA 02118, USA

Alwin Tilanus
Departamento de Medicina Interna/Infectologia, Hospital General de Medellin Luz Castro de Guti´errez, Carrera 48 # 32- 102, Medellin, Colombia

Patricia Van der Niepen and Karl Martin Wissing
Departement Interne Geneeskunde/Nefrologie, Universitair Ziekenhuis Brussel, Laarbeeklaan 101, 1090 Brussels, Belgium

Caroline Geers
Departement Anatomo-Pathologie, Universitair Ziekenhuis Brussel, Laarbeeklaan 101, 1090 Brussels, Belgium

Rachele Escoli, Paulo Santos and Sequeira Andrade
Department of Nephrology, Centro Hospitalar do M´edio Tejo, 2350-754 Torres Novas, Portugal

Fernanda Carvalho
Department of Nephrology, Centro Hospitalar de Lisboa Central, Hospital Curry Cabral, 1069-166 Lisbon, Portugal

Roshni Upputalla and Belinda Jim
Department of Nephrology/Medicine, Jacobi Medical Center, Albert Einstein College of Medicine, Bronx, NY 10461, USA

Robert M. Moore
Department of Obstetrics and Gynecology, Jacobi Medical Center, Albert Einstein College of Medicine, Bronx, NY 10461, USA

Aiyu Zhao, Maybel Tan, Aung Maung, Moro Salifu and Mary Mallappallil
State University of New York Downstate Medical Center, 450 Clarkson Avenue, Brooklyn, NY 11203, USA

Ryan Burkhart
Department of Internal Medicine, William Beaumont Army Medical Center, 5005 N. Piedras Street, El Paso, TX 79920, USA

Nina Shah
Department of Nephrology, William Beaumont Army Medical Center, 5005 N. Piedras Street, El Paso, TX 79920, USA

Michael Abel
Department of Rheumatology,William Beaumont Army Medical Center, 5005 N. Piedras Street, El Paso, TX 79920, USA

James D. Oliver III
Nephrology Service,Walter Reed National Military Medical Center, 8901 Rockville Pike, Bethesda, MD 20889, USA

Matthew Lewin
ProPath Services, LLP, 1355 River Bend Drive, Dallas, TX 75247,USA

Rima Abou Arkoub
Division of nephrology, The Ottawa Hospital,Ottawa, ON, Canada K1H 7W9

Don Wang
Division of Anatomical Pathology, Department of Pathology and Laboratory Medicine,The Ottawa Hospital and Kidney Research Centre of the Ottawa Hospital Research Institute, University of Ottawa, Ottawa, ON, Canada K1H 7W9

Deborah Zimmerman
Division of Nephrology,The Ottawa Hospital and University of Ottawa, Ottawa, ON, Canada K1H 7W9

Sandra Chomicki
Service de N´ephrologie, Centre Hospitalier Louis Pasteur, 4 rue Claude Bernard, 28 630 Le Coudray, France

Omar Dahmani
Service de N´ephrologie, Centre Hospitalier Louis Jaillon, 2 rue Hˆopital, 39 206 Saint-Claude, France

John Sy and Phuong-Chi T. Pham
Division of Nephrology and Hypertension, Department of Internal Medicine, UCLA-Olive View Medical Center, 14445 Olive View Drive, 2B-182, Sylmar, CA 91342, USA

Cynthia C. Nast
Cedars Sinai Medical Center, Department of Pathology, Los Angeles, CA 90048, USA

Phuong-Thu T. Pham
David Geffen School of Medicine at UCLA, Kidney and Pancreas Transplant Program, Los Angeles, CA 90095, USA

Fareed B. Kamar
University of Calgary, Suite G15, 1403-29 Street NW, Calgary, AB, Canada T2N 2T9

Rory F. McQuillan
University of Toronto and University Health Network, Toronto General Hospital, Room 8N-842, 200 Elizabeth Street, Toronto, ON, Canada M5G 2C4

Osman Zikrullah Sahin
Department of Nephrology, Recep Tayyip Erdogan University Medical School, 53100 Rize, Turkey

Teslime Ayaz, Suleyman Yuce and Fatih Sumer
Department of Internal Medicine, Recep Tayyip Erdogan University Medical School, 53100 Rize, Turkey

Serap Baydur Sahin
Department of Endocrinology and Metabolic Disease, Recep Tayyip Erdogan University Medical School, 53100 Rize, Turkey

Seongseok Yun
Department of Medicine, University of Arizona, Tucson, AZ 85721, USA
Department of Medicine, Arizona Health Sciences Center, 6th Floor, Room 6336, 1501 N. Campbell Avenue,Tucson, AZ 85719, USA

Beth L. Braunhut
Division of Pathology, University of Arizona, Tucson, AZ 85721, USA

Courtney N. Walker, Waheed Bhati and Amy N. Sussman
Department of Medicine, University of Arizona, Tucson, AZ 85721, USA

Faiz Anwer
Division of Hematology, Oncology, Blood & Marrow Transplantation, Department of Medicine, University of Arizona, Tucson, AZ 86721, USA

Kwok-Ying Chan, Mau-Kwong Sham, Benjamin Hon-Wai Cheng, Cho-Wing Li, Yim-Chi Wong, and Vikki Wai-Kee Lau
Palliative Medical Unit, Grantham Hospital,Wong Chuk Hang, Hong Kong

Terence Yip
Renal Unit, Department of Medicine, Tung Wah Hospital, Sheung Wan, Hong Kong

Erkan Dervisoglu and Mehmet Tuncay
Department of Nephrology, School of Medicine, Kocaeli University, 41000 Kocaeli, Turkey

Murat Ozturk
Department of Otorhinolaryngology, School of Medicine, Kocaeli University, 41000 Kocaeli, Turkey

Gulhatun Kilic Dervisoglu
Department of Neurology, Kandira Government Hospital, 41600 Kocaeli, Turkey

Yesim Gurbuz
Department of Pathology, School of Medicine, Kocaeli University, 41000 Kocaeli, Turkey

Serhan Derin
Department of Otorhinolaryngology School of Medicine, Mu˘gla Sıtkı Koc¸man University, 48000 Mu˘gla, Turkey

Sridhar R. Allam, Balamurugan Sankarapandian, Imran

A. Memon and Patrick C. Nef
Tarrant Nephrology Associates, 1001 Pennsylvania Avenue, FortWorth, TX 76104, USA
Division of Transplant Nephrology, FortWorth Transplant Institute, Plaza Medical Center, 900 Eighth Avenue, FortWorth, TX 76104, USA

Tom S. Livingston
Department of Interventional Radiology, Plaza Medical Center, 900 Eighth Avenue, FortWorth, TX 76104, USA

George Rofaiel
Division of Transplant Surgery, FortWorth Transplant Institute, Plaza Medical Center, 900 Eighth Avenue, FortWorth, TX 76104, USA

Youngho Kim
Division of Nephrology, Department of Internal Medicine, University of New Mexico, 901 University Boulevard SE, Suite 150, MSC 04-2785, Albuquerque, NM 87106, USA

Aurore Berthe-Aucejo and Emilia Perrier-Cornet
Service de Pharmacie, Hˆopital Robert Debr´e, 48 boulevard S´erurier, 75019 Paris, France

Mathieu Sacquépée
Service de N´ephrologie, Centre Hospitalier Territorial de Nouvelle Cal´edonie, Gaston Bourret, BP J5, 98849 Noum´ea, New Caledonia

Marc Fila and Georges Deschênes
Service de N´ephrologie P´ediatrique, Hˆopital Robert Debr´e, 48 boulevard S´erurier, 75019 Paris, France

Michel Peuchmaur
Laboratoire d'Anatomopathologie, Hˆopital Robert Debr´e, 48 boulevard S´erurier, 75019 Paris, France

Véronique Frémeaux-Bacchi
Laboratoire d'Immunologie, Hˆopital Europ´een Georges-Pompidou, 20-40 rue Leblanc, 75015 Paris, France

Susan Ziolkowski and Catherine Moore
University of Rochester Medical Center, 601 Elmwood Avenue, P.O. Box MED, Rochester, NY 14642, USA

Yasuyuki Nakada, Nobuo Tsuboi, Yasuto Takahashi, Hiraku Yoshida, Yoriko Hara, Hideo Okonogi, Tetsuya Kawamura and Takashi Yokoo
Division of Nephrology and Hypertension, Department of Internal Medicine,The Jikei University School of Medicine, 3-25-8 Nishi-Shinbashi, Minato-ku, Tokyo 105-8461, Japan

Yoshihiro Arimura
Department of Internal Medicine, Kyorin University School of Medicine, Tokyo, Japan

Fernando Caravaca, Victor Burguera, Milagros Fernández-Lucas, José Luis Teruel and Carlos Quereda
Department of Nephrology, Hospital Ram´on y Cajal, 28034 Madrid, Spain

Patrick Hamilton, Olumide Ogundare, Ammar Raza, Arvind Ponnusamy, Julie Gorton, Philip A. Kalra and Hana Alachkar
Renal Department, Salford Royal NHS Foundation Trust, Salford, Greater Manchester M6 8HD, UK

Jamil Choudhury
Histopathology Department, Salford NHS Foundation Trust, Salford, Greater Manchester M6 8HD, UK

Jonathan Barratt
JohnWalls Renal Unit, Leicester General Hospital, Gwendolen Road, Leicester LE5 4PW, UK

Faraz Jaffer and Vijay Chandiramani
University of Arizona, South Campus, Tucson, AZ 85715, USA

Adaobi Solarin
Department of Paediatrics, Babcock University Teaching Hospital, PMB 21244, Ilishan-Remo, Ogun State, Nigeria

Priya Gajjar and Peter Nourse
Renal Unit, Red Cross Children's Hospital, Cape Town, South Africa

Kana N. Miyata
Division of Nephrology and Hypertension, Harbor-UCLA Medical Center, 1124W. Carson Street, Torrance, CA 90502, USA
Division of Nephrology, Department of Medicine, Tokyo Metropolitan Tama Medical Center, 2-8-29 Musashidai, Fuchu-shi,

Hiromi Kihira, Manabu Haneda and Yasuhide Nishio
Division of Nephrology, Department of Medicine, Tokyo Metropolitan Tama Medical Center, 2-8-29 Musashidai, Fuchu-shi, Tokyo 183-8524, Japan

Giles Walters
Department of Renal Medicine, Canberra Hospital, Garran, ACT 2605, Australia
Australian National University Medical School, Canberra, Australia

Faisal A. Choudhury and Budhima Nanayakkara
The Canberra Hospital, Australia

Jan Van Keer and Daan Detroyer
Department of Nephrology, Dialysis and Renal Transplantation, University Hospitals Leuven, Herestraat 49, 3000 Leuven, Belgium

Bert Bammens
Department of Nephrology, Dialysis and Renal Transplantation, University Hospitals Leuven, Herestraat 49, 3000 Leuven, Belgium

Department of Microbiology and Immunology, KU Leuven, Minderbroedersstraat 10, 3000 Leuven, Belgium

Sreeja Nair, Jacob George, Sajeev Kumar and Noble Gracious
Department of Nephrology, Medical College, Thiruvananthapuram, Kerala 695011, India

Mohammed Muqeet Adnan and Tanzeel Iqbal
Department of Internal Medicine, University of Oklahoma Health Sciences Center, Oklahoma City, OK 73117, USA

Usman Bhutta
Department of Internal Medicine, University of Oklahoma Health Sciences Center, Oklahoma City, OK 73117, USA
Department of Nephrology, University of Oklahoma Health Sciences Center, Oklahoma City, OK 73117, USA

Sufyan Abdul Mujeeb
University of Illinois at Chicago, Chicago, IL 60607, USA

Lukas Haragsim
Department of Nephrology, University of Oklahoma Health Sciences Center, Oklahoma City, OK 73117, USA

Syed Amer
Department of Internal Medicine, Mayo Clinic Hospital, Phoenix, AZ 85054, USA

Fernando Caravaca-Fontan, Olga Martinez-Saez, Maria Delgado-Yague,
Estefania Yerovi and Fernando Liaño
Department of Nephrology, Hospital Universitario Ram´on y Cajal, Carretera de Colmenar Viejo, Km. 9100, 28034 Madrid, Spain

Santosh Kumar, Shivanshu Singh and Aditya Prakash Sharma
Department of Urology, Postgraduate Institute of Medical Education and Research, Chandigarh 160012, India

Manish Rathi
Department of Nephrology, Postgraduate Institute of Medical Education and Research, Chandigarh 160012, India

Amin Bagheri, Reza Khorramirouz, Sorena Keihani, Mehdi Fareghi and Abdol-Mohammad Kajbafzadeh
Pediatric Urology Research Center, Pediatrics Center of Excellence, Children's Hospital Medical Center, Tehran University of Medical Sciences, Tehran 1419433151, Iran

Cem Sahin, Hasan Tunca, Emine Koca and Mustafa Levent
Department of Internal Medicine, School of Medicine, Mugla Sıtkı Kocman University, Orhaniye Mahallesi ˙Ismet Catak Caddesi, 48000 Mugla, Turkey

Bulent Huddam
Department of Nephrology, Mugla Sitki Kocman University Education and Research Hospital, 48000 Mugla, Turkey

Gulhan Akbaba
Department of Endocrinology, School of Medicine, Mugla Sıtkı Kocman University, 48000 Mugla, Turkey

B. Jayakrishnan, Jamal Al Aghbari, Dawar Rizavi and Dawood Al Riyami
Department of Medicine, Sultan Qaboos University Hospital, 123 Muscat, Oman

Sinnakirouchenan Srinivasan
Department of Anaesthesia, Sultan Qaboos University Hospital, 123 Muscat, Oman

Ritu Lakhtakia
Department of Pathology, College of Medicine andHealth Sciences, Sultan Qaboos University, 123 Muscat,Oman

Nikos Sabanis and Sotirios Vasileiou
Department of Nephrology, General Hospital of Pella, 58200 Edessa, Greece

Eleni Paschou
Department of General Practice and Family Medicine, General Hospital of Pella, 58200 Edessa, Greece

Eleni Gavriilaki
Medical School, Aristotle University ofThessaloniki,Thessaloniki, Greece

Maria Mourounoglou
Department of General Surgery, General Hospital of Pella, 58200 Edessa, Greece

Nicolas De Schryver and Xavier Wittebole
Department of Intensive Care, Cliniques Universitaires Saint-Luc, Universit´e Catholique de Louvain, 1200 Brussels, Belgium

Peter Van den Bergh
Centre de R´ef´erence Neuromusculaire, Cliniques Universitaires Saint-Luc, Universit´e Catholique de Louvain, 1200 Brussels, Belgium

Vincent Haufroid
Louvain Centre for Toxicology and Applied Pharmacology, Cliniques Universitaires Saint-Luc, Universit´e Catholique de Louvain, 1200 Brussels, Belgium

Eric Goffin
Department of Nephrology, Cliniques Universitaires Saint-Luc, Universit´e Catholique de Louvain, 1200 Brussels, Belgium

Philippe Hantson
Department of Intensive Care, Cliniques Universitaires Saint-Luc, Universit´e Catholique de Louvain, 1200 Brussels, Belgium

Elena Gkrouzman
University of Connecticut Health Center, 263 Farmington Avenue, Farmington, CT 06030-1235, USA

Kyriakos A. Kirou
Division of Rheumatology, Hospital for Special Surgery, 535 East 70th Street, New York, NY 10021, USA

Surya V. Seshan
New York-Presbyterian Hospital, 525 East 68th Street, Starr Pavilion 1009, New York, NY 10021, USA

James M. Chevalier
Rogosin Kidney Center, 505 East 70th Street, New York, NY 10021, USA
Egemen Cebeci, Meltem Gursu, Abdullah Sumnu, BarJs Doner, Serhat Karadag, Sami Uzun, Ahmet Behlul, Oktay Ozkan and Savas Ozturk
Department of Nephrology, Haseki Training and Research Hospital, 34087 Istanbul, Turkey

Secil Demir and Mehmet Yamak
Department of Internal Medicine, Haseki Training and Research Hospital, 34087 Istanbul, Turkey

Yosuke Kawamorita, Yoshihide Fujigaki, Atsuko Imase, Shigeyuki Arai, Yoshifuru Tamura, Masayuki Tanemoto and Shunya Uchida
Department of Internal Medicine, Teikyo University School of Medicine, 2-11-1 Kaga, Itabashi-ku, Tokyo 173-8605, Japan

Hiroshi Uozaki
Department of Pathology, Teikyo University School of Medicine, 2-11-1 Kaga, Itabashi-ku, Tokyo 173-8605, Japan

Yutaka Yamaguchi
Yamaguchi's Pathology Laboratory, 20-31-1 Minoridai, Matsudo-shi, Chiba 270-2231, Japan

Saika Sharmeen and Esra Kalkan
Department of Medicine, Mount Sinai St. Luke's-Roosevelt Hospital Center, New York, NY 10025, USA

Chunhui Yi
Department of Pathology, Mount Sinai St. Luke's-Roosevelt Hospital Center, New York, NY 10025, USA

Steven D. Smith
Department of Medicine, Division of Nephrology, Mount Sinai St. Luke's-Roosevelt Hospital Center, New York, NY 10025, USA

Diana Yuan Yng Chiu, Darren Green and Philip A. Kalra
Vascular Research Group, Institute of Population Health, The University of Manchester, Manchester Academic Health Sciences Centre, Manchester M13 9PL, UK
Department of Renal Medicine, Salford Royal NHS Foundation Trust, Stott Lane, Salford M6 8HD, UK

Nik Abidin
Department of Cardiology, Salford Royal Hospital, Salford Royal NHS Foundation Trust, Stott Lane, Salford M6 8HD, UK

Ozlem Beyler Kilic and Ali Kemal Oguz
Department of Internal Medicine, Ufuk University School of Medicine, 06520 Ankara, Turkey

Ihsan Ergun
Division of Nephrology, Department of Internal Medicine, Ufuk University School of Medicine, 06520 Ankara, Turkey

Dilek Ertoy Baydar
Department of Pathology, Hacettepe University School of Medicine, 06100 Ankara, Turkey

Meltem Ayli
Division of Hematology, Department of Internal Medicine, Ufuk University School of Medicine, 06520 Ankara, Turkey

Amudha Palanisamy, AmberM. Reeves-Daniel and Barry I. Freedman
Department of Internal Medicine, Section on Nephrology, Wake Forest School of Medicine, Winston-Salem, NC 27103, USA

Paul Persad, Patrick P. Koty, Michael W. Beaty, Mark J. Pettenati, Samy S. Iskandar and David D. Grier
Department of Pathology, Wake Forest School of Medicine, Winston-Salem, NC 27103, USA

Laurie L. Douglas and Bayard L. Powell
Department of Internal Medicine, Section on Hematology and Oncology, Comprehensive Cancer Center of Wake Forest University, Winston-Salem, NC 27103, USA

Robert J. Stratta, Jeffrey Rogers, Giuseppe Orlando, Alan C. Farney and Michael D. Gautreaux
Department of General Surgery, Wake Forest School of Medicine, Winston-Salem, NC 27103, USA

Scott A. Kaczmorski and William H. Doares
Department of Pharmacy, Wake Forest School of Medicine, Winston-Salem, NC 27103, USA

Ana Ratola, Maria Miguel Almiro, Rita Lacerda Vidal, Adelaide Bicho and Sofia Figueiredo
Pediatrics Department, Baixo Vouga Hospital Center, Avenida Artur Ravara, 3814-501 Aveiro, Portugal

Nuno Neves
Radiology Department, Baixo Vouga Hospital Center, Avenida Artur Ravara, 3814-501 Aveiro, Portugal

Sophie Van Haare Heijmeijer and Caroline Clerckx
Department of Nephrology, Clinique Saint-Pierre, Ottignies, Belgium

Dunja Wilmes
Department of Internal Medicine, Cliniques universitaires Saint-Luc, Universit´e catholique de Louvain, Brussels, Belgium

Selda Aydin
Department of Pathology, Cliniques universitaires Saint-Luc, Universit´e catholique de Louvain, Brussels, Belgium

Laura Labriola
Department of Nephrology, Cliniques universitaires Saint-Luc, Universit´e catholique de Louvain, Brussels, Belgium

Isabel Tavares
Department of Nephrology, Centro Hospitalar de S˜ao Jo˜ao, 4200-319 Porto, Portugal
Nephrology and Infectious Diseases Research andDevelopment Group, INEB (I3S), University of Porto, 4150-180 Porto, Portugal

Luísa Lobato, Josefina Santos and António Castro Henriques
Department of Nephrology, Centro Hospitalar do Porto, Hospital de Santo Ant´onio, 4099-001 Porto, Portugal
Unit for Multidisciplinary Research in Biomedicine, Instituto de Ciˆencias Biom´edicas Abel Salazar, University of Porto, 4050-313 Porto, Portugal

Paul Moreira and Maria João Saraiva
Molecular Neurobiology, Institute of Molecular and Cellular Biology, University of Porto, 4150-180 Porto, Portugal

Carlos Matos
Department of Nephrology, Centro Hospitalar do Porto, Hospital de Santo Ant´onio, 4099-001 Porto, Portugal

Leyla Akdogan and Ali Kemal Oguz
Department of Internal Medicine, Ufuk University School of Medicine, Ankara, Turkey
Dr. Rıdvan EgeHospital, Konya Bulvarı No. 86-88, Balgat, C¸ankaya, 06520 Ankara, Turkey

Tarkan Ergun
Department of Radiology, Baskent University School of Medicine, Alanya, Antalya, Turkey
Baskent University School of Medicine, Alanya Research and Education Hospital, Alanya, 07400 Antalya, Turkey

Ihsan Ergun
Division of Nephrology, Department of Internal Medicine, Ufuk University School of Medicine, Ankara, Turkey

Ryan Burkhart and Nina Shah
William Beaumont Army Medical Center, 5005 N. Piedras Street, El Paso, TX 79920, USA

Matthew Lewin
ProPath Services, LLP, 1355 River Bend Drive, Dallas, TX 75247, USA

Reyner Loza
Unit of Pediatric Nephrology, Department of Pediatrics, Cayetano Heredia National Hospital, Avenida Honorio Delgado 265, SMP, Lima 31, Peru

Cayetano Heredia University, Avenida Honorio Delgado 430, SMP, Lima 31, Peru

Dimas Rodriguez
Unit of Pediatric Nephrology, Sergio Bernales National Hospital, Avenida Tupac Amaru 8000, Comas, Lima 7, Peru
Kalyana C. Janga, Tazleem Khan, Ciril Khorolsky, Sheldon Greenberg and Priscilla Persaud
Maimonides Medical Center, 4802 10th Avenue, Brooklyn, NY 11219, USA

www.ingramcontent.com/pod-product-compliance
Lightning Source LLC
Chambersburg PA
CBHW080527200326
41458CB00012B/4355